THE SEXUALLY TRANSMITTED DISEASES

A C

APPROACH

THE SEXUALLY TRANSMITTED DISEASES

A CURRENT APPROACH

GEORGE A. WISTREICH

East Los Angeles College

 Wm. C. Brown Publishers

Book Team

Editor *Colin H. Wheatley*
Developmental Editor *Jane DeShaw*
Production Coordinator *Kay Driscoll*

 Wm. C. Brown Publishers

President *G. Franklin Lewis*
Vice President, Publisher *George Wm. Bergquist*
Vice President, Operations and Production *Beverly Kolz*
National Sales Manager *Virginia S. Moffat*
Group Sales Manager *Vincent R. Di Blasi*
Vice President, Editor in Chief *Edward G. Jaffe*
Marketing Manager *John W. Calhoun*
Advertising Manager *Amy Schmitz*
Managing Editor, Production *Colleen A. Yonda*
Manager of Visuals and Design *Faye M. Schilling*
Production Editorial Manager *Julie A. Kennedy*
Production Editorial Manager *Ann Fuerste*
Publishing Services Manager *Karen J. Slaght*

WCB Group

President and Chief Executive Officer *Mark C. Falb*
Chairman of the Board *Wm. C. Brown*

Cover and interior design by Ophelia M. Chambliss-Jones

Copyedited by Jean E. Pascual

Library of Congress Catalog Card Number: 91–71197

ISBN 0–697–10976–3

Printed in the United States of America by Wm. C. Brown Publishers,
2460 Kerper Boulevard, Dubuque, IA 52001

10 9 8 7 6 5 4 3 2 1

DEDICATION

To my wife, Renee, and my sons, Eddie and Phil, for
all that was and for all that will be, I dedicate this
book.

CONTENTS

PREFACE

Today, as throughout history, few events generate so much attention, concern, and fear as epidemics—especially when these are severe, mysterious in origin, and carry a high death rate. When sexual behavior is involved, as with the Acquired Immune Deficiency Syndrome (AIDS), public interest, stimulated by the news media with their moral and political overtones, rises even higher.

The global impact of the AIDS epidemic has captured the interest and concern of the world. It also has, unfortunately, clouded the status of several sexually transmitted diseases (STDs), such as syphilis, genital herpes, and genital warts. Many of these diseases are increasing in incidence and may actually be contributing to the transmission of human immunodeficiency virus (HIV) infection.

There is no question that the sexually transmitted diseases have become a major health priority. During the past twelve or so years, emphasis and concern has shifted from the traditional so-called venereal diseases of syphilis and gonorrhea to the more increasingly recognized bacterial and viral diseases such as chlamydial infections, genital herpes, genital warts, and of course the fatal conditions caused by the human immunodeficiency viruses. The severity of the current situation can be appreciated from the fact that over 13 million Americans, most of whom are of reproductive age, acquire STDs each year. The number of such infections on a global scale is overwhelming. This book presents the sexually transmitted diseases in the context of social, public health, and educational problems, and answers questions such as: *What are the risks?*, *Who is at risk?*, and *What can be done?* As research into the cause, diagnosis, treatment, and prevention of STDs continues, there is a definite need to communicate this information to the public, to health care professionals, and to all other individuals who have a significant role to play in limiting the spread of infection.

The major emphasis in *The Sexually Transmitted Diseases: A Current Approach* is on information and its application. One of the important strengths of the book is that it approaches these diseases as a comprehensive and integrated topic. By thoughtfully selecting pertinent and useful information from the biological sciences, social sciences, and clinical medicine, the reader is provided with the "big picture" of diseases, and not only the sexually transmitted ones.

ORGANIZATION OF THE TEXT

The Sexually Transmitted Diseases: A Current Approach is organized into four parts. As the following description shows, the arrangement of the parts and the chapters within them allows for flexibility in the use of the book, so that instructors are free to design a course that meets the particular needs of their students.

Part 1, *Causes, Detection, and Control of Infectious Diseases*, begins with a chapter that draws the reader's attention to the features of infectious diseases and the types of microscopic life known to cause them. Chapter 2 includes a brief consideration of epidemics, past and present. It also discusses disease transmission, sources of disease agents, and approaches to disease reporting. In addition, approaches used in the control of diseases are presented.

Part 2, *The Well-Established Sexually Transmitted Diseases (STDs)*, provides a useful description of the general features of the sexually transmitted diseases, with the exception of human immunodeficiency virus (HIV) infection. As an introduction to the general topic of STDs, chapter 3 presents the human reproductive system not only from an anatomical and physiological point of view, but from the standpoint of an individual in need of information about his or her body. Attention also is given to what goes on during a physical examination for a possible sexually transmitted disease. In addition, this chapter contains a *genital self-examination procedure* which an individual can use to detect the signs that might indicate the presence of an STD. The information in chapter 3 serves as an important frame of reference for several of the remaining sections of this book. Chapter 4 introduces the sexually transmitted, or venereal, diseases. While many of these diseases have been associated with humans for thousands of years, newer infections previously considered to be of a nonvenereal nature have been added. Consideration also is given to sexual practices and the control and prevention of STDs. Chapter 5 deals with two of the "traditional" venereal diseases, syphilis and gonorrhea. In the United States these two infections currently outnumber, on a yearly basis, the cases of measles, mumps, scarlet fever, strep throat, and tuberculosis. Other countries have similarly disturbing statistics. Chapter 6 covers several other bacterial STDs, including chlamydial infections and chancroid. These diseases, like syphilis and gonorrhea, have increased in incidence as a result of changes in sexual behavior. Chapter 7 presents the features of the herpes viruses and the various diseases they are capable of causing. Chapter 8 deals with several other viral STDs, including genital warts, molluscum contagiosum, and hepatitis B infection. The far-reaching implications of these diseases also are discussed. Chapter 9, the last chapter in part 2, covers the areas of yeast and protozoan infections, and the problems caused by crab lice and the scabies mite. All chapters in this portion of the text contain **SIGNS & SYMPTOMS BOXES.** These boxes include approaches to the treatment and control of the STDs discussed.

Part 3, *The Spectrum of Human Immunodeficiency Virus (HIV) Infection*, begins with chapter 10, which provides a general description of the immune system, its functions, and types of disorders associated with it. The information and concepts in the chapter provide a foundation useful to understanding how HIV and related disease agents establish themselves. Chapter 11 explains the nature of a "compromised host" and a representative number of opportunistic disease agents that prey on such an individual. Chapter 12 describes HIV and other retroviruses. Chapter 13 gives special attention to AIDS and other conditions associated with the human immunodeficiency virus. Special consideration is given to pediatric AIDS. Chapter 14 concentrates on the area of research dealing with HIV vaccine development. An explanation of vaccine categories, and obstacles for an AIDS vaccine as well as for similar preparations for other STDs, are also included in the discussion. Chapter 15 surveys the risks for HIV infection in and out of the workplace, and the approaches to disease control and prevention. Most of the subject matter discussed here can be applied to everyday living. Attention also is given to the dilemma confronting many day-care centers, namely, casual contact as a factor in disease transmission.

Part 4, *Public Health Challenges and Society's Responsibilities,* considers some of the problems and social obstacles that have interfered with overcoming AIDS and STDs in general. Chapter 16 examines some economic, ethical, and political issues raised by AIDS. Despite the remarkable progress made in the research arena, a number of social and political issues have posed problems in developing workable public health policies. Chapter 17 primarily concentrates on STD prevention through education, with a special emphasis on the problems and challenges. Chapter 18 represents a glimpse of the future, not only with respect to HIV infection, but to all STDs.

DISTINCTIVE FEATURES

The Sexually Transmitted Diseases: A Current Approach includes a number of learning tools designed to help the reader absorb, review, and retain its content. Some of these tools and distinctive features are the following:

- Each chapter begins with an overview that orients the reader to the topics to be covered.
- Within most chapters, carefully selected **diagrams** and **photographs** are used to illustrate the concepts and features of the diseases presented.
- A total of four pages consisting of **twenty-nine color photographs** of sexually transmitted disease cases and related topics, together with appropriate and functional captions, have been incorporated into a separate section of the book. All color photos are coordinated and keyed to the subject matter in the text. Several of these illustrations have never before appeared in books.
- **Phonetic pronunciations** of most scientific and medical terms are given the first time mention is made of such words in a chapter. Knowing how to pronounce a term generally tends to increase its use.
- Specially developed **SIGNS & SYMPTOMS BOXES** have been incorporated into the chapters describing specific sexually transmitted diseases. Emphasis is placed on the easily seen symptoms which can be of value to the early detection of an STD.
- **STD FACT FILES** are functional summaries of specific STDs. They should serve to reinforce what the reader has learned.

- Much attention also has been given to assure that correct terms are clearly defined and accessible to help the reader develop and retain a useful vocabulary. Key terms initially appear in **boldface** type, and secondary terms in *italics*. Genus names will always appear in italics.
- A **glossary** with phonetic pronunciations is contained in a separate section at the end of the text. It will prove useful not only to readers unfamiliar with medical and related terms, but will serve as a convenient reference for others who wish a quick review of terminology. Most words appearing in the glossary are in **boldface** type in the text for easy reference.
- **Abbreviations** used in relation to sexually transmitted diseases and related topics are included on the inside back cover of the text.

A FINAL WORD

It is apparent that there is no scarcity of interest in sexual behavior, nor is there a lack of concern about sexually transmitted diseases and their control. The availability of this book should greatly stimulate the teaching about STDs at various levels of instruction and may prove to be a potent incentive to start such courses where none presently exist.

ACKNOWLEDGMENTS

Sexually Transmitted Diseases: A Current Approach was greatly influenced by the many concerns and inquiries of students, and by the wise guidance and counsel offered by many instructors and professionals, in particular the comments of the reviewers whose names follow this preface.

The author would also like to thank Ms. Jane DeShaw and other members of the editorial and production staffs of Wm. C. Brown Publishers for their untiring and imaginative efforts expended in the preparation of this text and the accompanying supplementary materials. I am also indebted to Ms. Sylvia Fernandez for the care and attention given to the typing of the manuscript.

The author also would like to especially acknowledge the contribution and support of Mr. Colin Wheatley, senior editor, who devoted a great deal of time, patience, and support for *Sexually Transmitted Diseases: A Current Approach.*

Special thanks also is extended to the many contributors here and abroad who willingly provided excellent photographs and diagrams.

Finally, the author would like to acknowledge and thank the following persons for reviewing the manuscript and offering valuable suggestions: Professor Francis M. Maxin, M.S., MPH, Community College Allegheny, Co.; Lois M. Bergquist, Ph.D., Los Angeles Valley College; Lynda J. Dimitroff, SUNY College at Brockport, Student Health Services; Edmund E. Bedecarrax, City College of San Francisco; Eleanor K. Marr, Dutchess Community College.

Phonetic Pronunciation Guide

This book is written for the individual who wants to obtain a broad understanding of the sexually transmitted diseases and some insight into the approaches used for their prevention, treatment, and control. To make *The Sexually Transmitted Diseases: A Current Approach* an effective and informative learning tool, phonetic pronunciations of the biological and/or medical terms are provided throughout the text. Taking time to sound out new terms and to say them aloud once or twice will help you to learn and build a powerful STD vocabulary. The following key explains the system used for the pronunciations.

Pronunciation Key

1. The strongest accented syllable appears in CAPITAL LETTERS (e.g., **syphilis,** SIF–i–lis).
2. A syllable that has a secondary accent is marked by a single quote mark ('), (e.g., **syphilitic,** sif'–i–LIT–ik).
3. Vowels pronounced with long sounds are indicated by a line above the vowel and are pronounced as in the following common words.

   $\bar{a}$ as in *māke*

   $\bar{e}$ as in *bē*

   $\bar{i}$ as in *īvy*

   $\bar{o}$ as in *pōle*
4. Vowels not marked for long sounds are pronounced with the short sound, as in the following words.

   e as in *bet*

   i as in *sip*

   o as in *not*

   u as in *bud*
5. Other phonetic symbols are used to indicate the following sounds.

   a as in *above*

   soo as in *sue*

   kyoo as in *cute.*

   oy as in *oil*

PART | 1 | CAUSES, DETECTION, AND CONTROL OF INFECTIOUS DISEASES

The first cases of the disease that later came to be known as **acquired immune deficiency syndrome (AIDS)** were officially reported in June of 1981. Today, some ten years later, AIDS is a well-known word, the subject of intense scientific research and steadily increasing economic, public, and social concern. The disease claims not only a significant share of space in medical and related publications but makes its presence known by the consistent coverage in newspaper and on television and radio.

The stunning rapidity with which the AIDS epidemic seized global attention is without parallel. It reflects, in part, the frightening and still largely inevitable lethal effects of the AIDS virus infection, and the size of the ever-increasing circle of victims.

Initially, the AIDS virus, now known as the **human immunodeficiency virus (HIV),** was transmitted only by individuals practicing various types of high-risk behavior. AIDS has now penetrated all facets of society. In addition to the tremendous challenge presented by AIDS, another major threat to public health and well-being has been posed by newer, as well as the older, sexually transmitted diseases, or STDs. Public embarrassment and hush-hush attitudes about this group of diseases have made them a "silent epidemic." The STDs, of which **syphilis** (SIF-i-lis) and **gonorrhea** (gon'-o-RĒ-a) are but two of over twenty-five diseases, come close to being the number one communicable disease problem in most modern nations of the world. It is estimated that over 10 million individuals annually visit physicians in the United States for treatment of a sexually transmitted disease. Several of these diseases, as later portions of this book will show, have a relationship to the spreading of AIDS.

The chapters in part 1 are designed to provide a general understanding of diseases (especially infectious diseases), their causes, treatment, detection, and control. The basic information presented serves as a firm foundation with which to approach the main topic of this book, the STDs.

Examples of the variety of press reports dealing with AIDS.

AIDS: $1.2-Billion Funding Bill Wins House Approval

Continued from Page 1

their addresses, said Rep. William
E. Dannemeyer (R-Fullerton).
Before the final vote, the House
soundly (_____ amendment
backed b _____
Bill McC _____
doctors t _____
effort" _____
people _____
AIDS vi _____
"I ca _____
importa _____
of fight _____
"It's bi _____
spousa _____

to speed up testing of new drugs
that might help combat AIDS.
The Senate bill, which does not
address confidentiality and testing
issues, focuses on research.
Few House members disagreed

AIDS: Congress Votes Bill Limiting Confidentiality

Continued from Page 1

n here, but we still have a job to
?," he said, vowing that House
embers would take up legislation
xt year mandating the confiden-
ity of AIDS test results and
e with the disease
on.

e, Congress
t $250 mil)
rograms
ps and
The
a
amir
idr cases

the names of those tested, even to
government health officials. He
said that the epidemic poses a
national health risk and supersedes
the concerns of individuals involved.
Waxman and others have con-
tended, however, that individuals
who have AIDS or are at risk of
-eloping the deadly disease may
forward for testing unless
that their identi-
confidence.
ta, they
ient will
e the full

nting Wax-
. M. Kennedy

AIDS Battle Lines Are Drawn Again in State

Major Health Organizations Attack Prop. 102,

Cultures Conflict Over Medicine

Total Number of AIDS Cases Put at 111,854 Worldwide

GENEVA—A total of
orted around
onth, raising
y as of

AIDS: Risk Cited in Cutoff of Funds for Condom Study

Continued from Page 1

disease.
But now federal officials say that
the effect _____
blocking _____
through ar _____
compromis _____
with high i _____
geles, San _____
Miami and _____
The fede _____
million in g _____
have paid f _____
condoms b _____
Los Angele _____
signed to r _____
condoms ar _____
of the hun _____
virus (HIV _____
sex. HIV is _____
AIDS.

'Ethical P

But in a Jo _____
of the UCL _____
Institutes c _____
"potential e _____
study were a _____
project, beg _____
received sli _____
million in fe _____
ready has pr _____
oratory test _____
of condoms i _____
brands, in _____
AIDS transm _____
The study _____
involved test _____
people.
The head of _____
Roger Detels _____
discuss the go _____
But Dr. Jeff _____
of contraceptive evaluation for the
National Institute of Child Health
and Human Development, a branch
of the NIH, said the cutoff stemmed

four other cities, the risks in such
sex, even with condom use, appea
overwhelming

32

les County Department of
be still be
Part 1/Sunday, October 2, 1988 ★ ★

use in high-infection areas appear
with earlier policies
Surgeon General C.
who has consistent-
people

AIDS: No on 102

The opposition to Proposition 102, the AIDS
reporting initiative, is almost unanimous among
health-care providers, public-health worker
and business and religious leaders—and for goo
reason. The initiative would mandate an end to t
nationally endorsed programs now in place, and
the same time would require a massive diversior
scarce funds into activities that have never b
tested and may well be of no value.
A few doctors have been attracted to the
tiative, arguing that it would command th
porting procedures already required of many
communicable diseases. So why not AIDS
answer lies in the unique aspects of this c
above all in the fact that no cure is yet
That is why the Presidential Commissio
Human Immunodeficiency Virus Epide
California AIDS Leadership Committee,
of the Centers for Disease Control, pub
experts at UCLA and UC Berkeley a
researchers at UC San Francisco all su
existing program, including its reliance
tary cooperation. Indeed, the single mo
instrument for reaching high-risk po
the anonymous test center that would
by this initiative.
The initiative not only would dest
ing demonstrably effective programs

AIDS: Ban on Bias Among Bills Vetoed by Governor

Continued from Page 1

Republican governor, who in 1986
had already surpassed his two
predecessors—Republican Ronald
Reagan and Democrat Edmund G.
Brown Jr.—in total number of
vetoes.
About 1,200 of the bills were
passed in the last weeks of the
session, which ended Sept. 1, and
Deukmejian chided lawmakers for
that as well.
Deukmejian's veto of the antidiscrimination bill appears to run
counter to the position of several of
his Republicans allies, including
Vice President George Bush and
California Sen. Pete Wilson, both of
whom have called for laws to
protect individuals who have been
exposed to the virus. Similar recommendations are contained in a
report by the Presidential Commission on AIDS.
In vetoing the measure, Deukmejian took great pains to explain
that AIDS patients are already
protected by the Fair Employment
and Housing Act, which bars housing and employment discrimination
against people with physical handi-
caps.
Deukmejian
said it would be

virus. Prison inmates are also allowed to request testing of fellow
inmates.
A second bill, by Sen. John
Doolittle (R-Rocklin), makes it a
felony for prostitutes to continue
working after knowing they have
been exposed to the virus. It would
also have financed education programs for victims and perpetrators
of sex offenses. But Deukmejian cut
$1.5 million from a $2-million ap-
propriation meant to underwrite
the program, saying he believed
$500,000 is sufficient.
The third AIDS bill, by Sen. Gary
K. Hart (D-Santa Barbara), loos-
ens the state's confidentiality laws,
allowing physicians to tell other
doctors, nurses and health workers
whether a patient has AIDS or has
tested positive for the virus. The
California Medical Assn. had complained that without the information, health care workers do not
know when to take steps to protect
themselves.

Bill on Toy Guns

In the area of law enforcement,
the bill signed by Deukmejian to
outlaw the manufacture, sale, or
distribution

risks of condom failure and subsequent AIDS transmission to study
volunteers were unacceptably
high

2

Memorial quilts serving as reminders of the lives lost to AIDS.
Each panel shown represents a person who died of this disease.
(Courtesy of World Health Organization)

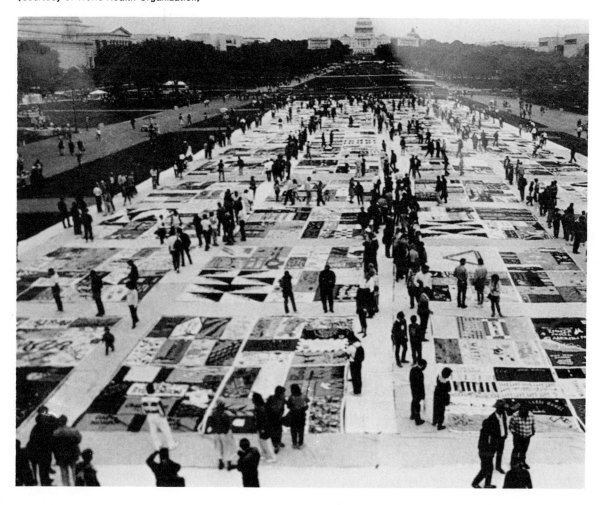

CHAPTER | 1

AN INTRODUCTION TO INFECTIOUS DISEASES

Diseases are more easily prevented than cured, and the first step to their prevention is the discovery of their exciting causes.

—William Farr

According to an ancient Greek myth there was once a Golden Age when humans lived completely free of illness, which continued until the curious Pandora opened the box containing the world's evils and allowed diseases to escape. Whether it was the Golden Age or the Garden of Eden, it is quite obvious that there is no chance of return to a mythical disease-free existence. Disease has always been a part of all forms of life, and always will be. Fossil remains clearly provide evidence that diseases such as smallpox (fig. 1.1), **poliomyelitis** (pol'-ē-ō-mī-el-ī-tis), cancer, and even tooth decay have afflicted humans since the earliest of times. This chapter briefly focuses on the question, What is disease?, and then concentrates on the categories of diseases with a major emphasis on infectious diseases and their causes.

FIGURE 1.1

Events in the plagues of history. The head of the mummy of Pharoah Ramses V, who reportedly died in 1157 B.C. of an illness resembling the viral disease smallpox. (Courtesy of World Health Organization)

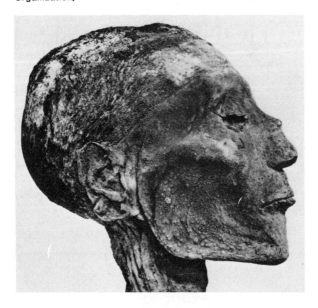

WHAT IS A DISEASE?

Viewpoints about the nature of disease date back to ancient times. Most of such theories generally fall into two views of the world: the *natural* and the *supernatural*. According to the supernatural position, the earth and everything it contains are controlled by gods, ghosts, or other supernatural forces. Thus, human fortunes and misfortunes, including disease, are directly under the influence of these sources. The natural viewpoint holds that there are no gods or supernatural forces in control, and the world around us is the sum total of reality. Moreover, diseases are caused by various natural factors, including chemicals, genetic defects, and microorganisms or microscopic forms of life such as viruses (fig. 1.2).

A *disease* may be defined as any interference with the normal functioning of body organs or systems. It is the pattern of response shown by a living organism to the development of some form of injury.

While conditions such as a broken bone, a wound, or a sprain of a joint involve the destruction of body tissue, they are not considered examples of diseases.

SIGNS, SYMPTOMS, AND SYNDROMES

Human diseases may be caused by environmental factors, defects of body structures or functions, activities of infectious microorganisms, or any combination of these agents. Most diseases are recognized by their *signs* or *symptoms*. A *sign* is a more or less observable and obvious feature of a disease and includes such things as diarrhea, a rash, or the unusual peeling of the skin (fig. 1.3). Certain diseases may be associated with structural changes called **lesions** (LĒ-zhuns) that are typically found in or on various body parts. For example, in the case of the sexually transmitted disease **syphilis** (SIF-i-lis), a hard, painless lesion (sore) known as a **chancre** (SHANG-ker) develops at the original site of *infection* (fig. 1.4). An infection is caused by a disease-causing agent and results from the ability to invade and multiply in the tissues of the host.

A *symptom* refers to any change in a body structure or function that can be observed or felt by the individual. In contrast to signs, symptoms are more subjective in nature, and include characteristics of a disease such as shortness of breath, pain, and general weakness. Some diseases may develop without the appearance of symptoms, thus not causing the affected individual any discomfort or disability. Such conditions are referred to as being **asymptomatic.** A disease is often asymptomatic in its early stages. If left untreated, the disease may progress to the stage where it causes symptoms and injury.

A combination of signs and symptoms occurring in a typical pattern is known as a **syndrome.** Syndromes are of value in diagnosis and in determining the distribution as well as the causes, or **etiology** (ē-tē-OL-ō-jē), of diseases. In order to better understand and eventually control a disease, it helps to know its cause.

FIGURE 1.2

Viruses are exceptionally small forms of life. This comparison view seen through an electron microscope shows influenza viruses (arrows) attached to the surfaces of human red blood cells.

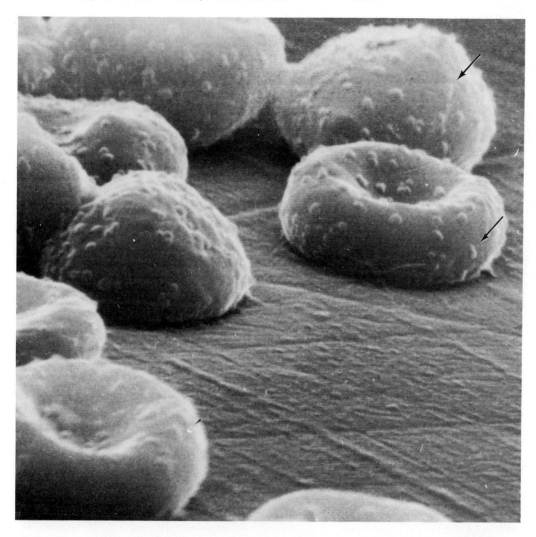

The outcome of a disease depends on several factors which not only include those associated with the individual, such as genetic (inherited) characteristics, age, nutritional status, prior exposure to infectious disease agents, and the resulting levels of body protection or immunity produced, but those related to the environment, such as sanitation and various socioeconomic influences. The interplay of these and other factors determines whether a disease results in complete recovery or causes a temporary period of disability, serious injury, or death. Even after recovery some diseases leave aftereffects, called **sequelae** (se-KWE-le). For example, viral infections of the liver can result in the loss of functioning liver cells and an interference with the flow of blood through this organ. In addition, syphilis, if

FIGURE 1.3

Signs of disease. (a) The rash. Rashes may result from a variety of causes. In this case, the rash is one of the typical signs of secondary syphilis, an STD known from ancient times. (b) The peeling of skin and the involvement of the toes here also may be found with individuals having syphilis. This statement, however, should not be taken to mean that anyone with skin peeling on the feet has syphilis. (Courtesy of Dr. Z. Starzycki)

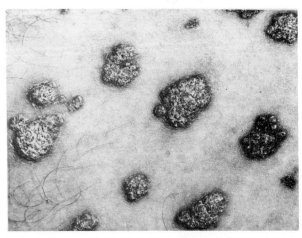

a

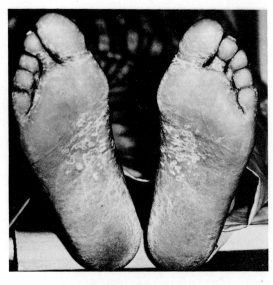

b

left untreated, often causes permanent damage to the heart, blood vessels, and the brain. The term **prognosis** (prog-NŌ-sis) is used to predict the course and outcome of a disease.

TYPES OF DISEASES

A large number of diseases are known. Arranging them according to their respective causes is helpful in systematizing existing knowledge. On this basis diseases can be placed into the following descriptive groups:

1. hereditary and congenital diseases
2. degenerative diseases
3. neoplastic diseases
4. metabolic diseases
5. immunological diseases
6. infectious diseases

FIGURE 1.4

A syphilitic chancre on the lip (arrow).

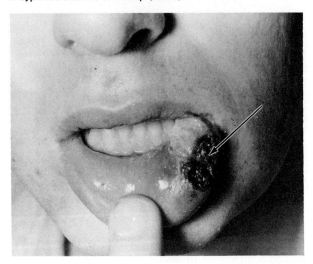

FIGURE 1.5

A child with Down's syndrome. This disease is a genetic disorder.

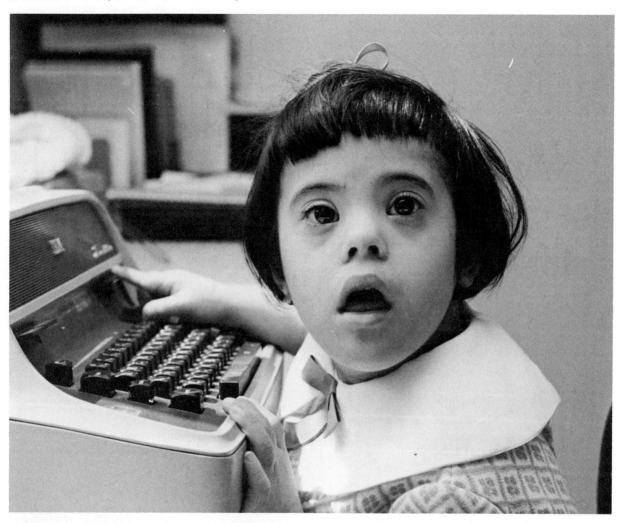

HEREDITARY AND CONGENITAL DISEASES

Hereditary diseases are caused by errors in the information present in an abnormal gene or genes. The resulting developmental disorders may be caused by abnormalities in the number and distribution of chromosomes, or the interaction of genetic and environmental factors. Down's syndrome (fig. 1.5), a well-known hereditary disease, results from an abnormal distribution of chromosomes. Individuals with this inherited disease have a characteristic facial expression, a mental deficiency, and defects involving the heart and other body organs. The features of several hereditary diseases do not fully develop until some time after birth.

Abnormalities that develop between the time of fertilization (conception) and birth are generally divided into two categories based on whether they start during the **embryonic** (em-brē-ON-ik) **period** (the first eight weeks of pregnancy), or during the **fetal period** (the time from the ninth week of pregnancy to birth). Changes occurring in the embryonic period produce visible deformities of organs or other body structures. These malformations are referred to as *embryonic,* or *congenital,* defects and are present at birth.

Drugs, excessive X-ray exposure, or certain infections may disrupt the development of an embryo or fetus. The effects of injury vary and depend on the agent and on the stage of pregnancy. The embryo is the most vulnerable to injury during the period from the third to eighth week after conception. This is the time when the embryo's organ systems are forming.

Certain infections acquired by the mother may injure the developing fetus and cause a number of congenital defects such as mental retardation, blindness, severe injury to the brain, and death. German measles (rubella), and the STDs syphilis and genital herpes are among this group of diseases.

DEGENERATIVE DISEASES

In the United States the average life span of women is about seventy-seven years, while that of men is approximately seventy-two. Given the remarkable medical and scientific advances currently being made it is anticipated that the longevity of the average individual may well extend beyond these ages. In degenerative diseases the primary abnormality is the breakdown of various body parts. Degenerative diseases are among the factors that pose barriers to extending life. Some of these conditions are associated with aging and are known to cause long-lasting (chronic) illnesses and to account for a significant number of deaths each year. These include heart attacks and strokes (bleeding and/or blockages in blood vessels of the brain).

In a number of cases, degeneration of body parts is more advanced and occurs earlier than would be expected if it were age related. Hardening of the arteries and certain forms of arthritis or degenerating joints are common examples of this group of diseases.

NEOPLASTIC DISEASES

These diseases are associated with abnormal cell growth that leads to the formation of various types of harmless (benign) and cancerous (malignant) tumors (fig. 1.6). Common forms of cancers involve the breast, the large intestine, the lungs, the stomach, and the uterus. In the United States, one in five persons dies of some form of cancer. These diseases have several possible causes including chemicals, physical agents such as various types of radiation which include sunlight and X-rays, and viruses. The **papilloma** (pap-i-LŌ-ma) viruses, which cause genital warts, also have been associated with the development of cervical cancer.

METABOLIC DISEASES

Metabolic diseases include a variety of disorders in which the body's production of chemical products essential to its functioning either are nonexistent or defective. Examples of such chemicals are **hormones** and **enzymes** (EN-zīms). A hormone is a chemical product of a body organ or gland, which is carried by the blood to another body site where it stimulates a particular function. Examples of hormones include insulin, adrenalin, and thyroid hormone. An enzyme is a complex protein produced by cells, that causes changes in other substances without being changed in the process. Activities in which enzymes are key factors include the formation of proteins, and the digestion of sugars, proteins, and fats.

While most metabolic diseases have a hereditary (genetic) basis, infections, tumors, and tissue degeneration also are recognized as possible causes. This group of diseases may be listed at times as **endocrine** (hormonal), kidney, or digestive system disorders to emphasize the specific body part involved.

IMMUNOLOGIC DISEASES

Immunological diseases result from the improper or impaired functioning of the body's immune system. This system provides protection against various disease agents and other factors in an individual's environment. A number of external and internal body structures, secretions, and related processes provide such protection by destroying or neutralizing disease agents and factors considered to be foreign by the immune system. These include the skin, tears, body temperature, various types of white blood cells, gastric secretions, and inflammation. **Inflammation** is a response to tissue injury. The associated signs and symptoms generally include *swelling, redness,*

FIGURE 1.6

An abnormal growth or neoplasm in the mouth. Growths of this type, also called *tumors*, develop from abnormal cell development or multiplication. They may or may not be life threatening.

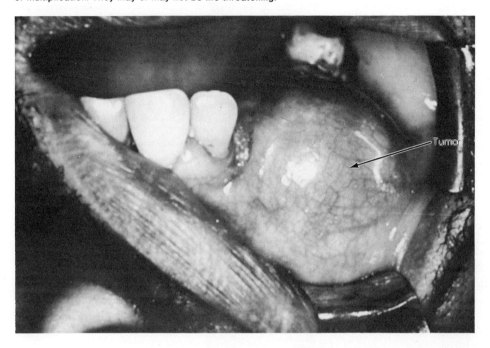

local heat, pain, and *abnormal functioning of the region or part involved.*

Immune responses and associated reactions usually are protective and helpful. In certain situations, however, they cause tissue injury and may even be life threatening. Immunologic diseases can be grouped into two categories: **primary** and **secondary immunodeficiencies.** Primary immunodeficiencies usually arise from an inherited lack of development of one or more parts of the immune system. Secondary immunodeficiencies occur more frequently than the primary ones and result from many factors that suppress an individual's immune responses to such events as an infection. AIDS is one consequence of a viral infection involving certain cells of the immune system called T lymphocytes. This disease is an example of a secondary immunodeficiency. Chapter 10 describes the various features of the immune system and some associated defects.

INFECTIOUS DISEASES

Various microscopic forms of life, or microorganisms, live on the skin (fig. 1.7), in the mouth, the large intestine, and other body locations. These microscopic forms are the body's **microbiota** (MĪ-krō-bī-ō'-ta), or resident microbial population. While most of them are harmless, some of them, if given an opportunity, have the capacity to cause a disease, and then are referred to as **opportunists.** Failure of the immune system to function normally leads to opportunistic infections in persons with AIDS and other immunodeficiencies. (Chapter 11 presents a general view of opportunists and the diseases they cause.) Still other microorganisms cause severe problems upon gaining entrance to host tissues (fig. 1.8). These forms are called **pathogens** (PATH-ō-jens), while the process associated with the development and eventual production of a disease is referred to as **pathogenesis** (path'-ō-JEN-ē-sis). The

FIGURE 1.7

The appearance of bacteria (spherical forms) on the skin's surface.

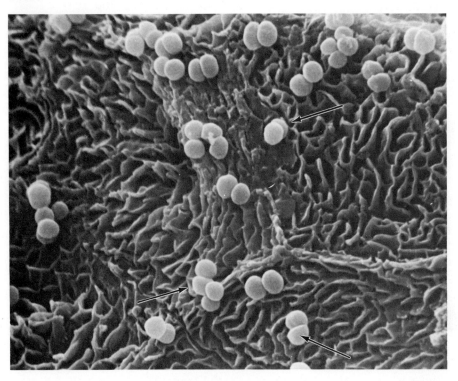

disease-producing capability of a pathogen is called **pathogenicity** (path'-ō-je-NIS-i-tē). It depends on the ability of a disease agent to invade a host, multiply in the host, and avoid being damaged by the host's defenses. The degree or intensity of pathogenicity is called **virulence** (VIR-ū-lens).

An infection usually is associated with the process by which pathogens gain entrance to the body, multiply, and spread to different regions of the body where they cause harmful effects. Hence the use of the term *infectious disease.* Infectious diseases are caused by infectious agents (pathogens) such as **bacteria, fungi, protozoa** (prō-tō-ZŌ-a), **viruses** (VĪ-rus-es), and **helminths** (HEL-minths) or worms. Noninfectious diseases are caused by any factor or agent other than an infectious organism.

Contagious and Noncontagious. Certain infectious diseases can be spread from person to person, and are said to be **communicable** (ko-MŪ-ne-ka-b'l) or **contagious.** The flu and measles are examples of highly communicable diseases. The STDs gonorrhea and syphilis also are communicable since they can be spread among sexual partners. There are also **noncommunicable diseases.** They are caused by infectious agents, but are not spread from person to person. Noncommunicable disease agents are acquired in some way from the environment. For example, lockjaw (tetanus) is a bacterial infection usually acquired by introducing the disease agent into a wound. A wooden splinter, piece of glass, nail, or rose thorn can serve this purpose.

FIGURE 1.8

Infectious diseases affect both young and old. (a) A young child with a severe virus skin infection. (Courtesy of Todd Wien, M.D.).

(b) A case of the virus disease known as shingles. The same virus also causes the childhood disease chicken pox.

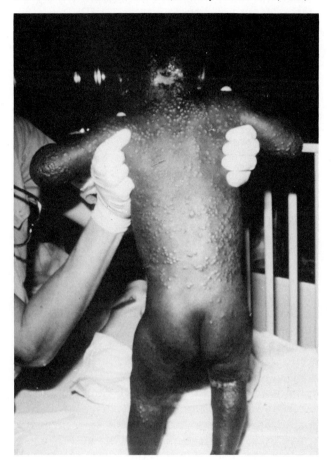

a

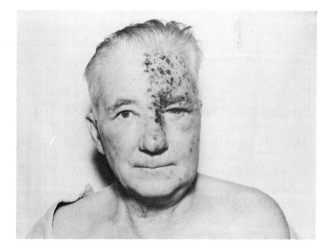

b

THE COURSE OF AN INFECTIOUS DISEASE

Most diseases caused by an infectious disease agent tend to pass through a fairly standard series of stages or phases. These include:

- *the incubation period:* the time between the multiplication of the pathogen and the appearance of signs and symptoms.
- *the prodromal phase:* the early stage of some diseases in which nonspecific symptoms such as headache and general weakness appear.

- *the invasive phase:* the period during which pathogens invade and cause tissue damage. Signs and symptoms of the disease appear at this time.
- *the convalescence (kon'-val-ES-ens) phase:* the time period during which recovery occurs, and includes healing, regaining strength, and the disappearance of symptoms. In some diseases even though signs and symptoms disappear, individuals can still spread the infectious disease agent to others.

Infectious diseases, as well as other types of diseases, can occur in **acute** (a-K$\overline{U}$T) and **chronic** forms. An acute disease occurs rapidly and sometimes with intense symptoms. A chronic disease develops more slowly and lasts for a longer, indefinite, period of time.

THE CONCEPT OF INFECTIOUS DISEASE

The concept of infectious disease appeared in human history long before the discovery of the microorganisms. As a remarkable example of human intellect reaching beyond existing knowledge, Girolamo Fracastorius, a Franciscan monk, in 1546 distinguished several ways in which infectious diseases could be spread. Based on long and detailed observations of diseases that periodically devastated major cities and small towns in Italy, he concluded that there were three specific types of transmission. These were: *contact with a sick person; contact with objects close to the sick person;* and *the air of the sickroom, which contained minute, invisible bodies called germs that were capable of passing into the body through pores.* The latter means of transmission formed the basis of Fracastorius's "germ theory" which was used to explain the nature of certain diseases.

After the recorded discovery of microorganisms in the late 1600s by the Dutchman Anton van Leeuwenhoek, a number of people suspected but could not prove that these microscopic forms of life could infect humans and other animals. Even with the development in the late 1800s of more effective methods with which to grow microorganisms and better microscopes with which to see them, it took over two hundred years to show the specific relationship of a pathogen to a specific infectious disease.

In 1876 the German bacteriologist Robert Koch provided the first convincing proof of Fracastorius's "germ theory of disease." He clearly demonstrated that a specific bacterium was the specific cause of anthrax, a serious and sometimes fatal disease of sheep, cattle, and even humans. Koch's historic milestone introduced the application of a set of experimental steps, which later was formalized and became known as **Koch's Postulates.** With relatively few exceptions, the causal relationship between pathogenic bacteria and a specific disease has been shown according to the dictates of Koch's postulates.

At the time when Koch's postulates were formulated, true viral pathogens were unknown. In 1937 T. M. Rivers established a similar group of experimental steps to show the causal relationship of viruses to infectious diseases.

There is no question that both groups of postulates have not only helped prove the microbial basis of a number of infectious diseases, but freed society from many superstitions and myths that had prevailed for centuries.

FACTORS CONTRIBUTING TO THE SUCCESS OF AN INFECTIOUS DISEASE

Whether or not an infectious disease develops is decided by the outcome of a battle involving the actions of pathogens and the ability of a host to deal with them. Pathogens act in certain ways that enable them to cause disease. Such actions include gaining access to the host, attaching to and reproducing on cell surfaces, invading body tissues, and producing poisonous substances known as *toxins* and other products such as enzymes which contribute to the breakdown of tissues and body defenses. Certain pathogens may even release toxic substances that often cause allergic responses in the host. The general characteristics of microorganisms and worms, some of which are the major contributors to the development of an infectious disease, are described in the next section.

AN INTRODUCTION TO THE MICROBIAL WORLD

The world of microorganisms includes bacteria, fungi, protozoa, and viruses. At first, these microscopic forms of life were thought to be mysterious oddities of little practical importance. However, the work of many individuals, such as Louis Pasteur and Robert Koch, drastically changed this limited view of microbes during the late nineteenth century. For the first time, the world became aware of the desirable and undesirable effects of microorganisms on the environment—including spoilage, disease, and death.

Microorganisms perform many activities that are beneficial. For example, these microscopic forms of life manufacture antibiotics and vitamins, decompose sewage and solid and industrial wastes, and are essential to the formation of foods such as cheeses, yogurt, bread, pickles, and sauerkraut. Many of these microbial products are of commercial importance.

Despite the established useful functions and the potentially valuable activities of microorganisms, these microscopic forms of life may be best known as causes of diseases including the flu, measles, and the sexually transmitted diseases. An understanding of these and other activities of microorganisms can best be accomplished with an examination of the microbial world. The following section also contains a brief consideration of worms since these forms of animal life can cause infectious diseases.

BACTERIA

Bacteria form a large mixture of single-celled microorganisms. This group of microscopic forms of life includes beneficial, harmful, and harmless members. Bacteria are differentiated from one another by several factors, including shape, color reactions when they are subjected to certain standard staining procedures, chemical composition, growth (nutrient) requirements, and responses to various chemicals such as antibiotics. Some of these factors are briefly described here.

Shape. Three basic shapes found among the bacteria are: 1) the *coccus* (KOK-us) or spherical form, (plural, *cocci,* KOK-sī); 2) the *bacillus* (ba-SIL-us) or rod, (plural, *bacilli,* ba-SIL-ī); and 3) the twisted or bent *spirillum* (fig. 1.9) (plural *spirilla* spī-RIL-a). Several different arrangements of these shaped cells are possible. For example, a spirillum that is compressed into a tighter corkscrew form is known as a **spirochete** (SPĪ-rō-kēt). The causative agent of the STD syphilis is a spirochete.

FIGURE 1.9

A scanning electron microscopic view of spiral-shaped bacteria. Note the coiling or twisting feature of these microorganisms.

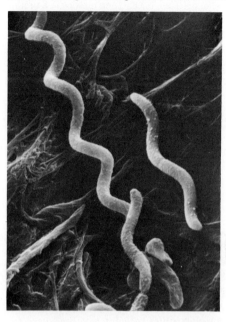

Isolation and Growing Bacteria (Culturing). In order to identify or to show the relationship of a *bacterium* to a particular process such as an infection, it must be isolated and grown in a particular nutrient preparation referred to as a *medium*. While a wide variety of these media are used, two general forms are recognized. These are broth or liquid, and the solid or **agar** (A-gar) forms of media, all of which contain a variety of nutrients such as sugars, proteins, fats, vitamins, and minerals.

In a broth culture, bacteria generally are distributed within the medium, while on an agar medium, bacteria aggregate and form *colonies*, which consist of thousands of cells (fig. 1.10). Media also can be used to test the sensitivies of bacteria and other microorganisms to various types of drugs and chemicals such as antibiotics (fig. 1.11).

In some cases preparations of animal and/or plant tissues known as *tissue cultures,* and whole animals such as mice, chicken embryos, and plants also may be used for the isolation and study of bacteria.

FIGURE 1.10

Bacteria and media. (a) A scanning electron micrograph of bacteria taken from a small portion of a bacterial colony. (b) The appearance of bacterial colonies. (c) Bacteria growing in a broth medium.

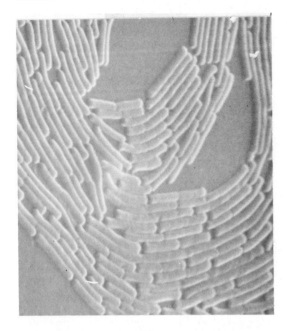

a

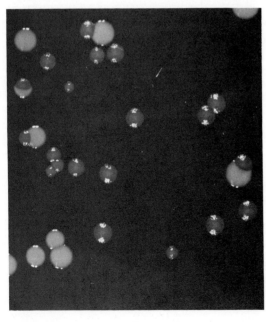

b

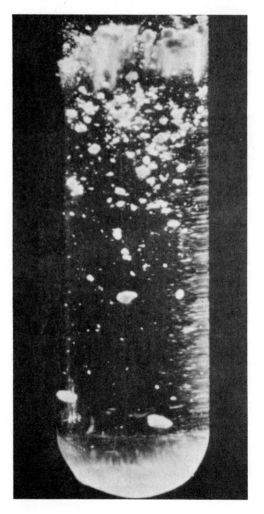

c

FIGURE 1.11
The testing of bacterial sensitivities. The small disks contain a substance to which growing bacteria are sensitive. This effect is obvious from the fact that no bacterial colonies are in the areas immediately surrounding the disks.

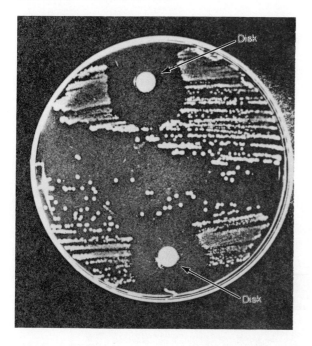

FUNGI

The fungi represent a group of single- and multicellular forms of life and include **yeasts** (yēsts), **molds,** and **mushrooms** (fig. 1.12). The majority of fungi are involved with the natural decomposition of rotting and decaying plant and related material. Several are of use in the commercial production of bakery goods, cheeses, antibiotics, alcoholic beverages, and certain chemicals. Still others are known for their destructive effects on plants, humans, and other animals. While some fungi can attack the skin, nails, and hair, causing different forms of ringworm such as athlete's foot (fig. 1.13), others can cause certain STDs such as yeast infections of the reproductive tract. Some fungi also are opportunists.

PROTOZOA

Protozoa are a group of single-celled animal-like microorganisms. Most of them are harmless and are found in great numbers in soil and water environments. Some protozoa cause diseases such as malaria, the brain infection African sleeping sickness (fig. 1.14), and amebic dysentery (a -MĒ-bik, DIS-enter-ē). Some of these microorganisms also are opportunistic and cause STDs.

VIRUSES

Viruses cannot be seen with an ordinary light microscope. An electron microscope must be used. Hence, these forms of microorganisms are referred to as being *submicroscopic.*

Viruses are known to cause a large number and variety of diseases including the childhood diseases chicken pox (fig. 1.15) and the more recently discovered range of conditions caused by the human immunodeficiency virus (HIV) which includes AIDS. There is no form of life that is free from possible viral infection. In addition, several tumors or neoplasms and cancers are believed to be caused by viruses.

Structure and Shape. One of the most important features to note about viruses is that they are not cells, thus differing in appearance from other microorganisms. While different viruses vary greatly in their general shapes, they have certain similarities. Individual virus particles, or **virions** (VI-re-ons), contain a single type of nucleic acid, either **deoxyribonucleic acid (DNA)** or **ribonucleic acid (RNA),** but never both. For many virions their nucleic acid component or core is enclosed in a protein coat known as a **capsid** (KAP-sid). In some cases the capsid may be covered by an envelope. The importance of viral parts (fig. 1.16) will be emphasized in the various chapters dealing with viral STDs (fig. 1.16b).

FIGURE 1.12

Microscopic views of two types of fungi showing their single and multicellular features. (a) The thin strands of a mold, together with round reproductive units called *spores*. (b) The single round cells of a yeast.

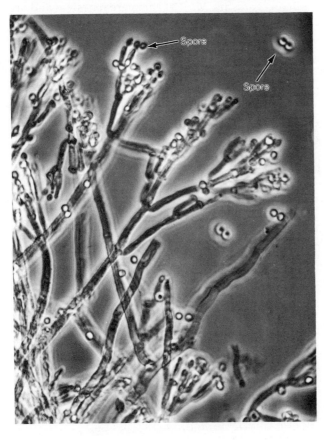

a

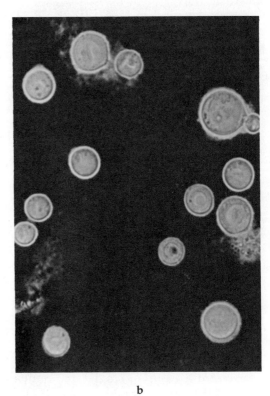

b

Cultivation. Another distinguishing characteristic of viruses is that they can only replicate (multiply) in living cells. Preparations of cells in the form of tissue cultures or living laboratory animals such as mice and chicken embryos are used for animal virus cultivation. Plants and their tissues are used for the cultivation of plant viruses.

HELMINTHS (WORMS) AND DISEASES

From a medical standpoint, helminths (worms) causing most human diseases belong to two large groups, the flatworms and the roundworms. Worms generally are not associated with STDs. However,

FIGURE 1.13

A case of athlete's foot.

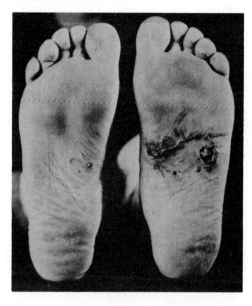

FIGURE 1.14

African sleeping sickness. (a) A victim of this protozoan disease. (b) A scanning electron microscope view of the causative agent of African sleeping sickness (arrow). Several red blood cells also are shown.

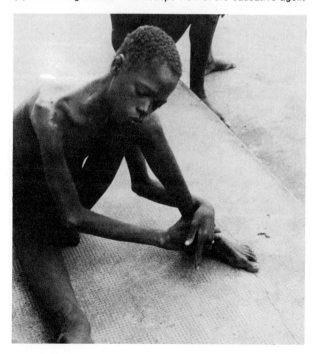

a

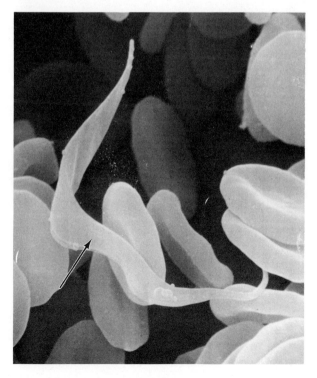

b

reports have appeared that indicate certain round-worm infections such as pinworm were sexually transmitted.

HOST-MICROORGANISM RELATIONSHIPS

This chapter provided an overview of diseases with a special emphasis on infectious diseases and their causes. **Microorganisms** display a variety of inter-relationships with other microorganisms, and with larger life forms such as humans that serve as hosts for them. Whether a **pathogen** causes disease in a host is a matter of whether the pathogen or the **host** wins the battle they wage against each other. The pathogen has certain invasive capabilities at its disposal, and the host has certain defenses against them. Later chapters in this text explore the outcome of such host-microorganism relationships.

FIGURE 1.15

The appearance of chicken pox. Note that the pox are scattered over the chest of this individual.

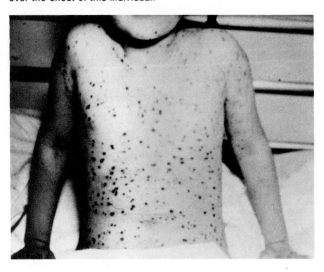

FIGURE 1.16

Two electron micrographs showing the features of virus particles. (a) Virions of a pox virus. The nucleic acid core in relation to other parts is shown. (b) The virus that causes AIDS. (Courtesy of Drs. T. Katsumoto and T. Kurimura)

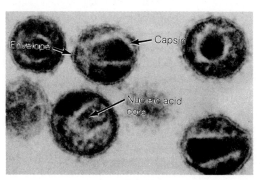

b

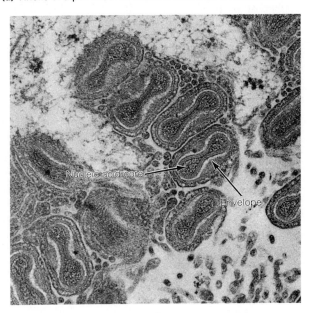

a

CHAPTER | 2

FACTORS IN THE SPREAD OF DISEASE

No easy thing seeing that there are above 1500 diseases to which Man is subjected.

—Sidney Smith, Letter to Lord Grey

So far as is known, all primitive and civilized societies have experienced diseases caused by pathogenic microorganisms. Frequently throughout history the results of such encounters have been disastrous as evidenced by the loss of human life in epidemics associated with smallpox, the bubonic plague (fig. 2.1), cholera, malaria, and yellow fever. The Renaissance period is a good example to show the devastating effects certain infectious diseases had on the populations of the world. The Renaissance, which was centered in Italy and spread throughout Europe in the fourteenth, fifteenth, and sixteenth centuries, was considered a Golden Age of not only art, but also of plague, syphilis (fig. 2.2), and murder. Interestingly, while people sang gloriously of love, of human possibilities, of life and beauty in the here and now, they also lived in fear of sudden death by poison in a palace, a dagger thrust in an alleyway, or any number of incurable diseases of the times. These included the bacterial diseases, typhus and typhoid fevers, which periodically swept through Europe, filling mass graves with their victims. However, the most dreaded of the incurable afflictions was the bubonic plague, or "Black Death", which in the fourteenth century claimed the lives of at least a quarter of all Europeans (fig. 2.3). Some historians place the death toll at 75 percent of the continent's population, in addition to the uncounted millions in Asia and Africa. The Black Death, which is now known to be a bacterial disease

FIGURE 2.1

This painting, "The Plague of Epirus," by Pierre Mignard, shows the confusion and destruction of human life caused by the bacterial disease that became known as the Black Death.

Records of this major epidemic, which occurred in the sixth century A.D., indicate that over 100 million people were killed by this plague within a 50–year period. (Courtesy of National Library of Medicine)

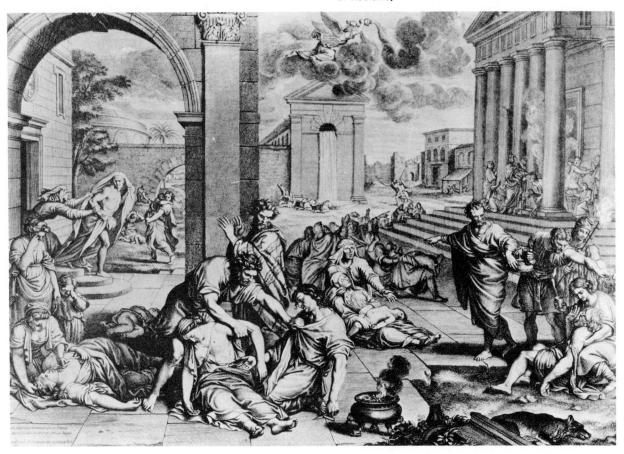

and spread by a rat flea (fig. 2.4), had been casting its devastating effects in Africa, Asia, and Europe for a thousand years. Physicians of the time were limited in their knowledge of the disease and how to treat it. No one had the foggiest idea of the enemy being fought. When the first signs of plague appeared in a European city, a physician who was brave enough to venture out on house calls to care for the infected usually wore a protective outfit of some type. A representative outfit consisted of a cloak tightly sewn with thread believed to be impenetrable to any contagious material from patients, a long birdlike beak made of leather and filled with sweet-smelling herbs to neutralize the

FIGURE 2.2

The appearance of sores that develop in the secondary stage of syphilis in some individuals. (a) This severe form of the sexually transmitted disease, which at times is described as early malignant syphilis, was commonly seen during the sixteenth century when a "new" disease referred to as the "great pox" made its appearance in Europe. (b) A magnified view. (From J. Lejman and Z. Starzycki, *British Journal of Venereal Diseases*, (1972) 48:194.)

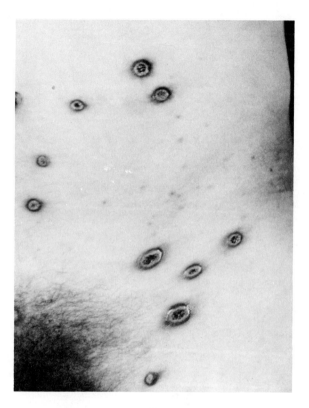

a

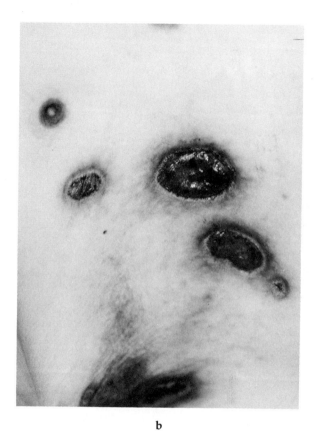

b

odors from decomposing bodies, and a metal mask to guard against the splattering of material into the eyes (fig.2.5).

The New World was not without its epidemics and loss of human life. Viral infectious diseases such as smallpox, measles, and influenza also took their tolls during the 1800s and 1900s. However, with a better understanding of the causes of diseases, and factors including improved nutrition, immunizations, rapid diagnostic tests, antibiotics, and other drugs for treatment and control, a significant reduction of disease cases has been achieved. Unfortunately, in some geographic regions, microbial-associated epidemics still claim large numbers of victims. One example here is AIDS, a contender for the title of a modern plague (fig. 2.6). In 1981, this disease was first officially recognized and added to the list of life-endangering virus infections. More than 50,000 new cases of the disease were diagnosed in the United States alone in

FIGURE 2.3
Burying victims of the Black Death of London of 1664 in mass graves.

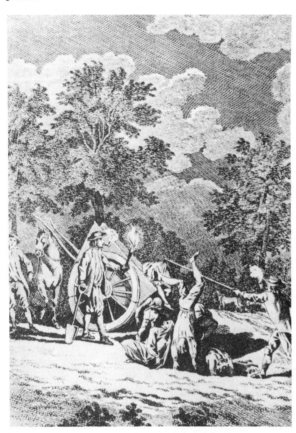

FIGURE 2.4
The main characters in the Black Death. (a) The rat, which carried the death-causing bacteria. (b) The spreader of the Black Death, the flea.

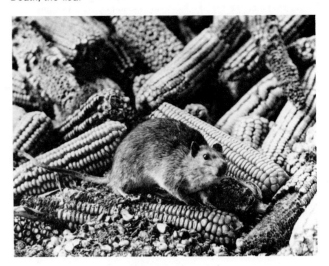

a

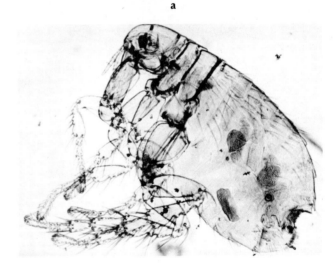

b

1988. As of February 1990, 1–2 million additional people were believed to be infected with the causative agent HIV (fig. 2.7). From a worldwide perspective, it is believed that the number of HIV-infected persons is currently around 5–10 million. Without effective measures for prevention, detection, and treatment, the number clearly would be expected to rise. Fortunately, there are preventative measures, methods for early detection, and a limited number of approaches for treatment. In addition, the search for better drugs and the development of an effective vaccine are ongoing.

Figure 2.5

The rather strange-looking clothing worn by Roman doctors during the 1656 outbreak of the plague. This outfit provided protection for the physician against the splattering of material from patients. The birdlike beak contained sweet-smelling herbs to neutralize the odors of decomposing bodies. The pointer was used to indicate to a patient which body part to move or to change position during the examination.

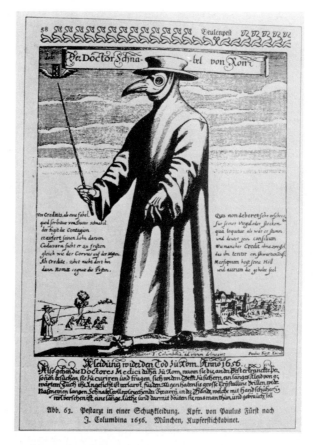

Central to the control and possible elimination of any infectious disease is the knowledge of factors that contribute to its occurrence and continuation within a population. This chapter presents selected aspects of **epidemiology** (ep-i-dē-mē-OL-ō-jē), an area of investigation that deals with factors that influence the frequency and distribution of diseases. Information gained through epidemiological investigations is used to find ways to control and to prevent the outbreaks of disease. Special attention is also given to the sources and transmission of infectious disease, and the reporting of and control of such diseases.

FIGURE 2.6

This sign was erected near a busy intersection in Los Angeles, California, in June, 1988. It registers the number of persons who died of AIDS in the United States as of the date shown.

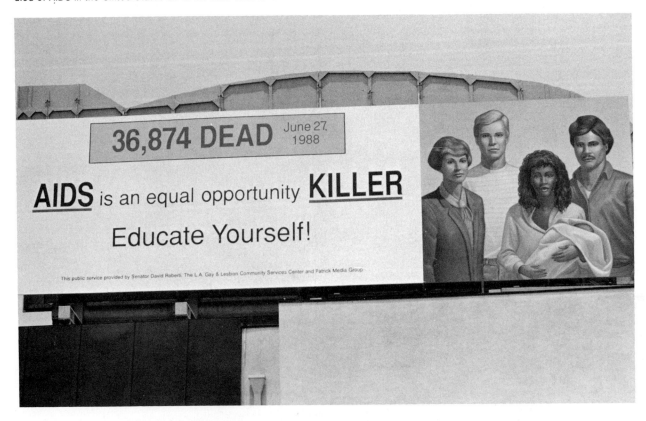

FEATURES OF EPIDEMIOLOGY

Epidemiology is concerned with disease as it applies to populations of individuals. It relies heavily on numerical information or statistics that indicate the frequency of both infectious and noninfectious diseases. Obtaining such information is not always a simple matter. It requires a familiarity with the specific signs, symptoms, and stages of a disease (fig. 2.8), and the relationships among pathogens, their hosts, and the environment.

PATTERNS OF DISEASE OCCURRENCE

The occurrence of a disease within a population may be quantified by determining its **incidence** and **prevalance.** The incidence of a disease is the number of new cases seen in a specific time period (fig. 2.9), while the prevalence of a disease refers to the total number of cases at any one time. It includes both old and new cases and is influenced by the duration of the disease. In various reports, the incidence of a

FIGURE 2.7

The AIDS virus, known also as the human immunodeficiency virus (HIV). Since the first report of this disease-causing agent over 1.5 million persons have been infected with it in the United States. The World Health Organization estimates that during the 1990s over 10 million will be infected on a worldwide basis.

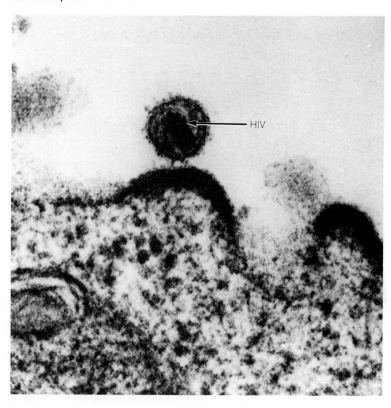

disease may be referred to as the **morbidity** (mor-BID-i-tē) **rate** and is expressed as the number of new cases per 10,000 in the population per year (fig. 2.10). The **mortality** (mor-TAL-i-tē) **rate** refers to the number of individuals that died as a result of a specific disease in a specific time period. Once epidemiological information of this type is gathered it is usually published. In the United States, one of the major sources of such information is the *Morbidity and Mortality Weekly Report* (fig. 2.11). Other countries use similar means to publicize statistical information related to disease occurrence and prevalence.

Occasionally, outbreaks of disease occur that are more or less limited to particular segments of a population. Consequently, morbidity and mortality rates may be calculated for that population segment alone. An infant mortality rate is an example.

ENDEMIC, EPIDEMIC, PANDEMIC, AND SPORADIC DISEASE PATTERNS

The patterns of occurrence among infectious and other types of diseases are influenced by the frequency of cases in populations, the size of the geographic area affected, and the degree of injury

FIGURE 2.8

Individuals reported to the Chicago Department of Health with confirmed measles infection in 1989. The graph is based on the age of the infected individual and the week the rash appeared. (From *Morbidity and Mortality Weekly Report* (1990) 39:317.)

FIGURE 1. Patients with confirmed measles, by age and by week of rash onset — Chicago, February 14–December 31, 1989

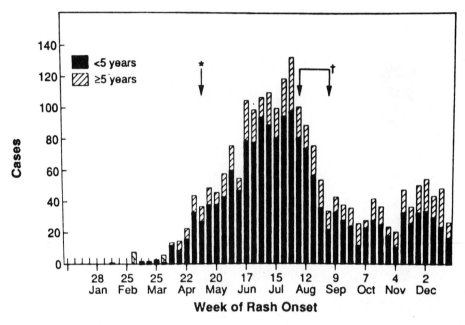

caused. On the bases of such factors, diseases can be categorized as being **endemic, epidemic, pandemic,** or **sporadic.** There terms are used to indicate the prevalence of diseases.

An *endemic disease* is constantly present in the population of a particular geographic area, but involves relatively few individuals. Since the severity of the disease is low, it does not present a major public health problem. Examples include the bacterial disease **tuberculosis** (tū-ber-kū-LŌ-sis) and the viral disease mumps. Both of these diseases are normally endemic to the entire United States. Various STDs such as **chancroid** (SHANG-kroyd) and gonorrhea have been endemic throughout the world for centuries.

An *epidemic* is an unusual occurrence of a disease involving large segments of a population for a limited period of time. An endemic disease can develop into an epidemic, especially when a particular harmful form of a pathogen appears on the scene or when a large segment of the population lacks resistance (immunity) to the disease agent. Influenza and childhood diseases such as measles (fig. 2.8) and chicken pox often give rise to epidemics.

A *pandemic* is a series of epidemics affecting several countries, or even major portions of the world. The influenza pandemic of 1918–1919 exhibited such a worldwide involvement. Currently, HIV infections and AIDS are following a similar path. The viral STDs genital herpes and genital warts also occur in epidemic proportions in the population.

FIGURE 2.9

The incidence of the viral disease measles in the United States for weeks 32–35 of 1989. The new cases are shown by individual states. (From *Morbidity and Mortality Weekly Report* (1989) 38:628.)

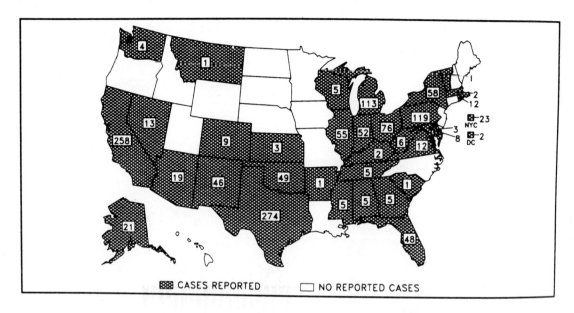

FIGURE 2.10

The rate per 100,000 women (morbidity rate) with the first two stages (*P*rimary and *S*econdary) of syphilis in New York City during the period 1983–1988. The incidence of congenital syphilis occurring during this time also is shown. Congenital syphilis cases refer to the infection in infants less than one year of age. (From *Morbidity and Mortality Weekly Report* (1989) 38:825–829.)

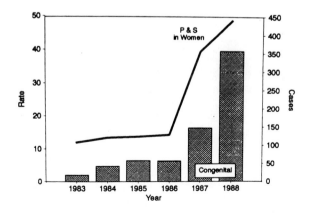

Sporadic diseases are uncommon, occur irregularly, and affect only a relatively few persons. Infections such as the bacterially-caused respiratory diseases **diphtheria** (diff-THĒ-rē-a) and **whooping** (HOOP-ing) **cough** occur sporadically. These and other infectious diseases may ordinarily be sporadic or endemic, but depending upon factors such as the immunity of the population, they can unfortunately, at times, become epidemic.

Infectious diseases, either endemic, epidemic, or pandemic, threaten human populations only when they can be spread from sources of the disease agents to susceptible hosts (fig. 2.12). Factors contributing to the transmission of infectious diseases include sources and reservoirs of disease agents, portals by which such agents leave and enter the body, and the mechanisms or means of transmission. The following section takes a look at these factors in more detail.

FIGURE 2.11

Examples of the *Morbidity and Mortality Weekly Report* (MMWR), prepared by the Centers for Disease Control in Atlanta, Georgia. This publication provides up-to-date articles, statistics, and information concerning notifiable diseases.

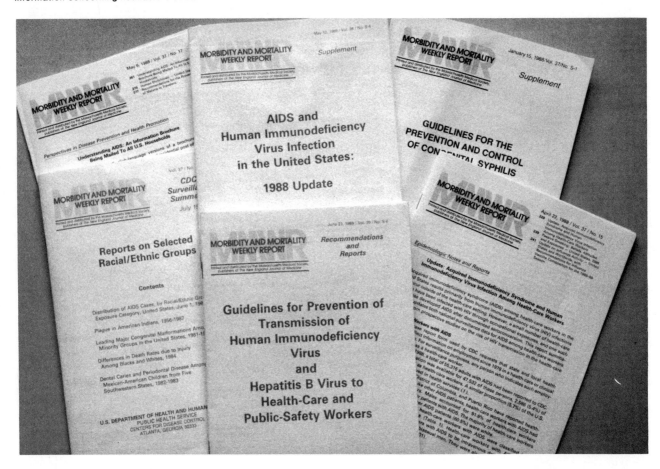

FIGURE 2.12

The epidemiological eyeglass model of an infectious disease. This model shows the interrelations between the factors involved with the transmission of an infectious disease from a source of the disease agent to a susceptible host. Knowing this information is of value in controlling the spread of a disease.

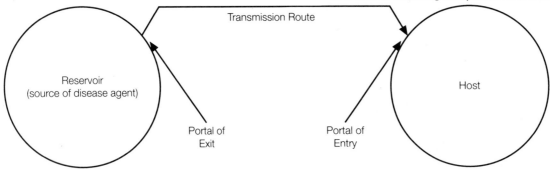

FACTORS IN THE SPREAD OF INFECTIOUS DISEASES

SOURCES

The sources of infectious disease agents are many and varied. Generally speaking, however, the most disabling and common infections among humans are caused by microorganisms capable of living and reproducing in human tissues. Most microorganisms capable of infecting humans cannot survive outside the body of a host long enough to serve as a source of infection. For example, **Treponema pallidum** (trep'-ō-NĒ-ma, PAL-e-dum), the cause of the STD syphilis (fig. 2.13), is restricted almost entirely to human beings, since this bacterium normally does not infect animals, and it cannot survive in the environment. Therefore, body locations where organisms can persist and maintain their ability to infect serve as potential sources of disease agents. These include body fluids and waste materials such as feces from the gastrointestinal tract, urine, semen, and discharges from genitourinary system, saliva from the mouth, mucus from the respiratory tract, blood, and discharges from sores and wounds on the skin and other areas (fig. 2.14).

RESERVOIRS OF INFECTION

A host or a local environment that supports the survival and multiplication of pathogens is referred to as a *reservoir of infection*. Living reservoirs include infected humans and other animals, whereas nonliving reservoirs include air, food, soil, water, eating utensils, and toothbrushes. Reservoirs of infection provide disease agents with a suitable environment for survival over a prolonged time and also provide opportunities for their transmission to others. Some diseases are transmissible before symptoms appear and even during the recovery period when symptoms are disappearing. Such situations can occur with several STDs, including syphilis and HIV infection.

A newly infected host may, in turn, become a new reservoir capable of infecting others, thus extending the chain of infection. Individuals who

FIGURE 2.13

The causative agent of syphilis, *Treponema pallidum*, in a specimen removed from the sore of an infected person. The bacteria (arrows) are magnified 1,800 times their normal size. (Courtesy of Dr. Z. Starzycki)

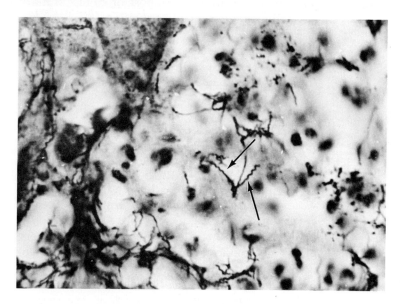

harbor pathogens transmissible to others are called **carriers.** A carrier who apparently suffers no ill effects is called a *healthy carrier.* The individual who is in an incubating state, undergoing the initial stages of a disease but without exhibiting symptoms, is referred to as an *incubatory carrier.* Such persons may be infectious during the last stages of their incubation period. Other categories of carriers include the *intermittent carrier,* who periodically releases disease agents, and the *convalescent carrier* who serves as a source of pathogens during the recovery period. Both reservoirs and sources of disease agents are important not only to the transmission of a disease agent, but also to the continuation of an infectious disease within a population.

How Do Pathogens Get Into and Out of the Body?

Portals of Entry. Pathogens enter the body through a small number of routes known as *portals of entry.* These include the skin, and the respiratory, gastrointestinal and genitourinary tracts. Injuries in the form of wounds (fig. 2.14) or animal bites also provide access routes into the body. A particular pathogen is generally restricted to a specific portal of entry. This is largely due to its ability to establish a disease process and the local defenses found in a particular part of the host's body.

The number of pathogens needed to initiate a disease process, known as the *infectious dose,* may be as low as one organism in some cases, or as many as hundreds of thousands in other situations. HIV infection, for example, requires large doses of the disease agent. The pathogen must be able to overcome the host's defenses in order to reproduce within the body. If this is not possible, the pathogen fails and eventually dies.

There is no question that the host defenses acting at the portal of entry, and the ability of a pathogen to overcome these defenses, influence the infectious dose required to start a disease process. However, other factors, such as malnutrition and the immunity of the host, are also important considerations. Chapter 10 concentrates on many of the immunity factors available to a host.

Portals of Exit. The sites at which organisms leave the body are called the *portals of exit.* In most cases pathogens are discharged with the body fluids and wastes described earlier as sources of disease agents. Actions of a host also help. For example, respiratory pathogens exit through the nose or mouth in fluids normally expelled during coughing, sneezing (fig. 2.15), or speaking.

With STDs such as gonorrhea and HIV infection, semen from males and discharges from the vagina from females are means by which pathogens can exit the body.

Mechanisms of Disease Transmission

The spread or transmission of a disease from its reservoir, or source, to a susceptible individual, or host, varies according to the particular features of the disease agent. It may occur in a variety of ways such as 1) direct contact with infected persons or carriers; 2) indirect contact with nonliving objects, or food or water contaminated by infected individuals; 3) inhalation of airborne dust or droplets of saliva, or other body fluids containing pathogens;

Figure 2.14

A case of syphilis of the finger. This infection was acquired through a cut coming into contact with a source of the disease agent. (Courtesy of Dr. Z. Starzycki)

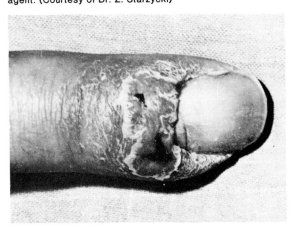

FIGURE 2.15

Sneezing. (a) Even this stifled sneeze produces many droplets. It is clear from this photo that the hands and arms can easily become contaminated with nasal secretions. (b) A full-blown, unstifled sneeze. Note the heavy cloud of material introduced into the air.

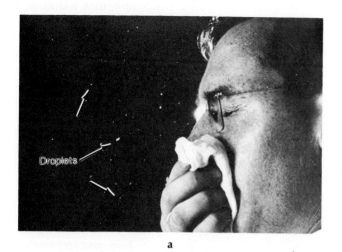

Droplets

a

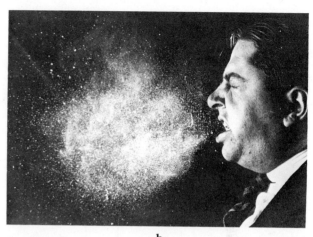

b

4) injection of body fluids containing disease agents; and 5) insects and related forms carrying pathogens.

For new cases of infectious diseases to develop, pathogens must be spread by some form of mechanism from portals of exit to portals of entry. Such mechanisms include *contact transmission, mechanical transmission,* and *biological transmission.*

Contact Transmission. Contact transmission may be either *direct* or *indirect*. Direct contact refers to the transmission of pathogens from person to person through close personal association. Examples include coughing, handshaking, kissing, sneezing, (fig. 2.16), and sexual activities. Indirect contact occurs when infectious agents are carried from one individual to another on contaminated, living or nonliving, objects. Contaminated nonliving objects other than food and water are called **fomites** (FŌ-mi-tēz). Eating utensils, toothbrushes, and hypodermic needles can serve as fomites. Certainly the washing of hands after blowing the nose, urinating, defecating, or working with infected persons helps to limit the spread of disease agents.

Mechanical Transmission. The mechanical means of transmission refers to situations involving the physical carrying of pathogens on or within contaminated materials such as food, water, or insects to other objects. This form of transmission makes use of the **five Fs: food, fingers, flies, feces,** and **fomites.** Diseases such as typhoid fever, certain types of food poisoning, chicken pox, and the common cold can be spread by these means.

The term **vector** is frequently used for forms of life that transmit disease to humans. Most vectors are arthropods, such as flies, ticks, cockroaches, and mosquitoes. Two categories of such transmitters are recognized: *mechanical vectors,* such as flies and cockroaches, which carry infectious agents on their bodies and are not used by the agents for multiplication and/or development; and *biological vectors,* which serve as reservoirs and are at times required by disease agents for their development, include but are not limited to arthropods such as bloodsucking ticks and mosquitoes. Currently there is no evidence to show that any STD can be spread by arthropod vectors.

FIGURE 2.16
Routes of infectious disease transmission.

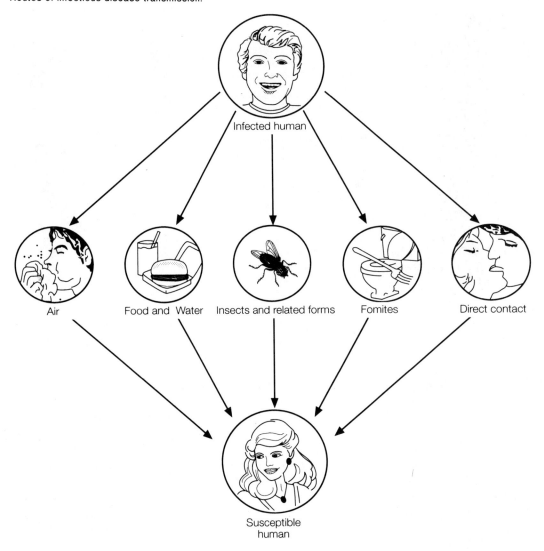

Infected human

Air

Food and Water

Insects and related forms

Fomites

Direct contact

Susceptible
human

Biological Transmission. In the biological means of transmission, a portion of the pathogen's development occurs in the form of life that serves to transmit the disease agent. The injection of blood or blood products, the bites of warm-blooded animals, and arthropods are examples of how pathogens are transmitted by this means. Malaria and rabies are examples of diseases transmitted by arthropod bites and warm-blooded animal bites respectively. Hepatitis and HIV infections have been transmitted by means of contaminated blood or blood products.

Horizontal and Vertical Transmission. Many diseases can be spread in a variety of ways within a population. These include *horizontal* and *vertical transmission*. Horizontal transmission is the transfer of disease agents in the population by air, physical contact, food, water, or vectors. Vertical transmission involves the transfer of infectious agents from parent to offspring by means of male and female sex cells or breast milk, or during pregnancy, which involves a mother infecting her unborn child. Maternal infections of unborn children are major public health problems and are dramatically increasing with STDs such as syphilis (fig. 2.10) and HIV infections.

GENERAL APPROACHES TO THE CONTROL OF CONTAGIOUS DISEASES

Several methods for the partial or full control of contagious diseases are available (fig. 2.17). They are directed toward reducing disease morbidity and mortality and include isolation, quarantine, elimination of vectors and sources of disease agents, and protection of susceptible hosts by increasing disease resistance through immunization.

FIGURE 2.17
General approaches to the control of contagious diseases.

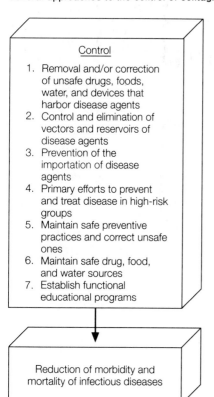

ISOLATION AND QUARANTINE

The isolation of an individual with a contagious disease prevents contact with the general population. This control method can not only minimize the spread of disease among susceptible persons, but can also protect infected individuals from exposure to other diseases.

The decision to isolate a patient may be based on a particular syndrome, or microorganism, or on the requirements of a specific hospital, or health care system. In some cases isolation practices are not without controversy. This has been especially true in the case of AIDS.

Quarantine is one of the oldest methods of controlling contagious diseases and involves the separation of humans and other forms of life from the general population when they either have a contagious disease or have been exposed to one. Neither isolation nor quarantine is used with STDs.

ELIMINATION OF VECTORS AND SOURCES OF DISEASE AGENTS

Elimination of vectors and sources of disease agents is an effective means of controlling contagious diseases. Incorporating functional sanitary measures, such as hand washing, the appropriate use of disinfectants, the spraying of insecticides, and the development and implementation of educational programs stressing preventative practices are effective measures to control certain diseases. Accurate detection and treatment of infected persons also are important aspects of disease control. Many of the following chapters will briefly describe the specific approaches used for treatment as they relate to specific STDs.

IMMUNIZATION

Before the discovery of the germ theory of infectious diseases, it was known that recovery from certain illnesses such as the viral disease smallpox was accompanied by an ability to resist reinfection. Thus in its infancy, this study of resistance, or *immunology*, was devoted almost exclusively to disease prevention by vaccination, or as it is commonly now referred to, *immunization*.

One of the greatest triumphs of modern medicine has been the elimination of smallpox everywhere in the world. Not one case has been reported since 1978. This is largely the result of a concentrated immunization campaign by the World Health Organization (WHO), a special agency of the United Nations. Because of this success, similar campaigns are under way to eliminate other infectious diseases such as polio and measles. Considerable effort is also being made to improve existing vaccines, develop new ones, and to increase their use. While there are no vaccines against STDs currently, numerous research efforts are under way to develop such preparations against many of these diseases. This is especially true for HIV infection, genital herpes, and gonorrhea. Chapter 14 describes the general nature of vaccines and the problems associated with the development of STD vaccines.

THE CHAIN OF EVENTS FOR AN INFECTIOUS DISEASE

This chapter has presented an overview of how pathogens are transmitted and how humans can serve as sources of disease agents. Clearly, individuals with infections are members of a population—they acquire disease agents and spread them within a population. Humans are the principal reservoirs for the microorganisms that cause STDs, and in most cases the reproductive system serves as both the portal of exit and the portal of entry.

PART 2 | SEXUALLY TRANSMITTED DISEASES

The causative agents of sexually transmissible or transmitted diseases, generally referred to as the **STDs,** cause not only discomfort and disability, but may result in death. These diseases have become a major worldwide health problem. This situation is especially evident among sexually active individuals in the age range of 15–24 years. It is increasingly common for young people to be sexually active. World Health Organization reports indicate that the median age at first intercourse or *coitus* (KŌ-i-tus) is as low as 14–15 years in Africa; 14–18 years in Sweden, the United States, Great Britain, and France; and 20 years in Canada. The age of coitus has been declining with time, as has the age of sexual maturity. Various studies show that most young people as well as older individuals are concerned and interested in learning about their sexuality. Receiving timely, relevant, and comprehensive information about sexually transmitted diseases also is of major interest. Toward this end, part 2 will present the major group of the well-established STDs. Parts 3 and 4 will focus on the spectrum of human immunodeficiency virus (HIV) infections, AIDS, AIDS-related complex (ARC), pediatric AIDS, and several of the associated problems and issues posed by these diseases.

"Fighting men" during World War II were warned to beware of the perils of venereal disease (VD) which "scarlet women," whether amateur or professional, were just waiting to inflict on them. Although an article on venereal diseases was finally published in the *Ladies Home Journal* in 1937, and premarital and prepregnancy blood tests were being given to women routinely just before the second world war, a chauvinistic attitude still prevailed. This poster was used to blame VD on an evil woman. The other two individuals shown represent the other two major enemies of the free world in World War II. (From A. M. Brandt, *Science* (1988) 239:375.) (Courtesy of Dr. Allan M. Brandt, Harvard Medical School)

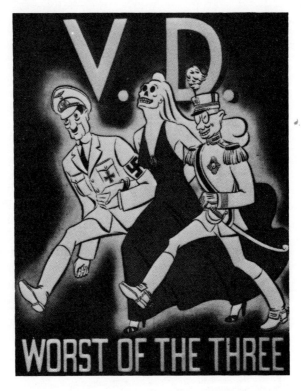

Chapter 3 presents a brief description of the anatomical and physiological features of the human reproductive system as a frame of reference with which to follow the effects of the STDs discussed in part 2. What goes on during a physical examination for an STD, and a genital self-examination, form a major portion of this chapter.

Chapter 4 begins its coverage by introducing the big picture of the STDs and related disorders. The remaining chapters present the general features, symptoms, and issues associated with individual diseases. **SIGNS & SYMPTOMS BOXES** and **STD FACT FILES** found in each of these chapters summarize main points.

Before going onto chapter 3, here is a **12 QUESTION STD CHALLENGE** to test your general knowledge of this group of diseases.

THE 12 QUESTION STD CHALLENGE

Test your general knowledge of STDs by answering the following questions. Indicate your responses by checking either the *true* or *false* box provided next to each question number. The answers and brief comments are given at the end of the test.

RESPONSE COLUMNS

TRUE   FALSE

QUESTION COLUMN

☐ ☐   1. The signs of certain sexually transmitted diseases (STDs) such as syphilis and chlamydial infection are not always obvious.

☐ ☐   2. In general, STDs can be acquired through casual contact situations such as shaking hands.

☐ ☐   3. Diagnostic tests are available for the detection of most STDs.

☐ ☐   4. Most STDs are treatable if detected early.

☐ ☐   5. Having an STD such as syphilis, chancroid, or genital warts can increase the possibility of human immunodeficiency virus (HIV) transmission.

☐ ☐   6. The proper use of latex condoms during sexually related activities, while not foolproof, is effective in preventing STD transmission.

☐ ☐   7. An infected mother can transmit certain STDs such as syphilis and HIV infection to her newborn.

☐ ☐   8. With the exception of hepatitis B virus infection, no immunizations (vaccines) are available for any STD.

☐ ☐   9. The use of oil-based lubricants such as Crisco and Vaseline can weaken condoms, making them useless as protection against STD transmission.

☐ ☐   10. Sexually transmitted diseases can be spread by women as well as men.

☐ ☐   11. An individual can acquire an STD by donating blood.

☐ ☐   12. Sexually transmitted diseases such as syphilis and gonorrhea can be spread by kissing.

ANSWERS

1. **TRUE.** Unfortunately, the signs of several STDs are not obvious and frequently go unnoticed by the infected person.

2. **TRUE.** Most STDs cannot be acquired through casual contact. However, with STDs such as syphilis, an infectious rash which can develop on the hands can be a hazard. In syphilis, infectious sores can also appear on the scalp. Other situations are described in later chapters.

3. **TRUE.** Diagnostic tests of various kinds are available for STDs. The approaches to STD detection and diagnosis are presented in the chapters of part 3.

4. **TRUE.** Most STDs, especially those caused by bacteria, yeasts, protozoa, and worms are treatable. *Cures* for virus-caused STDs currently are not available.

5. **TRUE.** STDs in which open sores develop are considered to be cofactors in HIV transmission.

6. **TRUE.** To be effective, condoms should be put on either before or during foreplay. This point also applies to oral sex.

7. **TRUE.** Pregnancy in an infected female does carry with it the increased risk of syphilis and HIV transmission to a fetus or newborn.

8. **TRUE.** Vaccines are under study for several STDs, but as yet none are available for immunizations.

9. **TRUE.** Oil-based lubricating materials applied to condoms may actually dissolve them. Water-based lubricants such as KY jelly do not destroy or weaken condoms.

10. **TRUE.** Both sexes can spread STDs.

11. **FALSE.** There is no evidence to show that donating blood carries any risk of acquiring any infectious disease.

12. **TRUE.** Sores containing the agents of syphilis and gonorrhea may be present in the mouths of infected persons.

CHAPTER | 3

AN EXAMINATION OF THE REPRODUCTIVE SYSTEM

What geography is to history, such is anatomy to medicine—it describes the theater.

—J. Fernel

General knowledge of the human reproductive system is important not only to understand the effects of sexually transmitted diseases, but also to comprehend how such diseases are detected and controlled. This chapter presents an overview of the reproductive system as well as other body structures associated with STDs. A section describing what is involved with a physical examination for STDs and a procedure for a simple *STD self-examination* also are included. The self-examination should be of particular importance in view of the fact that many people who have an STD do not know they are infected. With the STD self-examination procedure some of the obvious signs and symptoms that might indicate the possible presence of an STD can be found (fig. 3.1).

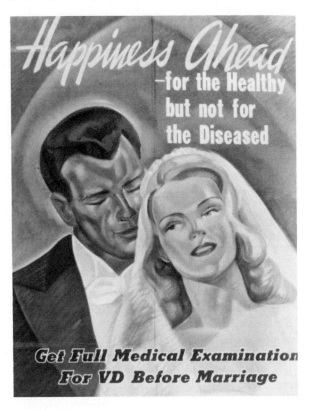

FIGURE 3.1

A poster used during the early 1940s to stress the importance of a physical examination before marriage. The main focus was on the prevention of venereal diseases, and especially syphilis. (Courtesy of Dr. Allan M. Brandt, Harvard Medical School)

THE HUMAN REPRODUCTIVE SYSTEM

OVERVIEW OF STRUCTURES AND FUNCTIONS

The adult human reproductive system produces, stores, nourishes, and transports sex cells, also known as **gametes** (GAM-ēts). This system includes the organs that produce the gametes and specific hormones; the channels, or ducts, that receive and transport gametes; and the accessory glands that secrete fluids into the ducts. Structures located outside of the body and related to the reproductive system are referred to as the **external genitalia** (gen-i-TĀ-lē-a).

In the adult male, the primary sex organs are the **testes** (TES-tēz). The testes produce large numbers of sex cells known as *sperm*. While moving through a long duct system the sperm are combined with accessory gland secretions, resulting in a mixture called **semen** (SĒ-men). The formed semen is expelled from the body through an external structure called the *penis* (PĒ-nis) during *ejaculation* (ē-jak-ū-LĀ-shun).

In a sexually mature female, the primary sex organs are a pair of **ovaries** (Ō-va-rēz). Normally, one ovary produces and releases only one mature sex cell, or *egg*, per month. The egg moves along one of two short uterine tubes, also known as the *oviducts*, that end in a muscular organ called the *uterus*. The uterus, in turn, is connected to the outside of the body by a short passageway, the *vagina* (va-JĪ-nah).

During sexual intercourse, semen and therefore sperm is introduced into the vagina. The sperm swim into the uterine cavity and toward the oviducts. In the event a sperm makes contact with an egg cell, the two may fuse to form a fertilized egg, or *zygote* (ZĪ-gōt). This process is called *fertilization*. The zygote divides several times, forming a cell mass that passes down the oviducts into the uterus and plants itself into the wall of this muscular organ. During the next three months the cell mass becomes an embryo, and then during the remaining months of pregnancy continues to develop as a fetus. At the end of its developmental period, the fetus travels downward, through and out of the vaginal canal into the external world as a newborn infant.

With this general overview of the structures and functions of the human reproductive system in mind, the next sections provide a more descriptive orientation to the male and female reproductive organs and related structures. This information will be a valuable frame of reference to the later discussions of the effects of specific sexually transmitted diseases.

THE MALE REPRODUCTIVE SYSTEM

The main parts of the male reproductive system are the testes, a number of ducts, accessory sex glands, and several supporting structures (fig. 3.2). The

FIGURE 3.2

The male reproductive system. (a) An external view showing the location of the scrotum and penis. (b) An internal view showing the system's parts and their relationship. Accessory glands and ducts associated with the urethra and urinary bladder are also shown. (From K. M. Van De Graaff and S. I. Fox, *Concepts of Human Anatomy and Physiology*, 2d ed., Wm. C. Brown, Publishers: Dubuque, Iowa.)

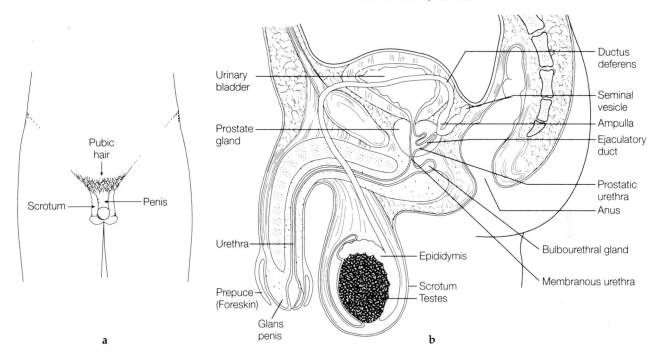

a

b

scrotum (SKRŌ-tum) is a fleshy pouch, or sac, situated in front of but between the thighs. It contains the two major organs, the testes.

Each **testis** (TES-tis) is composed of a large number of narrow, coiled, microscopic tubes called the *seminiferous tubules* (sem-in-IF-er-us, TŪ-būls). Male sex cells, or sperm, production takes place within these tubules. **Interstitial** (in-ter-STISH-al) cells scattered between the tubules manufacture male hormones, the most important of which is *testosterone* (tes-TOS-ter-ōn). This hormone is responsible for the initiation and the maintenance of body changes that occur during *puberty* in males. Puberty is the period of human development during which the reproductive organs become functional. In males it generally occurs between 12–14 years of age.

Testosterone increases the size of the testes and the accessory sex glands, the **seminal vesicles** (SEM-i-nal, VES-i-kls) and the **prostate** (PROS-tāt) gland. It also stimulates sperm production and the development of male secondary sex characteristics. Secondary sex characteristics are not essential for reproduction, and include the appearance of body hair patterns such as pubic, chest, and facial hair, enlargement of the voicebox causing a deepening of the voice, and muscle and bone development resulting in the formation of wide shoulders, narrow hips, and other changes in the body's physique.

In order for sperm to move to the other end of the male reproductive system, the penis, and to the outside of the body, they must move through a long channel or duct system (fig. 3.2). The sperm first are transported to the **epididymis** (ep-i-DID-i-mis), a long tube located at the top of each testis. This structure may store sperm for up to four weeks. After that, they are either expelled from the epididymis or reabsorbed. From the epididymis, sperm are propelled by the force of muscle contraction through the **vas deferens** (VAS, DEF-e-renz), which carries them into the pelvic region and around the urinary bladder into the next portions of the reproductive system before leaving the body. The **ejaculatory** (ē-JAK-ū-la-tō-rē) **ducts,** just prior to ejaculation, expel sperm into the **urethra** (ū-RĒ-thra), a tube which in the male is also used to eliminate urine. Three types of accessory sex glands, the two **seminal vesicles,** the **prostate gland,** and two bulbourethral (bul-bō-ū-RĒ-thral) glands secrete their respective fluids into the ejaculatory ducts and urethra. The resulting mixture, **semen,** is a combination of these glandular fluids and sperm. Semen passes to the outside of the body through an erect **penis.**

The penis consists of erectile tissue that surrounds the major portion of the urethra. When the erectile tissue becomes filled with blood, an erection occurs, causing the penis to become rigid. The expanded tip of the penis forms a soft, sensitive region called the **glans penis.** Ordinarily, a fold of skin, the **prepuce** (PRĒ-pūs), or **foreskin,** covers the tip of the penis. Circumcision (ser-kum-SI-zuhn), which literally means "cutting around" is the procedure by which the foreskin is removed, leaving the glans penis visible at all times. It is generally performed shortly after birth. Because the circumcised penis is easier to clean, secretions and other substances are less likely to collect under the prepuce.

The Accessory Sex Glands

The three accessory sex glands, the prostate gland, the seminal vesicles, and the bulbourethral glands, have important functions. They are also subject to the harmful effects of the sexually transmitted diseases.

The prostate gland is a small structure about the size of a large walnut. It consists of three parts and its base lies against the bottom of the urinary bladder (fig. 3.2b). The prostate gland produces a thin, milk-like fluid, the *prostatic fluid,* which contributes to sperm motility and protection against acidic secre-

tions of the female reproductive tract. Acidic secretions would inactivate and kill sperm if not neutralized. The prostatic fluid forms about 13–33 percent of the volume of semen. Contraction of muscle within the prostate gland empties the contents of the gland into the urethra, and contributes to the force needed to propel the semen during ejaculation.

The seminal vesicles are two sacs individually measuring about two inches in length. Each vesicle ends in a straight, narrow channel, which joins the tip of the vas deferens to form the ejaculatory duct. These structures secrete a thick, yellowish fluid which contains a variety of nutrients such as fructose, a sugar, that provides sperm with an energy source. Seminal vesicular fluid forms approximately 60 percent of the volume of semen.

The bulbourethral, or **Cowper's** (KOW-pers), glands are two pea-sized structures found on both sides of the urethra and beneath the prostate gland. Upon sexual arousal and before ejaculation, these glands are stimulated to secrete a clear, sticky fluid which coats the lining of the urethra to neutralize any remaining urine, and lubricates the tip of the penis in preparation for sexual intercourse. Although this fluid secretion must not be confused with semen, it may contain sperm.

The Female Reproductive Organs

Figure 3.3 shows the overall structure and organization of the female reproductive system. Its principal organs include the *ovaries, uterine tubes,* or *oviducts, uterus* (Ū-ter-us), and *vagina* (va-JĪ-na).

The ovaries, like the testes, have a dual function, namely, the production of sex or egg cells, and sex hormones. Sex hormones contribute to the development of and maintenance of female reproductive structures, secondary sex characteristics, and the breasts. Secondary female sex characteristics include the distribution of fat to the breasts, mons pubis, hips, and abdomen, voice changes, broadening of the pelvis, and appearance of body hair patterns.

In their normal position, the almond-shaped ovaries lie vertically on either side of the uterus. These

FIGURE 3.3

The important organs of the female reproductive system. (a) The system viewed from the side. (b) The deeper structures of the system, showing the relationship of the ovaries, uterine tubes (oviducts), uterus, cervix and vagina. (From K. M. Van De Graaff and S. I. Fox, *Concepts of Anatomy and Physiology*, 2d ed., Wm. C. Brown, Publishers: Dubuque, Iowa.)

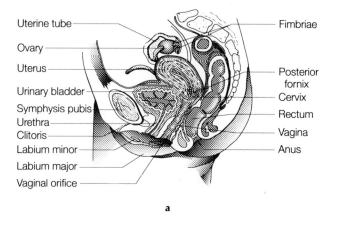

a

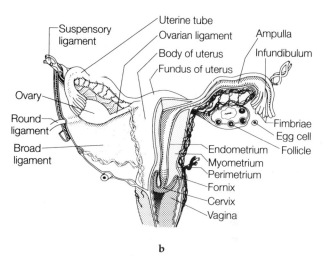

b

organs are held in place by a number of cordlike structures including the ovarian ligaments and are protected by a surrounding mass of fat.

In contrast to a testis, an ovary has no tubes leading directly out of it. An egg cell, or **ovum** (Ō-vum), leaves the organ by breaking through its surface. After its release, the ovum is caught in the fingerlike ends of a tube called the *oviduct*, one of which is near each ovary. These two oviducts, which measure about five-and-a-half inches in length, extend between the ovaries and the uterus. Muscular contractions and the action of *cilia*, little microscopic hairlike processes in the oviduct, help to move the ovum along. Fertilization normally takes place within the oviducts if sperm are present.

As indicated earlier, each oviduct leads into the cavity of the uterus. The typical uterus is a pear-shaped hollow organ with muscular walls. These muscular walls are richly lined with blood vessels. The uterus can be divided into an expanded upper portion known as the **body,** a narrowed region, the **isthmus** (IS-mus), and the lower part, the **cervix.** The cervix extends to the vagina, which opens to the outside of the body. As shown in figure 3.3a the vagina is bordered in front by the urethra and the urinary bladder, and in the rear by the rectum.

THE EXTERNAL GENITALIA

The area enclosing the female genitalia is called the **vulva** (VUL-va). Figure 3.4 shows the various parts of the region, which includes the **mons pubis,** (mons, PŪ-bis), the **major** and **minor lips** or **labia majora** and **labia minora,** (LĀ-bē-a, mā-JOR-a, LĀ-bē-a, mi-NOR-a), the **clitoris,** and the **vaginal opening** or entrance. The outer limits of the vulva are established by the mons pubis and the major lips. The mons pubis is a recognizable, prominent, rounded, elevated area covered with hair, while the major lips can be seen as two folds of skin that run down and back from the mons. The minor lips are two pinkish, hairless folds of skin located between the major lips. They enclose a space known as the **vestibule** into which the vagina, the urethra and the ducts of the two **Bartholin's glands** open. Secretions of the Bartholin's glands lubricate the vaginal opening during sexual excitement. Just in front of the urethral opening, the clitoris projects into the vestibule. The clitoris is considered to be the female equivalent of the penis. Since it contains erectile tissue, the structure can become engorged with blood and can become erect during sexual activities.

FIGURE 3.4
The female external genitalia.

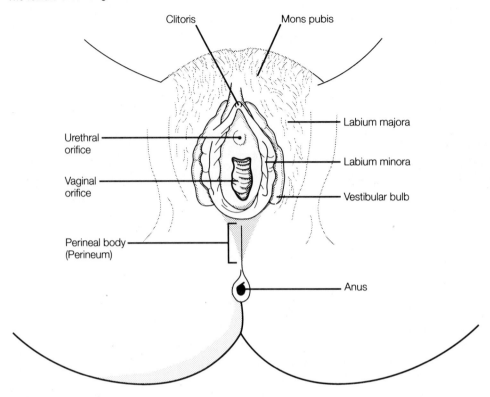

THE BREASTS (MAMMARY GLANDS)

The breasts are **mammary** (MAM-a-rē) **glands** that produce milk during and after pregnancy. Each of these accessory organs of the female reproductive system are located in the upper front portion of the chest. They contain fatty tissue, special milk-transporting channels, or ducts, and several cavities that carry milk produced in response to hormones to an opening, or *nipple*. The reddish-brown area surrounding the nipple of each breast is known as the **areola** (a-RĒ-ō-la). Figure 3.5 shows the general features of the breast.

WHAT IS INVOLVED IN A PHYSICAL EXAMINATION FOR STDs?

The physical examination for a sexually transmitted disease differs from those for other diseases in that there may be an extra sense of anxiety on the part of individuals to be examined. Feelings of fear, embarrassment, general discomfort, rejection, and perhaps even guilt can cause such persons to hesitate in visiting a physician or STD clinic. While in most cases the examination can be completed in only a

FIGURE 3.5

The general features of the human breast.

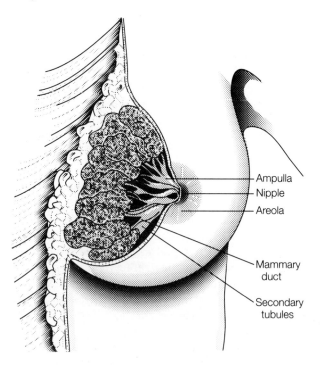

Ampulla
Nipple
Areola
Mammary duct
Secondary tubules

few minutes, not knowing what to expect, being inadequately informed, or having a limited vocabulary in relation to sexual matters may also add to an individual's anxiety and hesitation.

Physical examinations are performed as both a routine procedure to confirm the absence of an illness or a disorder and as a means to detect or diagnose certain diseases. The following sections describe the particular aspects of an examination that apply to STDs. If certain signs or symptoms noticed by the patient disappear before the exam, other tests, such as various blood tests, may be needed. Tests of this type are described in later chapters dealing with specific STDs.

THE CLINICAL HISTORY PHASE

The physician or other health professional who conducts the STD physical examination generally obtains a *clinical history* from the individual. This is done to pinpoint the source of the medical problem,

and to help arrive at a diagnosis. Many diseases have predictable courses and clinical histories. A clinical history includes such information about the person as age, sex, and ethnic background; the major complaint or complaints; history of the current problem (when did it begin?); family history; and social history. The social history of an individual concerns information about occupation, and such habits as cigarette, alcohol, and drug use. Previous medical problems and hospitalizations also are noted.

In the case of a female's examination, additional **gynecologic** (gī-nē-kō-LOJ-ik) history usually is needed. This includes information concerning the amount and length of time of the **menstrual** (MEN-stroo-al) flow, the presence of menstrual disturbances, such as pain, spotting (bleeding) after *menstruation* (men-stroo-Ā-shun), and the appearance of any unusual vaginal discharge (color photograph 1). A more thorough examination of the individual can be provided when this information is available.

GENERAL ITEMS CHECKED

There are two major differences in genitalia anatomy and examination between male and female patients. First, in the case of the male, the examination involves only a single genitourinary tract. In the female, there is a urinary tract and a separate genital tract to be examined. Two functions are combined in the male genitourinary tract, in which the urethra serves as a common channel for the excretion of urine and the delivery of semen.

The second major difference between males and females is that critical reproductive organs in the male are easily accessible for examination (fig. 3.2). In contrast, the female reproductive organs are located in the pelvis (fig. 3.3) and are not as easily examined as the comparable male organs. Thus, the examination of portions of the male urinary tract and the entire male genital tract is easily done and generally is straightforward.

In addition to examining the genitalia, other regions of the body are inspected for indications of a sexually transmitted disease. These include the skin surfaces of the palm and back of the hands and forearms (for rashes or blisters); the groin (for sores or swollen regions); the arm and leg joints (for tenderness or pain); and the pubic hairs (for crab lice or their egg cases). If oral sex is practiced, the lips and the inner surfaces of the mouth are examined for sores, isolated red or bleeding patches (fig. 3.6), and any oozing of fluid or other secretions.

PHYSICAL EXAMINATION OF THE MALE GENITALIA

Preparation of the Patient. Prior to the examination, the male patient generally is instructed to disrobe down to his shorts, which are later lowered to expose the genitalia. The examination generally begins with an inspection of the penis, the foreskin (if present), the glans, and the urethral opening. If a foreskin is present, it is necessary to retract or pull it back completely for the examination. Inability to retract the penile covering can occur and may result from some irritation or swelling of the foreskin related to vigorous sexual activity. The presence or absence of any open sores (fig. 3.7), scars, unusual growths, or discharge from the urethral opening is noted.

Next, the surface of the scrotum is inspected for the presence of sores, scars, discolored patches of skin, and abnormal growths. It is lifted to examine the undersurface for the same signs of possible infection. The scrotum may be felt or **palpated** (PAL-pāt-ed) to detect any internal lumps or masses. The thigh and upper leg areas also are generally inspected for any unusual bulges, sores, or blisters. Unusual bulges are not necessarily related to STDs, but they may be indications of cancer or a **hernia** (HER-nē-a), an abnormal extension of the intestine through the abdominal wall.

PHYSICAL EXAMINATION OF THE FEMALE GENITALIA

At the time the appointment is made, the woman is told not to **douche** (doosh) or to have sexual intercourse for twenty-four hours prior to the examination. The use of a douche involves the application of a stream of either plain or medicated water solutions to cleanse, deodorize, or treat the genitalia. These precautions are necessary for an accurate evaluation of any vaginal discharge and for obtaining functional specimens.

Positioning the Patient. Just before an examination takes place, the patient is instructed to empty her bladder and rectum, to completely disrobe, and to put on a gown. With the assistance of a nurse or

FIGURE 3.6

Some possible signs of infections involving the mouth. (a) A small red patch (arrow) on the roof of the mouth. Material from this area was found to contain the causative agent of syphilis. (b) The typical sores associated with herpes.

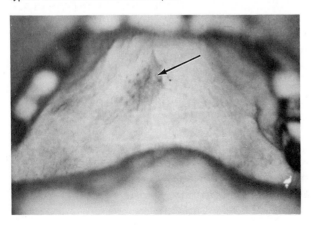

a

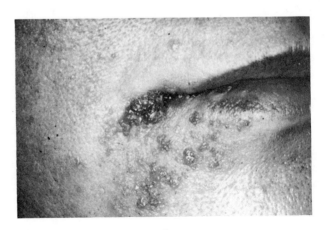

b

Figure 3.7

The presence of open sores such as the one shown can be easily detected during the physical examination. However, at times such lesions may heal and disappear before the exam takes place.

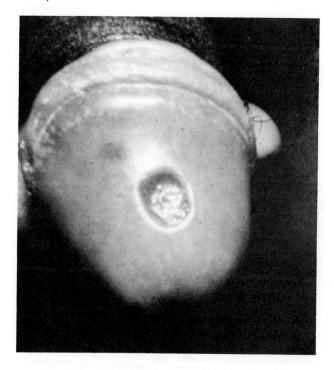

Figure 3.8

The lithotomy position used in the physical examination of the female patient.

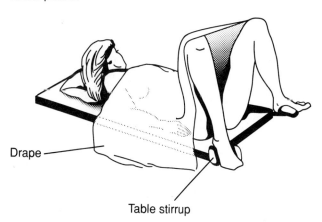

Drape

Table stirrup

other health care professional (who generally remains in the room during the examination), the woman is placed into a lithotomy (lith-OT-ō-mē) position (fig. 3.8). In this position the patient is on her back with the knees flexed, the arms are placed at the sides or are folded over the chest, and the buttocks are located slightly near the edge of the examining table. The feet are supported by the table **stirrups** (STIR-ups). A towel is placed under the patient's buttocks and a drape of some type, usually a sheet, is used to cover the abdomen and knees. The examining physician will move the drape away from the pubic area when the examination begins.

General Aspects of the Examination. The external genitalia is inspected first for scratches, sores, and crab lice or their eggs. Next, the labia and vaginal opening are examined for tenderness, swelling, open sores (fig. 3.9), warts, or blisters. Examination of the external genitalia also includes palpating the **Bartholin's** (BAR-tō-linz) glands and the area between the vagina and the rectum known as the perineal (per'i-NĒ-al) body. If the patient complains of burning or irritation on urination, the examiner inspects the urethra by spreading the labia with the thumb and the index finger of one gloved hand. Then, the gloved index finger of the other hand is inserted into the vagina and the urethra is gently pressed from the inside outward to obtain a specimen for laboratory study, which may include isolating the causative agent through culture.

Next, the examiner places two fingers inside the vaginal opening, and the patient is asked to push or bear down while a warmed vaginal **speculum** (SPEK-ū-lum) is inserted. This instrument is used for the inspection of the vaginal canal and the cervix (fig. 3.10). Both of these structures are checked for

FIGURE 3.9
Sores such as the one shown can be detected during the examination of the external genitalia. However, these lesions may heal rapidly and thus avoid detection, or they may be hidden by the pubic hairs.

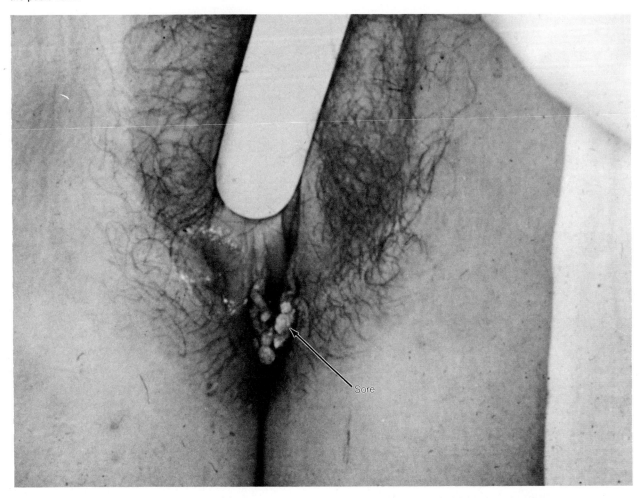

Sore

bleeding, open sores, and abnormal growths and discharges. During this part of the examination, it is customary to obtain cervical specimens for the detection of cervical cancer (fig. 3.11). This material, which may be collected by means of a brush or a **spatula** (SPACH-ū-la) is used for the well-known **Pap (Papanicolaou) test** or **smear.** Individuals having abnormal Pap smears may require additional visual examination with a magnifying instrument known as the **colposcope** (KOL-pō-skōp). Sores, abnormal growths, and genital warts can be readily seen with the colposcope. Color photograph 2 shows the colposcopic appearance of an abnormal cervix.

After the speculum is removed from the vagina,

FIGURE 3.10

The insertion of a vaginal speculum for the examination of the cervix and vaginal canal. A spatula for obtaining a specimen also is shown.

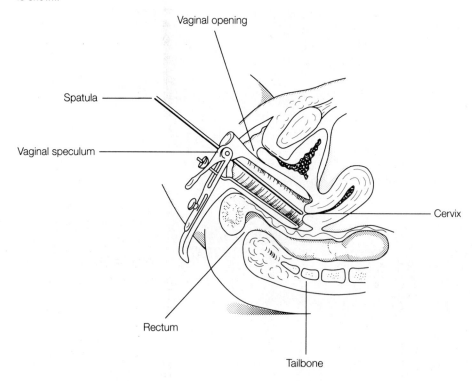

Vaginal opening

Spatula

Vaginal speculum

Cervix

Rectum

Tailbone

a **bimanual examination** of the uterus, the pelvic organs, the oviducts, and the ovaries generally is performed. In this procedure, the gloved middle fingers of one hand are lubricated and gently inserted into the vagina, and the outline of the uterus and the cervix is felt by the other hand through pressure applied externally on the abdominal area over the pelvic organs (fig. 3.12). This type of pelvic examination is done to check the position of the uterus and ovaries and for **pelvic inflammatory disease** (PID), and other infections of the female reproductive tract. PID is described in chapter 4.

THE RECTAL EXAMINATION

An examination of the rectum may follow the examination of the male and female genitalia.

The male rectum usually is checked with the individual in a standing position bending over an examining table. This position also allows the examiner to feel the prostate gland, which is checked for size, shape, and firmness. The anus is examined visually for redness, rashes, blisters, sores, or other unusual signs. The buttocks are spread to assist in viewing the anus. If any abnormalities exist such as discoloration, growths, cracks, sores, or tubelike holes the

FIGURE 3.11
The CERVEX-BRUSH, a modern device used to obtain cervical specimens. (Courtesy of Unimar, Inc.)

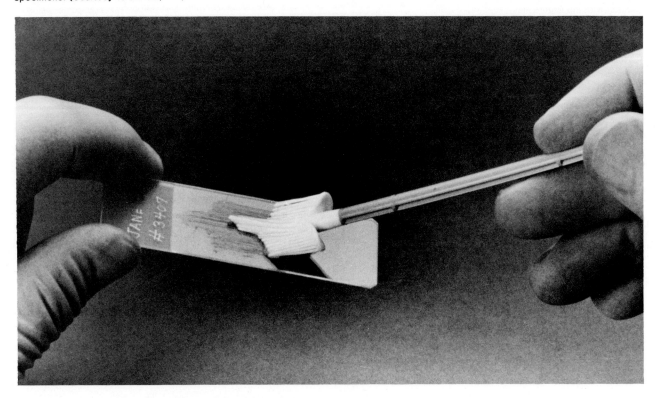

individual will feel pain. When the buttocks are spread, men having anorectal complaints may require an **anoscopic** ($\overline{\text{A}}$-n$\overline{\text{o}}$-skop-ik) examination. A lubricated **anoscope** ($\overline{\text{A}}$-n$\overline{\text{o}}$-sk$\overline{\text{o}}$p) is inserted a short distance into the anal opening to view the lining of the area. Specimens may be taken for the laboratory isolation of a causative agent.

In the case of the female, the rectum may be inspected while the individual is in the lithotomy position (fig. 3.8). The rear portion of the vagina and the front of the rectum are felt for the presence of any unusual lumps or growths. This is done by placing the index finger into the vaginal canal and the middle finger into the rectum. The anus also may be visually examined for the signs described for the male.

DIFFERENTIAL DIAGNOSIS (PUTTING THE FACTS TOGETHER)

Putting the complaints, the clinical history, and the physical findings together with the results of the physical examination, the physician considers all of the possible diseases or disorders that are the most probable cause of the patient's condition. This process is known as **differential** (diff-er-EN-shal) **diagnosis.** Confirmation of an STD diagnosis comes from laboratory tests.

FIGURE 3.12
The features of the bimanual pelvic examination. The hand pressing on the abdomen brings more of the pelvic contents into contact with the fingers inserted in the vagina.

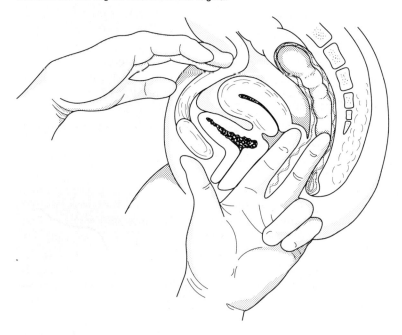

LABORATORY TESTS—SOME ROUTINE, SOME NOT

All individuals undergoing an examination for an STD should have a blood test. In several situations, signs of an STD are either not present or obvious. Moreover, specimens taken during the examination for the isolation and the growth, or culture, of a suspected disease agent may not be of any value. Blood tests, more specifically referred to as **serological** (sē-rō-LOJ-ik-al) **tests,** are particularly important in the diagnosis of certain STDs such as syphilis. These procedures depend on the presence of specific proteins called antibodies, or **immunoglobulins** (im'-ū-nō-GLOB-ū-lins) formed by the infected individual in response to the disease agent.

Other laboratory procedures exist to identify STD agents. These include special microscopic examinations and/or the staining of specimens obtained from patients during the physical examination (color photograph 3), or using combinations of nutrients called *media* to grow (culture) and to perform biochemical tests known to be characteristic of certain STD pathogens. Chapters in part 2 provide additional details of these laboratory identification approaches.

THE MALE SELF-EXAMINATION

The self-examination of the male reproductive system includes inspection of the entire length of the *penis,* extending from its base to the urinary or *urethral opening,* the *prepuce,* or *foreskin* (if present); the *glans,* or head, and the *scrotum.* The specific signs or symptoms that should be noted are bumps, pimples, blisters, warts, open sores, scars, or discharges. Since some of these signs may be difficult to see, the use of a strong light and mirror are recommended.

Once undressed, the man starts the self-examination by holding the penis in one hand. He inspects the head from the urinary opening to where it extends out slightly above the shaft (fig. 3.2). If there is a foreskin, he gently pulls it down to examine the head. He carefully looks for a discharge of any type from the urinary opening, and for the presence of flat, colored spots, bumps, blisters, fleshy warts, or sores. If any of these signs are present, he needs to seek medical attention.

The man continues the examination by inspecting the entire length of the penile shaft. He looks again for the presence of spots, bumps, blisters, fleshy warts, or sores. Next he separates the hairs at the base of the penis with the fingers to view the underlying skin. A good light source and mirror may be helpful here. The hair in the area should be checked for the presence of crab lice or their egg cases. Egg cases are attached to individual hairs and feel like pieces of sand. Any of the signs mentioned should be brought to the attention of a physician.

The last structure of the reproductive system to be examined is the *scrotum*. Not only should the top and undersurfaces of this organ be inspected for the presence of spots, blisters, and open sores, but each testis should be gently felt for the presence of any lump, swelling, or soreness. If any of these signs or symptoms is noticed, no matter how slight, a physician should be consulted as soon as possible. The presence of scrotal tenderness or unusual lumps may be an indication of testicular cancer. When the genital self-examination is finished, the hands should be washed and dried.

One other area of inspection remains. If oral sex is practiced, the mouth and lips need to be checked. A mirror and a flashlight are important here for an adequate examination. Particular signs to be noted include open sores, blisters, the presence of a thick, creamy film or deposit on the tongue, or reddened and/or bleeding patches on the inner sides of the mouth. Again, the presence of these conditions should be brought to the attention of a physician. The hands also should be washed after this examination.

THE FEMALE SELF-EXAMINATION

The self-examination of the female reproductive system is limited to the external genitalia and includes the *mons*, the outer and inner lips, or *labia majora* and *labia minora*, the *prepuce* or *hood*, a fold of the inner lips that covers the clitoris, and the urinary, or *urethral, opening*. The specific signs or symptoms to be noted during the examination include unusual growths, bumps, itchy rash, blisters, open sores, bleeding, an unusual discharge, and a foul odor. The use of a mirror and a strong light may be helpful in inspecting some areas of the genitalia.

Once undressed the woman starts the self-examination by inspecting the hair and underlying skin of the mons (fig. 3.4). She spreads the hair apart with her fingers and carefully looks for red spots, blisters, pimples, sores, and unusual growths (warts) or lumps, painful or not. If any of these conditions is found, she should seek medical attention. The woman continues the examination by looking for any unusual discharge from the vaginal area. Next, she carefully spreads the outer vaginal lips (labia majora) apart and inspects the prepuce or the hood of the clitoris, for blisters, sores, warts, or bleeding. She then examines both sides of the inner lips (labia minora) for any of the same signs.

The woman should inspect the area around the urinary opening and the vaginal opening. Again, she looks for the signs mentioned earlier. After completing this part of the self-examination, the woman should wash and dry her hands.

If oral sex is practiced, the mouth and lips need to be checked. A mirror and a flashlight are important here for an adequate examination. Particular signs to be noted include open sores, the presence of a thick, creamy film or deposit on the tongue, blisters, or reddened or bleeding patches on the inner sides of the mouth. Again, the presence of these conditions should be brought to the attention of a physician. The hands also should be washed and dried after this examination.

The breasts also need to be examined. The woman should use the right hand to examine the left breast and the left hand for the right breast. The surface and nipple of each breast should be checked for spots, blisters, pimples, or open sores. In certain sexually transmitted diseases, the infection may involve the breasts. The presence of any of the signs described should be brought to the attention of a physician.

A Reference for Later Chapters

The overview of the human reproductive system and the simple self-examination will be of value in following and understanding the signs and symptoms of the STDs presented in the following chapters.

CHAPTER | 4

AN INTRODUCTION TO SEXUALLY TRANSMITTED DISEASES

Some of Shakespeare's father-murder complex, some of Hamlet's horror of his mother, of his uncle, of all old men came from the feeling that fathers may transmit syphilis, or syphilis-consequences to children . . .

—*D. H. Lawrence*

Sexually transmitted diseases (STDs) are specific infections spread primarily during sexual contact. More than twenty-five different diseases currently are recognized STDs. Table 4.1 lists representatives of this group of diseases. Despite all the advances in modern medicine, STDs are among the most common of all public health problems. Unfortunately, the incidence of STDs continues to rise despite the efforts made by health authorities to inform and to educate the public about prevention. The high incidence may be the result of several factors, including the sexual revolution of the 1970s. During this time the age at which sexual intercourse first took place was earlier than in previous years, and the number of sex partners and premarital sexual activities increased dramatically. Other contributing factors include the introduction of contraceptives, and the sense of security provided by knowing of the availability of antibiotics, such as penicillin for the treatment of the so-called traditional venereal diseases: syphilis, gonorrhea, chancroid, **lymphogranuloma venereum** (lim-f$\overline{\text{o}}$-gran-$\overline{\text{u}}$-L$\overline{\text{O}}$-ma, veh-ner-$\overline{\text{E}}$-um), and **granuloma inguinale** (gran-$\overline{\text{u}}$-L$\overline{\text{O}}$-ma, IN-gwinal-$\overline{\text{e}}$). The term *venereal disease* comes from Venus, the Roman goddess of love. Beginning about 1950, this term slowly began to be replaced by *sexually transmitted diseases.*

TABLE 4.1

TABLE 4.1 | CURRENTLY RECOGNIZED SEXUALLY TRANSMITTED (TRANSMISSIBLE) DISEASES ACCORDING TO CAUSATIVE AGENTS[a]

BACTERIA

Balanitis (bal-a NĪ-tis)

Cervicitis (ser-vi-SĪ-tis)

Chancroid (SHANG-kroid)

Epididymitis (ep-i-DID-e-mī-tis)

Gonorrhea (gon-ō-RĒ-ah)

Granuloma inguinale
(gran-ū-LŌ-mah, IN-gwi-nal-ē)

Lymphogranuloma venereum (LGV)
lim-fō-gran-ū-LŌ-mah, veh-ner-Ē-um)

Nongonococcal urethritis (NUG)
(non-gon-ō-KOK-al, ū-rē-THRĪ-tis)

Nongonococcal pelvic inflammatory
disease

Pelvic inflammatory disease

Proctitis (prock-TĪ-tis)

Prostatitis (pros-ta-TĪ-tis)

Salpingitis (sal-pin-JĪ-tis)

Syphilis (SIF-i-lis)

Urethritis (ūr-ē-THRĪ-tis)

Vaginitis (vaj-in-Ī-tis)

Vaginosis (vaj-i-NŌ-sis)

Vulvitis (vul-VĪ-tis)

VIRUSES

Acquired immune deficiency syndrome
(AIDS)

AIDS dementia complex (ADC)

AIDS-related complex (ARC)

Cytomegalovirus infection
(sī-tō-meg-a-lō-VĪ-rus)

Epstein-Barr virus infection

Genital herpes or herpes progenitalis
(HER-pēz, pro-JEN-e-tal-is)

Genital warts or condylomata acuminata
(kon-di-LŌ-mata, a-KŪ-min-at-ah)

Hepatitis (hep-a-TĪ-tis)

Molluscum contagiosum (mo-LUS-kum, kon-TĀ-jē-
ō-sum)

Vulvitis (vul-VĪ-tis)

FUNGI

Infective balanitis

Vulvovaginal Candidiasis
(vul-vō-VAJ-i-nal, kan-di-DĪ-a-sis)

PROTOZOA

Amebiasis (am-e-BĪ-a-sis)

Giardiasis (jē-ar-DĪ-a-sis)

Infective balanitis

Trichomoniasis (trik-ō-mō-NĪ-a-sis)

Vulvovaginitis (vul-vō-vaj-i-NĪ-tis)

WORMS

Pinworm:

ECTOPARASITES

Balanitis	Scabies (SKĀ-bēz)
Pediculosis (pē-dik-ū-LŌ-sis)	

ᵃRefer to specific chapters in the text for a description of these diseases.

While estimates often vary depending on the sources of information it is generally agreed that over 10 million persons in the United States visit doctors' offices and clinics every year for treatment of some STD.

NEWER STDs

In recent years several newer STDs have been recognized (fig. 4.1). These include bacterial infections caused by *Chlamydia*, and the viral diseases Acquired Immune Deficiency Syndrome (AIDS), genital warts (caused by human papilloma viruses), genital herpes, and hepatitis B. The range of STDs does not end here; since the late 1960s in the United States certain

sexual practices such as anal intercourse and oral sex or **fellatio** (fel-Ā-shē-ō), brought a new group of sexually transmitted diseases onto the scene. These diseases which are associated with the gastrointestinal system, have become a major group of STDs in various segments of the population. They include viral hepatitis, protozoan infections, such as **amebic dysentery** (a-MĒ-bik, DIS-en-ter-ē), and worm infections such as pinworm. Infestations by pubic lice and mites also pose additional problems. It should be noted that several of the newer infections are not always directly transmitted through sexual intercourse but are closely related to, or are the indirect result of, some other form of sexual activity.

FIGURE 4.1

The approximate annual incidence of selected sexually transmitted diseases in the United States. Note the large number of chlamydial infections.

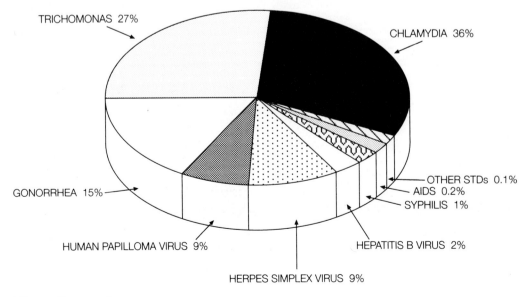

Consequences of STDs

Collectively, the STDs are the direct cause of immense personal, biologic, and economic costs to individuals, families, potential families, and society as a whole. The consequences of this group of diseases, as later chapters indicate, go far beyond the early symptoms or effects on sexual life. In the case of fetuses or infants, for example, the major consequences of STDs include severe infection involving the eyes, brain, and other body organs, birth defects, spontaneous abortion, and stillbirth. Infected adults may experience infertility, severe destructive infections of the reproductive system (color photographs 4 and 5), and in some situations a predisposition to some forms of cancer. It should also be pointed out here that although STDs in the past were considered to be most often afflictions of men, the picture has changed. Young women, their fetuses, and their newborn children are experiencing the most severe symptoms and consequences of many of the more recently recognized infections. It is quite apparent that the influence of the STDs extends to many aspects of human life and society.

This chapter presents some of the general conditions caused by the agents of STDs, some approaches to their control, and related topics. The remaining chapters of part 2 discuss specific STDs.

STDs as Increased Risk Factors for HIV Infection

Since the discovery of AIDS and later the human immunodeficiency virus (HIV), a number of factors have been identified as being capable of influencing the spread, the pace, and the course of HIV infection. The most often used terms for such contributing situations are *risk factors* and *cofactors*. Examples include continued drug abuse, poor nutrition associated with protein or vitamin deficiencies, and infections with certain STD agents. Most of these risk factors interfere in some way with the working of an individual's immune system, thus lowering resistance to HIV infection. Table 4.2 lists the recognized factors as well as the mechanisms believed to be operating in each.

There is significant documented evidence that the risk of HIV infection is increased by the presence of certain STDs including chancroid, syphilis, and genital herpes. The added risk is probably due to breaks in the skin or the surface linings (mucosa) of various parts of the reproductive system and **anorectal** (ā-nō-REK-tal) areas. These STDs cause genital sores, or ulcers (fig. 4.3 and color photographs 6 and 7). In response to the injury, large numbers of specific white blood cells, such as macrophages and

---

Focus on STDs	**An Italian Mummy and Syphilis**

Although the exact origin and subsequent spread of syphilis is still a matter of heated debate among medical historians, it is generally accepted that this STD did not become widespread until the early sixteenth century. Information and evidence on the roots of syphilis are limited to the skeletal remains of those who possibly were infected. Recently, researchers at the University of Pisa, Italy, uncovered a specimen still containing tissue. The mummy of Italian noblewoman Maria d'Aragona was exhumed in 1984, some 450 years after her death (fig. 4.2). Famed for her beauty, this noblewoman mingled in Italy's intellectual and religious circles, even rubbing elbows with Michelangelo's friends. Unfortunately, those elbows were rotting with the late stages of syphilis. Both of d'Aragona's arms were found to have open sores containing the syphilis-causing spirochetes. This finding is the first demonstration of syphilis in the soft tissues of ancient human remains.

TABLE 4.2	RECOGNIZED RISK FACTORS (COFACTORS) IN HUMAN IMMUNODEFICIENCY VIRUS (HIV) TRANSMISSION

RISK FACTOR (COFACTOR)	POSSIBLE OPERATING MECHANISMS
Continued intravenous and other forms of drug abuse such as alcohol and marijuana	May interfere with the immune system's protective function; increases chance for infections through shared contaminated needles and syringes.
Malnutrition	General resistance to infections is lowered when protein, vitamin, and mineral deficiencies exist.
Presence of active STD (such as chancroid, syphilis, or genital herpes)	These STDs cause genital ulcers (breaks in skin or mucosal surfaces lining the vagina and anorectal area) and may increase the risk of HIV infection and AIDS.
Hidden or inapparent viral infections	Certain viruses such as hepatitis B, cytomegalovirus, and the Epstein-Barr may interact with the HIV to lower the effectiveness of the immune system and thereby hasten the development HIV infection and AIDS.

FIGURE 4.2

The mummy of Maria d'Aragona found to be infected with syphilis, then called the "Neopolitan disease." (a) The full view of the mummy. (b) An open sore on the arm of the mummy found to contain evidence of syphilitic infection. (From G. Fornaciari and Associates, *Lancet* (1989) 614: September 9.)

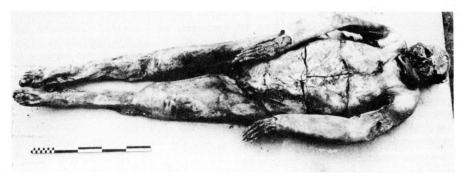

a

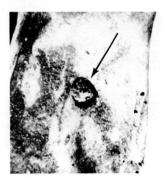

b

FIGURE 4.3

An example of genital ulcers (arrows), found with a case of chancroid. Other features of this sexually transmitted disease are described in chapter 6. (Courtesy of Centers for Disease Control)

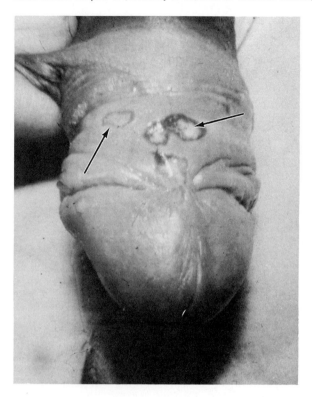

FIGURE 4.4

The condom or so-called rubber has been a taboo term in polite society. However, times have changed, as evidenced by this New York City poster used in a safe-sex education campaign. (Courtesy of GMHC, New York)

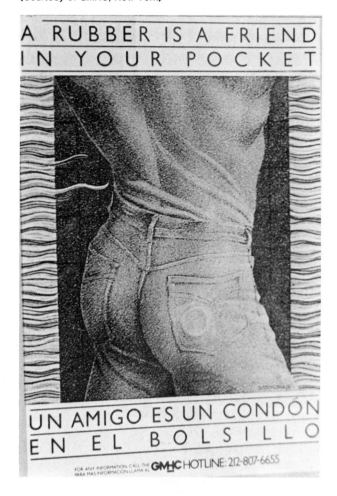

A RUBBER IS A FRIEND IN YOUR POCKET

UN AMIGO ES UN CONDÓN EN EL BOLSILLO

FOR ANY INFORMATION CALL THE **GMHC** HOTLINE: 212-807-6655
PARA MAS INFORMACION LLAMA AL

a certain type of lymphocyte, known to be HIV targets, flock to the area. HIV infection is described in chapter 13. Thus it appears that these genital ulcer-causing diseases could raise the risk of HIV infection by increasing the ineffectivity of the *index sex partner* (the person with the ulcer) by HIV excretion from the ulcer or by increasing the susceptibility of sexual partners through exposure to the discharge or open surface of an ulcer.

Reduction of STD risk factors can be accomplished in several ways, including avoidance of sexual activities with infected persons, the use of condoms (fig. 4.4) during sex, and the use of appropriate antibiotics for the STDs that are treatable by such means.

A number of factors are important to the prevention and control of STDs. These include early detection, treating infected persons and their sexual partners, and increasing the knowledge and awareness of the general public and even of health care personnel as to the characteristics of STDs, sex practices that contribute to STD spread and available preventative or "safer sex" practices. Safer sex refers to sexual activities without the exchange of potentially infectious body fluids such as semen, vaginal secretions, and blood. This section deals with some of these areas.

Figure 4.5

The appearance of a sexually transmitted disease is not always as obvious as this view of secondary syphilis (arrows). Frequently, the first signs are overlooked. The features of most sexually transmitted diseases are presented in part 2. (From K. Lejman and Z. Starzycki, *British Journal of Venereal Diseases* (1977) 53:195.)

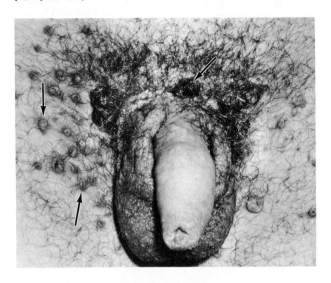

A Word about Symptoms

Depending on an individual's level of anxiety and general knowledge of the reproductive system, the presence of an unusual discharge, abnormal growths, or other symptoms may be interpreted as indications of an STD. While certain STDs have definite recognizable physical symptoms associated with the external genitalia (fig. 4.5), some normal conditions can resemble other STDs. For example, groups of painless, small, yellow spots may be present on the inner side of the prepuce or on the vulva. These are not genital warts, they are surface oil or **sebaceous** (sē-BA-shus) **glands.** Other forms of growths, some of which are pigmented, may develop on the penis, the scrotum, and in and around the vagina and the anus. While these growths are quite common and usually are considered to be harmless or benign, they should be brought to the attention of a physician.

Several signs of STDs can be detected by a self-examination of the genitalia as described in chapter 3. If symptoms are present, medical attention should be sought immediately. *Individuals should not take a chance. STDs do not go away.* Although the obvious signs and symptoms of some STDs such as syphilis and others disappear, the infection does not disappear. Confirmation and treatment are only possible with additional medical examination and appropriate laboratory tests.

Diagnosis

A definite diagnosis of an STD requires specific laboratory procedures and tests. The approaches used for this group of diseases are similar to, if not the same as, those for other infectious diseases. Basically, they include techniques for : (1) isolating and growing the causative agent from specimens; (2) direct microscopic demonstration of the agent or agents in specimens (fig. 4.6); or (3) determining the infected person's response to the STD agent by **serological** (sē-rō-LOJ-ik-al), or blood tests (fig. 4.7). Serological tests are used to demonstrate the presence of specific proteins called antibodies, or **immunoglobulins** (im-ū-nō-GLOB-ū-lins) which are formed by the infected individual in response to the causative agent. The laboratory approaches used to diagnose STDs accompany the descriptions of the diseases in later chapters.

FIGURE 4.6

Examples of laboratory findings. Specimens stained by specific procedures can be used to show the presence of STD agents. (a) The clinical view of an STD involving a woman's genitalia. Specimens from the infected sites were examined by laboratory procedures. (b) A stained preparation showing the causative agent of lymphogranuloma venereum. This is a chlamydial infection. Blood tests are not needed to confirm these findings. (From A. L. De Boer, F. de Boer, and J. V. Van der Merwe, *ACTA Cytologica* (1983) 28:126.)

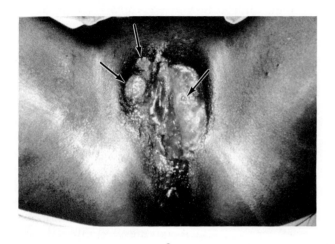

a

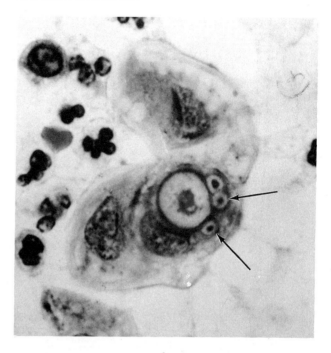

b

TREATMENT

In 1909 Nobel prize winner Paul Ehrlich announced the discovery of Salvarsan, a cure for syphilis. His discovery marked a major breakthrough in the history of modern medical science. For the first time, a specific chemical had been found to kill a specific pathogen. Ehrlich referred to his chemical as a "magic bullet," a drug that would seek out and destroy its target. He also predicted that during the twentieth century other magic bullets would be developed to cure *all* diseases. Indeed a significant number of effective drugs have been found, and newer ones are under study and development. For a drug to be useful, it must kill or stop the growth of the disease agent while causing little or no injury to the host.

Curing and preventing the spread of STDs, as well as other infectious diseases, require accurate diagnosis and effective treatment. This involves selecting the correct drug or drugs if they are available, and performing follow-up examinations and appropriate laboratory tests to determine if the treatment is effective. In addition, the sexual partners of infected individuals must be identified so that they can be examined and treated if necessary.

Education also plays an important role in STD treatment and control. Infected persons and sexual contacts should be counseled on how to avoid *reinfection* and on how to recognize the signs and symptoms of infections. (See chapter 3 for features of a genital self-examination.)

It should be noted here that while drugs for bacterial, fungal, and protozoan STDs are available, treatment may be ineffective. Failures may be due

FIGURE 4.7

The importance of blood testing for venereal disease before marriage during the 1940s. Blood tests were only available for syphilis. (Courtesy of Dr. Allan M. Brandt, Harvard Medical School)

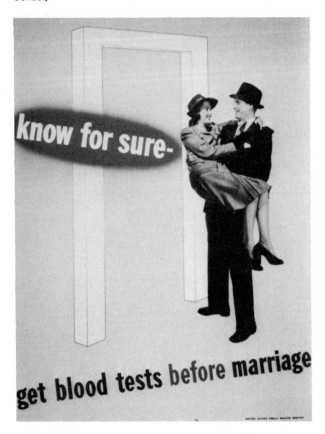

host cell functions. To date, only a handful of antiviral drugs have been approved for use in the United States (table 4.3). While the severity of some of the symptoms associated with viral STDs can be decreased with the use of certain antiviral drugs, cures are currently not available.

APPROACHES TO PREVENTING THE SPREAD OF STDs

Many infectious disease agents can be spread through unprotected sexual contact. STDs can be transmitted *man to woman, woman to man, man to man, and woman to woman.* Oral-genital and oral-rectal sexual practices often lead to sexually transmitted infections caused by pathogens normally associated with the mouth and gastrointestinal tract.

STDs represent a major, largely preventable health threat that endangers men, and women, and their fetuses. The continued life-threatening actions of HIV and AIDS have renewed the interest in measures with which to prevent all STDs. Such preventative or *safer sex* measures, include (1) not having sex when genital sores, abnormal discharge, or a body rash are present; (2) using a condom (fig. 4.8) for all forms of sexual activities, but especially for those involving oral, vaginal, or anal contact; and (3) regular physical examinations and related blood tests for the presence of STDs. Table 4.4 lists a number of principles for prevention and their applications.

to (1) the use of too little medication (either in duration of the treatment or the dosage used), or (2) the development of resistance toward the drug by the STD-causing pathogen.

Some Problems with Treatment. Many of the bacterial, fungal, and protozoan STDs can be effectively treated with antibiotics. Unfortunately, this is not the case with virus-caused infections. To multiply, viruses must take over the internal workings of the invaded host cell. This fact has major significance for the development and designing of antiviral drugs, since most drugs that interfere with viral activities would also interrupt and interfere with

CONDOM

The use of barrier methods such as condoms appears to offer the greatest possibilities for effectively reducing the incidence of STDs. The advantages of the condom over other protective methods are its:

1. relative low unit cost, thus making it within the financial reach of most at-risk individuals;
2. availability without a prescription;
3. use without side effects;
4. demonstrated effectiveness in preventing STDs when properly used.

TABLE 4.3	EXAMPLES OF ANTIVIRAL DRUGS

DRUG	DISEASES TREATED	ACTION(S) OF DRUG
Acyclovir	Herpes virus infections (cold sore, genital herpes) having leukoplakia[a]	Interferes with viral nucleic acid formation
Amantadine	Influenza	Prevents virus from entering cell and/or from beginning its cycle inside the infected cell
Dideoxycytidine	HIV	Interferes with viral and related nucleic acid formation
Interferon	Genital warts, HIV infection, influenza	Interferes with viral multiplication
Iodoxuridine	Herpes virus eye infections	Interferes with viral nucleic acid formation
Ribavirin	Influenza, HIV infections	Interferes with viral nucleic acid formation
Trifluridine	Herpes virus eye infections	Interferes with viral nucleic acid formation
Vidarabadine	Herpes virus eye infections, chicken pox, shingles, and herpes virus infections of the brain	Interferes with viral nucleic acid formation
Zidovudine (formerly known as AZT, azidothymidine)	Kaposi's sarcoma, HIV infection	Interferes with viral multiplication

[a]An infection involving the tongue and believed to be caused by the Epstein-Barr virus. The condition is found in some HIV infections.

Despite the reliability and safety of the condom as a technique for STD prevention, motivating sexually active persons to use them has been and continues to be a major challenge. Certain beliefs are held by individuals which tend to serve as barriers to condom use. These include:

1. Condom use is unnatural.
2. The use of a condom offends one's sex partner.
3. The use of a condom interferes with the pleasure of sexual intercourse.
4. A condom is a birth control device rather than an STD barrier.

To be effective, condoms must be used correctly. They must be applied before genital contact and must remain intact during such activity. Table 4.5 summarizes the guidelines for the handling, application, and disposal of condoms.

FIGURE 4.8
A condom display in a local pharmacy. These items are easily obtained and in plain view.

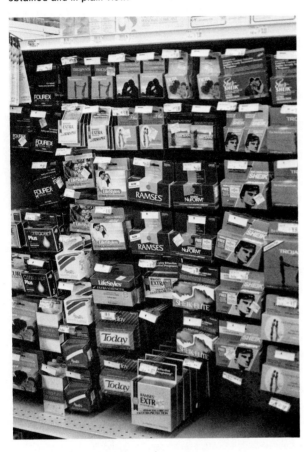

STDs AND PREGNANCY

STDs not only can complicate pregnancy for a woman, but they also can cause significant injury to her unborn child and sexual partner(s). The practice of safer sex is especially important to the pregnant woman in any of the following situations:

1. A woman whose sexual partner has a history, recent diagnosis, or obvious signs of an STD.
2. A woman who is diagnosed during her pregnancy as having an STD.
3. A woman whose sexual partner is an intravenous drug user or who is bisexual.
4. A woman who is likely to have more than one sexual partner during her pregnancy.
5. A woman whose partner is likely to have several sexual partners.

NONSPECIFIC GENITAL INFECTIONS

Several nonspecific genital infections also occur with some degree of frequency in the general population. While many of these are caused by the agents of the better-known STDs, it should be noted that other pathogens such as those responsible for urinary tract infections, may be involved. Examples of

---

FOCUS ON STDs

A NEW CONDOM FOR WOMEN

A new barrier contraceptive device for internal use by women is undergoing end-stage development work in the United States. The condom for women, designated WPC-333 (Wisconsin Pharmacal Company, Jackson, WI) is for one-time use and is designed to help reduce the risks of pregnancy and sexually transmitted diseases. It consists of a tightly fitting polyurethane sheath and two diaphragm-like flexible polyurethane rings. One ring lies inside the sheath and serves as an insertion mechanism and internal anchor. The other ring remains outside the vagina once the device is inserted. The outer ring protects the labia and the base of the penis.

An artificial intercourse model was used in testing for the possibility of viral leakage. After three different trials no leakage was detected. The use of this device, which can be controlled by the woman, may reduce the incidence of sexually acquired HIV and CMV infections.

TABLE 4.4 | PRINCIPLES AND APPLICATIONS FOR PERSONAL STD PREVENTION

PRINCIPLES	APPLICATION(S)
Critical considerations of sexual activities	Abstinence or restricting sexual activity to a single (uninfected) partner reduces the risk of STD infection to a minimum. Risk of infection increases with additional partners, especially unfamiliar ones. Long-term monogamy (having one partner) generally is the safer relationship. Knowing the health status of sex partners is of major importance. This includes frank discussions as to mutual health histories and using preventative measures during sexual activities.
Use of condoms, combined with sperm killing agents (spermicides)	The correct use of condoms together with spermicides reduces the risk of STD transmission during sexual intercourse. It should be noted that condoms will not work if open sores or infectious secretions are present on body surfaces around the genitalia.
Avoiding "unsafe sex" practices	Avoid activities or actions that cause local skin or membrane lining injury and increase the direct contact with STD disease agents. Such activities include oral–anal contact, receptive anal intercourse and actions that cause bleeding or local injury.
Avoiding other high-risk and related behavior	Avoid the use of shared needles. If infected with an STD, do not donate blood. Practice sexual activities that do not involve exchange of body fluids. If the infected individual is a female, avoid pregnancy. **Safer sex** always should be practiced to avoid STDs.
Local application of antimicrobial agents (drugs)	The use of antiseptic agents before and immediately following sexual intercourse may reduce the risk of gonorrhea, syphilis, and other STDs.
Selective use of antibiotics (if effective against the disease agent)	Can be used when diagnostic tests are not available, or risk of exposure is high. A full course of treatment is necessary for best results.
Periodic examination (screening) for STDs	Periodic examinations should be performed according to degree of risk or problem (*e.g.*, known exposure to an STD, multiple sex partners, and other types of high risk behavior).
Sexual partner compliance with diagnosis and follow-up treatment available for STDs	Once a treatable STD is detected, treatment should be given to all individuals involved regardless of the presence or absence of signs and symptoms.

TABLE 4.5	FACTORS TO BE CONSIDERED FOR THE EFFECTIVE AND PROPER USE OF CONDOMS

MATERIAL AND PACKAGING

1. Latex (rubber) condoms should be used instead of membrane condoms since they provide greater protection against viral STDs.

2. The package should state that the condoms are for disease prevention.

3. Some condom packages have the words "DATE MFG" followed by a date on them. This refers to the date when the condoms were made, and is not an expiration date.

4. All condoms to which a spermicide has been added must have an expiration date for the spermicide.

5. The use of condoms containing spermicides may provide additional protection against STDs.

6. Do not purchase condoms from a vending machine located where it may be exposed to extreme temperatures or direct sunlight.

7. Condoms in damaged packages or those that are sticky, discolored, or brittle SHOULD NOT BE USED. THEY ARE NOT SAFE.

STORAGE

1. Store condoms in a cool, dry place, and away from direct sunlight.
2. Condoms should not be kept in a pocket, wallet, or purse for more than a few hours at a time.

HANDLING AND USE

1. Condoms should be handled carefully to prevent punctures. DO NOT USE teeth, sharp fingernails, scissors, or other sharp objects.

2. After opening the package, inspect the condom top for obvious damage such as holes and brittleness.

3. Use a new condom for each time of sexual intercourse. Discard used condoms.

4. A condom should be put on before any genital contact to prevent any exposure to infectious agent-containing body fluids.

5. Put on a condom when the penis is erect.

6. To put on a condom, hold the tip of the condom and unroll it onto the erect penis and all the way to the base of the penis. Leave a small empty space about a half-an-inch at the tip to collect semen. Some condoms have a small, empty nipple (a reservoir tip) that will hold semen. DO NOT PULL THE CONDOM TIGHTLY AGAINST THE TIP OF THE PENIS.

7. If a lubricant is needed or desired, use only water-based materials such as contraceptive jelly. DO NOT USE PETROLEUM OR OIL-BASED LUBRICANTS, SUCH AS PETROLEUM JELLY, COOKING OILS, SHORTENING OR LOTIONS, since they damage latex.

8. DO NOT USE SALIVA TO MOISTEN A CONDOM since it may contain HIV.

9. If the condom should break during sexual intercourse, stop and withdraw immediately. Put on a new condom.

10. After ejaculation, withdraw the penis while it is still erect. Hold onto the rim of condom during withdrawal to prevent it from slipping off.

11. Discard the used condom in a tissue, and throw it in the trash where others will not handle it.

12. Wash the penis and the genital/vaginal/rectal areas with soap and water.

13. Wash hands with soap and water.

FIGURE 4.9

The appearance of a clue cell. This type of cell is a typical finding in bacterial vaginosis. The infection is associated with the bacterium *Gardnerella vaginalis*.

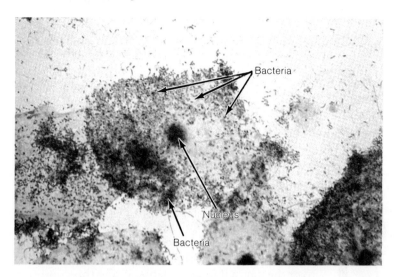

common nonspecific genital infections in women include pelvic inflammatory disease (PID), nonspecific vaginitis, and vaginosis. Two common nonspecific diseases found among men are urethritis and prostatitis.

In women the general symptoms of many of these nonspecific STDs include a vaginal discharge, with or without external itching, burning, or other forms of irritation, and genital sores. In men, the general symptoms are urethral discharge and genital ulcers. Additional symptoms are given in the following section and in the **SIGNS & SYMPTOMS BOXES** accompanying each nonspecific STD described.

NONSPECIFIC GENITAL INFECTIONS OF WOMEN

Vaginal Infections — A General Note. Inflammation of and a discharge from the vagina are the most noticeable and common signs of a vaginal infection, or *vaginitis*. The population of microorganisms or *microbiota* (mī-krō-bī-Ō-ta), normally found in the vagina varies according to hormone-directed changes that occur in this region of the body. The microbiota consists of a mixture of many dynamic microorganisms that vary without any particular one

predominating with the female's menstrual cycle. However, changes in the vaginal environment favor the selection of different microorganisms and depending on the ones present, may result in the development of an infection (fig. 4.9).

Pelvic Inflammatory Disease. Pelvic inflammatory disease (PID) is caused by pathogenic microorganisms moving from the lower genital tract through the cervix into the uterus, the uterine tubes, and the neighboring structures of the reproductive system. Most cases of PID occur following sexual contact. A small percentage of cases develop following certain surgical procedures, such as *dilation and curettage* (scraping the walls of the uterus), and the insertion of an intrauterine device (IUD), a form of birth control. The agents responsible for PID come from the large number of bacteria found in the individual's vagina or cervix.

PID is by far the most serious infectious disease and complication of STDs affecting 15-to-25-year-old women. The economic costs associated with PID are staggering. Annually, PID accounts for over 1 million cases requiring more than 212,000 hospital admissions, 115,000 surgical procedures, and 2.5 million physician visits. The amount of effort and money needed to diagnose and to treat PID is enormous and is increasing yearly. Current estimates indicate that over 3.5 billion dollars will be needed on a yearly basis by 1992.

Women with PID exhibit a range of symptoms, the most common of which is lower abdominal pain. This pain usually is continuous, found on both sides, and increases with movement of the body. Changes in the vaginal discharge is yet another common complaint. The general characteristics of PID can be found in the accompanying **SIGNS & SYMPTOMS BOX.**

The diagnosis of PID usually is based on a careful physical examination (such as the one described in chapter 3), and laboratory procedures that identify the specific bacteria in the cervical discharge obtained from the infected individual. Distinguishing PID from other conditions with similar symptoms may require the use of a **laparoscope** (LAP-a-rō-skōp). This instrument allows for the examination of the oviducts and associated structures.

PID generally is treated with specific antibiotics, usually for ten days. Some cases may require hospitalization. It should be noted that sexual partners of women with PID also should be examined and treated accordingly.

Nonspecific Vaginitis. Inflammation of the vagina, known as vaginitis, causes pain or burning on urination and the need to urinate more frequently. In most instances individuals with vaginitis say the burning sensation occurs as urine passes over the vaginal folds, or labia. While this condition is common among women seeking treatment for STDs, it should be kept in mind that there are other causes.

Other common symptoms of vaginitis are an unusual vaginal discharge or a change in the amount of discharge. These situations may not be abnormal symptoms, but actually may result from the normal secretion of glands in the cervix, or the influence of pregnancy or oral birth control pills (see **SIGNS & SYMPTOMS BOX**).

The diagnosis of vaginitis is based on the findings of a carefully performed physical examination and or laboratory tests that identify specific pathogens in vaginal specimens.

Treatment of the condition should be based on laboratory findings. These usually result in the prescription of specific antibiotics. Sexual partners also should be treated. Condoms or other safer sexual practices should be followed to prevent the spread of the causative agents.

THE SIGNS AND SYMPTOMS BOX	**DISEASE** PELVIC INFLAMMATORY DISEASE (PID) **INCUBATION PERIOD** 1-3 WEEKS

First Symptoms Usually Appear: 1–3 Weeks

Signs
1. Abnormal bleeding
2. Increased vaginal discharge
3. Displacement of the cervix from its normal position
4. Growths on the ovaries and/or uterine tubes

Symptoms
1. Lower abdominal pain; usually continuous, dull and increases in intensity with body movements
2. Fever
3. Pain during sexual intercourse
4. Nausea and vomiting (usually late symptoms)
5. Painful and frequent urination
6. Menstrual changes (irregularities)

Complications
1. Liver involvement resulting in an inflammation of the organ.
2. Upper abdominal pain and tenderness caused by the spreading of the infection.
3. Infertility

<table>
<tr><td rowspan="2">

**THE SIGNS
AND
SYMPTOMS
BOX**

</td><td>

DISEASE
NONSPECIFIC VAGINITIS
(vaj-in-$\overline{\text{I}}$-tis)
</td></tr>
<tr><td>

INCUBATION PERIOD
VARIABLE
</td></tr>
</table>

First Symptoms Usually Appear: 1–4 Weeks

Signs
1. Some bleeding

Symptoms
1. Increased vaginal discharge, which varies according to its cause; may be thin to thick and range in color from clear to yellowish-green
2. Vulvar and vaginal itching
3. General discomfort

Complications
If a pregnant woman has vaginitis, her newborn may develop mouth and throat infections.

<table>
<tr><td rowspan="2">

**THE SIGNS
AND
SYMPTOMS
BOX**

</td><td>

DISEASE
VAGINOSIS
(vaj-i-N$\overline{\text{O}}$-sis)
</td></tr>
<tr><td>

INCUBATION PERIOD
VARIABLE
</td></tr>
</table>

First Symptoms Usually Appear: Variable, But Usually Occurs Within 2–10 Days.
Signs
1. Large amounts of milky white discharge

Symptoms
1. Odor usually appears after sexual intercourse
2. General discomfort

Complications
1. Pelvic Inflammatory Disease (PID)
2. Infection of the ovaries
3. Urinary tract infection
4. In the case of pregnancy, premature labor

Bacterial Vaginosis. Bacterial vaginosis is a disease that results from the massive overgrowth of the vaginal bacterial population. While the exact cause of the condition is unknown, most women experience a chemical change in the vaginal environment resulting in a noticeable milk-like discharge and odor (see **SIGNS & SYMPTOMS BOX**). In addition, the bacteria associated with vaginosis attach to the surfaces of the vaginal lining resulting in "clue" cells (fig. 4.9) which is of value in diagnosing the condition. If bacterial vaginosis is left untreated, serious consequences can develop including an inflammation of the uterine tubes known as **salpingitis** (sal-pin-J$\overline{\text{I}}$-tis) and PID.

Although sexual transmission of vaginosis has not been proven, antibiotic treatment of sexual partners is considered advisable. The role of STD agents in vaginosis is explored in later chapters.

NONSPECIFIC GENITAL INFECTIONS IN MEN

Prostatitis. An infection of the prostate gland, or prostatitis (pros-ta-T$\overline{\text{I}}$-tis) can be associated with specific as well as nonspecific sexually transmitted agents, and with urinary tract infections. Prostatitis can appear suddenly (the *acute* form) or it can develop slowly and last for a long time (the *chronic* form). Common symptoms include a burning feeling on urination, the frequent need to urinate, fever, and some lower abdominal pain. Other features of prostatitis are given in the accompanying **SIGNS & SYMPTOMS BOX.**

<table>
<tr><td rowspan="2">

**THE SIGNS
AND
SYMPTOMS
BOX**

</td><td>

DISEASE
PROSTATITIS (pros-tah-TĪ-tis)
INCUBATION PERIOD
VARIABLE

</td></tr>
</table>

First Symptoms Usually Appear: Acute Form: Within One Week After it Starts.
Chronic Form: Variable.

Signs	Symptoms
Acute Form None	1. Painful urination (usually burning sensation) 2. Frequent need to urinate 3. Fever 4. Pain in and around anus
Chronic Form Blood in urine	1. Pain in areas such as the tip of the penis, the scrotum, lower back, and thighs 2. Pain on ejaculation 3. Painful (burning) urniation 4. Frequent need to urinate

Complications
Low sex drive or libido (li-BĒ-do)

The diagnosis of prostatitis involves a physical examination and laboratory examination of a urine sample. Antibiotics are used for treatment.

Urethritis. An inflammation of the urethra, or urethritis (ū-rē-THRĪ-tis), is a very common condition that also is associated with both nonspecific genital infections and specific STDs. After an incubation period of one to three weeks, the infected individual notices a burning sensation on urination and the presence of a sticky, thick urethral discharge, usually occurring in the morning. While these are typical symptoms, it is possible for infected persons to be *asymptomatic*, or without symptoms.

Although urethritis occurs in both men and women, the condition is generally diagnosed only in men. When urethritis is found in women and it is not associated with a urinary bladder infection, or **cystitis** (sis-TĪ-tis), the term *urethral syndrome* is used. The particular features of urethritis are given in the accompanying **SIGNS & SYMPTOMS BOX.**

Diagnosis of urethritis generally is based on the individual's personal history, the symptoms noted, a thorough physical examination, and the results of laboratory diagnostic tests to identify the causative agent.

Treatment includes the use of antibiotics and follow-up examinations. Sexual partners also need to be contacted, examined, and treated. This is especially important because the woman's reproductive organs can be severely damaged by urethritis. A partner experiencing such symptoms as pain during intercourse, lower abdominal pain, or unusual bleeding should seek medical attention as soon as possible.

TABLE 4.6 | EXAMPLES OF FACTORS THAT CAN INFLUENCE SEXUAL BEHAVIOR

PERSONAL FACTORS	INTERPERSONAL FACTORS
Knowledge of STD infection and transmission, effects, and prevention	Recognizing the viewpoints of friends, family, and society-at-large in relation to risky sexual practices. Do these groups approve?
Recognizing one's limitations and susceptibility to infection, i.e., *This can happen to me!*	Knowing the limits of social support; specifically,
Understanding the true costs, and more importantly the benefits of STD infection prevention	1. Who will provide the needed support and care?
Recognizing one's skills and abilities to:	2. What types of support can be expected? Money, housing, medical, or just plain caring?
1. reduce or even eliminate the use of alcohol and/or drugs.	
2. effectively use a condom, if appropriate.	
3. openly discuss and/or arrange for safer sexual practices with a sex partner.	
4. adjust to safer sexual practices.	

WHAT'S NEEDED TO REDUCE THE NUMBER OF STD CASES?

The behavior of infected individuals clearly is the key to STD prevention and control. The recognition of viral STDs such as genital herpes, hepatitis B, and HIV infection highlight the importance of the infected in disease transmission. Reducing or even eliminating risky sexual practices is the essential element in the prevention and ultimate control of STDs. Such changes obviously do not occur overnight. Moreover, they will require knowledge of life-style choices, personal, and interpersonal factors that can influence sexual behavior (table 4.6), reinforcing healthful living habits, and adopting as well as promoting safer sex.

CHAPTER | 5 | SYPHILIS AND GONORRHEA

In one day: 2,700 Americans discover that they have gonorrhea. Two hundred discover that they have syphilis.

—Tom Parker, In One Day

From the sixteenth century until well into the nineteenth century, most doctors assumed that **syphilis** (SIF-i-lis) and **gonorrhea** (gon'-ō-RĒ-a) were one and the same disease. It was not until 1837 that the specific natures of these two bacterial infections were established. This chapter presents the distinctive features of these two important STDs.

FIGURE 5.1

Syphilis. (a) A magnified view of the causative agent of syphilis *Treponema pallidum*, as seen through an electron microscope. The corkscrew-shaped agents (arrows) are attached to host cells. (From E. E. Quist, L. A. Repesh, R. Zeleznikar, and T. J.

Fitzgerald, *British Journal of Venereal Diseases* (1983) 59: 11–20.) (b) The primary sore, or chancre, of syphilis is on the lower lip. This typical lesion contains hundreds of the causative agent. (Courtesy of U.S. Public Health Service)

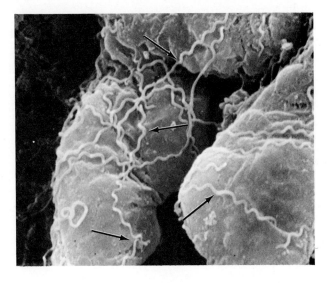

a

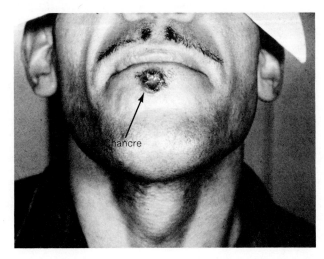

b

SYPHILIS—THE TIMELESS SCOURGE

CAUSE AND TRANSMISSION

Syphilis is a long-lasting, contagious infection caused by the bacterium **Treponema pallidum** (trep'-ō-NĒ-ma, PAL-i-dum). This microorganism is called a **spirochete** (SPĪ-rō-kēt), because of its rather corkscrew appearance (fig. 5.1a). It is usually spread through sexual activities and causes an extraordinary variety of signs and symptoms (fig. 5.1b). Infected, expectant mothers may also transmit syphilis to their unborn.

BACKGROUND

Medical historians have traced syphilis from Spain throughout Europe and Asia and have discovered the disease to be what distinguished physician Sir Willaim Osler once described as "The most formidable enemy of the race, an enemy entrenched behind the strongest human passions and the deepest of social prejudices." It is apparent from the list of famous syphilitics (table 5.1) that this disease did not recognize any international barriers nor leave any generation untouched.

TABLE 5.1 | VICTIMS OF SYPHILIS THROUGH THE YEARS

CROWNED HEADS OF EUROPE

Charles VII of France	Frederick the Great
France's Henry III	Russia's Peter the Great
Ivan the Terrible	

ARTISTS

Albrecht Durer	Benvenuto Cellini
Paul Gauguin	Vincent van Gogh

WRITERS

Guy de Maupassant	Christopher Marlowe
Heinrich Heine	Oscar Wilde

MUSICIANS

Robert Schumann	Niccolò Paganini
Ludwig van Beethoven	Hugo Wolf

PHILOSOPHERS

Arthur Schopenhauer	Friedrich Nietzsche

CRIME FIGURES

Al Capone

Among the intriguing questions raised by medical historians are how and why syphilis suddenly appeared in Europe in the late 1400s. A few possible answers to these questions are discussed here.

One commonly held view is that syphilis was brought to Europe by Columbus and his crew after their first voyage to the West Indies. It is true that within a few years of Columbus's return from his first voyage to the New World, epidemics of the disease spread across Europe with devastating effects. History suggests that the Spaniards introduced the disease to the Italians while fighting beside the troops of Alfonso II of Naples. Then, in 1495, an army of mercenaries fighting for Charles VIII of France conquered Naples. As they returned home through France, Germany, Switzerland, Austria, and England, they carried along the disease. By 1496, syphilis was so uncontrolled in Paris that strict laws were passed banishing anyone with the disease from the city. In 1498, Vasco de Gama and his Portuguese crew carried syphilis to India, and from there it spread to China. Outbreaks of syphilis in Japan soon followed the visits of European ships.

Another view holds that syphilis arrived in Spain and Portugal with slaves imported from Africa in the mid-1400s. Another bacterial disease found in Africa, called **yaws** (yawz), which is quite similar to syphilis in several respects, is believed by certain historians to have flared in the form of syphilis in the late 1400s. They further speculate that the army of Charles VIII provided a highly susceptible population that spread the disease wherever they went.

STD FACT FILE

DISEASE
SYPHILIS (SIF-i-lis)
CAUSE
THE BACTERIUM TREPONEMA PALLIDUM (trep-ō-NĒ-mah, PAL-i-dum)

Source/Transmission
Infected humans; sexual intercourse and/or other activities involving direct contact with syphilitic sores or lesions; infant infection can also occur during pregnancy.

Epidemiology
Disease is found worldwide.

Control
1. Injections of the antibiotic penicillin, or the antibiotics erythromycin or tetracycline (tet'-ra-SĪ-klen) for individuals allergic to penicillin
2. Tracing, contacting, and treating sexual partners
3. Follow-up for the effectiveness of treatments. Infected persons should be checked periodically after treatment.

Prevention
1. Use of barrier devices such as condoms for prevention of the disease's spread.

Physicians in the early sixteenth century did not have a name for the disease we now call syphilis. However, its obvious devastating effects through the years inspired a number of epithets. The Italians referred to it as the Spanish disease, while the French called it the Neapolitan disease. As syphilis spread to many countries it acquired the name of French sickness, a name that lasted for about a century.

The term syphilis was introduced by the Italian physician Girolamo Fracastorius, who wrote a poem about a shepherd boy named Syphilus. Apparently, Syphilus left a flock of sheep belonging to the Greek god Apollo for some sexual activity. As punishment for leaving the sheep unattended, he developed the horrible sores of the disease.

EPIDEMIOLOGY NOTES

The incidence of syphilis is on the rise. Once believed to be nearly eradicated, this disease is again a major concern. The results of various studies in 1988 show a steady increase of syphilis among prostitutes, drug users and their sexual contacts, and newborn infants in various parts of the United States. These findings, which may be an indication of a widespread phenomenon, have important global implications for the control of not only syphilis, but other STDs, including human immunodeficiency virus (HIV) infections. This is largely because the genital ulcers found with a syphilitic infection (fig. 5.2) greatly increase HIV transmission possibility. A general summary of syphilis is given in the accompanying **STD FACT FILE.**

Figure 5.2

Example of the destructive, open sores of early syphilis, commonly called *malignant syphilis*. (a) The presence of blisters (pustules) and open sores appearing on the genitals in a first infection. (b) Ulcerated syphilides (some covered with dark crusts) observed with the same individual experiencing a reinfection. (From K. Lejman and Z. Starzycki, *British Journal of Venereal Diseases* (1978) 54:278.)

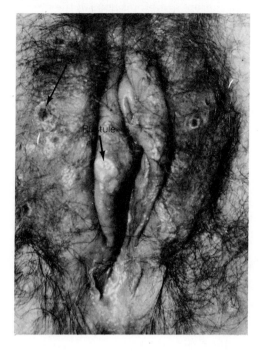

a

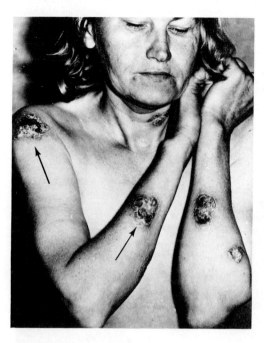

b

FOCUS ON STDs

SYPHILIS AND ART

Rembrandt van Rijn certainly is considered to be one of the world's greatest artists. "Nightwatch" and "Aristotle Contemplating the Bust of Homer," which are among his better known masterpieces, have been viewed and enjoyed by thousands. Recently, one of his creations attracted particular attention because the subject of the painting, a seventeenth century gentleman, appears to have the obvious signs of late congenital syphilis (fig. 5.3). These signs include deep grooves extending from the corners of the eyes and the mouth and a characteristic saddle nose.

Rembrandt painted this portrait of Gèrard de Lairesse, a Flemish painter, in 1665. The painting is currently in the *Robert Lehman Collection of the Metropolitan Museum of Art* in New York City.

FIGURE 5.3

A portrait of Gerard de Lairesse painted by the artist Rembrandt van Rijn in 1665. G. de Lairesse was a famous painter in his own right and was known for his luxurious tastes and unpleasant appearance. His face, as this figure shows, was marred by the gross signs of late syphilis. (From G. Borrini, *American Journal of Dermopathology* (1988) 10:448–450.)

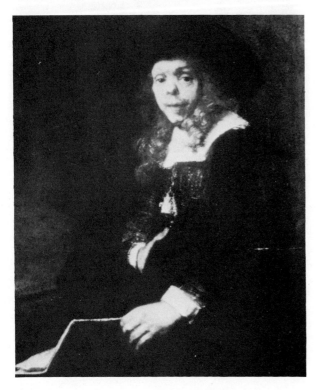

SIGNS AND STAGES

Physicians in the early 1500s recognized syphilis as an STD. Unfortunately, a French physician who named the infection *morbus venereus* in 1527 unwittingly injected himself with a specimen containing the causative agents of both syphilis and gonorrhea. His descriptions of what he thought was syphilis alone were a major source of confusion until 1837, when the two diseases were identified as separate and distinct conditions. This section will describe the established stages of syphilis.

Incubation Period. The time from exposure to the appearance of syphilis symptoms ranges from ten to ninety days. Most incubation periods fall between twenty-one and thirty-five days. In general, the shorter the time before symptoms appear, the greater the infectious dose of *Treponema pallidum* to which the individual has been exposed.

Syphilis is divided into the three stages: *primary, secondary,* and *late.* In an infection these stages do not necessarily follow an orderly progression, in fact they may overlap. Moreover, all stages do not always develop. A summary of the features of syphilis infection is given in the accompanying **SIGNS & SYMPTOMS BOX.**

Primary Syphilis. The first physical sign of primary syphilis is a hard sore or chancre (SHANG-ker) which develops at the site of injury or inoculation. This lesion begins as a small, elevated, reddened area, that eventually breaks down into an open sore, or ulcer (fig. 5.4). These events usually take about three to seven days. Fully developed chancres range in size from a few millimeters to several centimeters in diameter. The chancre usually is painless, and without treatment takes from one to six weeks to heal. Some individuals may have two or more such lesions, and in about 20 to 30 percent of cases, the chancres go unnoticed.

Chancres can be expected to occur at any point of effective body contact. In men and women, these sites are located on the genitalia. Extragenital locations include the fingers, lips, breasts, and armpits. With individuals practicing oral or anal sex, lesions may be found in the mouth and around the anus.

Secondary Syphilis. Secondary syphilis generally develops six weeks to six months after the appearance of the primary lesion. Infected individuals frequently experience symptoms similar to those associated with a case of the flu. These include muscular aches and pains, an occasional sore throat, low-grade fever, and general discomfort. In the secondary stage, the spirochetes invade the circulatory system and thereby can gain access to any body organ.

<table>
<tr><td rowspan="2">

THE SIGNS AND SYMPTOMS BOX

</td><td>

DISEASE
SYPHILIS (SIF-i-lis)
INCUBATION PERIOD
10–90 DAYS (USUALLY 3 WEEKS)

</td></tr>
</table>

First Symptoms Usually Appear: 10 Days to 3 Months After Exposure

Signs	Symptoms
Primary Stage	
Men	
1. Usually a single chancre (a firm, painless open sore on the genitals or mouth)	1. Generally no noticeable symptoms
2. Swollen glands in the surrounding regions of the genitalia	
Secondary Stage	
1. Patchy hair loss	1. Slight fever
2. Skin rash, and red patches in the mouth (highly infectious in most cases)	2. Sore throat
3. Swollen glands	3. Headache
4. Inflammation of the liver, anus, and rectum	4. Weight loss

Latent Stage
Generally no major symptoms, however, the infected individual can be contagious for 4 years if treatment is not given.

Tertiary Stage	
1. Difficulties in speaking, and memory recall	1. Unable to concentrate
2. Shaking (tremors) of lips and/or hands	2. Personality changes
	3. Alternating moods of depression and well-being (happiness)
Primary Stage	
Women	
1. Usually a single chancre appears around the genitals, mouth, or breast; genital chancres may be difficult to detect	1. Generally no noticeable symptoms

Secondary Stage
Similar to the signs and symptoms listed for men.

Latent Stage
Similar to the signs and symptoms listed for men.

Tertiary Stage
Similar to the signs and symptoms listed for men.

Complications

Men and Women
1. Infection and destruction of the heart, blood vessels, and brain
2. Paralysis
3. Insanity

Newborns
1. Congenital defects include deafness, blindness, and the abnormal development of various body structures, and the central nervous system

FIGURE 5.4

An example of primary syphilis on a body location away from the genitalia (extragenital site). Primary syphilitic chancres on the fingers result from direct contact with genital lesions. (Courtesy of Dr. Z. Starzycki)

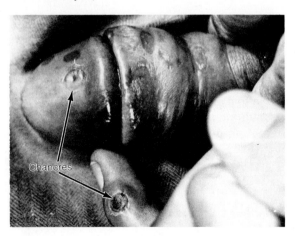

FIGURE 5.5

The appearance of secondary syphilis. The rash is infectious.

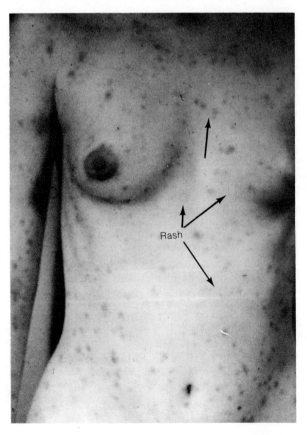

A particular feature of the secondary stage of syphilis infection is the development of a discrete brownish or copper-colored rash in about 80 percent of the cases. The rash involves the face, palms of the hands, soles of the feet, and eventually most of the body's surface (fig. 5.5). The rash tends to disappear spontaneously within four to twelve weeks.

FIGURE 5.6

The appearance of moth-eaten-like skin eruptions, syphilides. These skin conditions may accompany secondary syphilis. (a) A syphilide on the neck. (From Z. Starzycki, *Acta Dermatology and Venereology* (1989) 69:173.) (b) A similar eruption on the left arm of the same patient. (Courtesy of Dr. Z. Starzycki)

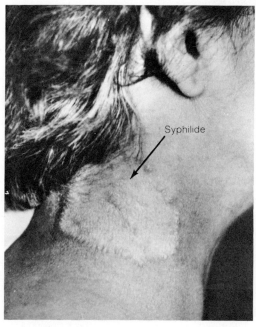

a

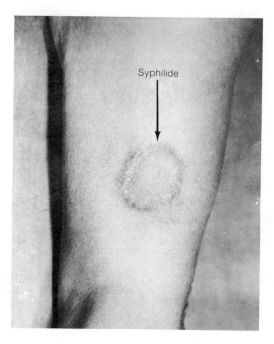

b

Unfortunately, however, about 25 percent of infected individuals experience relapses of this rash.

Other features of secondary syphilis include: swollen lymph glands in the regions of the groin, thigh, armpits, and collarbone; the presence of highly infectious, moist, flat patches (called **condylomata lata**) that have a tendency to run together in skin folds of the genital and anal areas; hair loss; spirochete-containing mucous patches in the mouth; and funguslike skin eruptions called **syphilides** (SIF-il-ids) (fig. 5.6).

Latent Syphilis. By definition, individuals with historical evidence of syphilis, or a positive blood test, but with no clinical signs of disease (figs. 5.4 and 5.5) have hidden or **latent syphilis.** Clearly the destructive spirochetes of *T. pallidum* have a remarkable capacity to resist the actions of a host's immune system to eliminate them. However, it is believed that latent syphilis is due to the immune system's control of active infection. Latent syphilis may be divided into early latency and late latency on the basis of time when treated individuals are likely to experience spontaneous relapses and develop lesions.

Late Syphilis. The various symptoms and consequences of late syphilis can be conveniently grouped under the three headings of **benign tertiary syphilis, cardiovascular syphilis,** and **neurosyphilis.**

Benign tertiary syphilis includes the symptoms and consequences that develop after the secondary stage, with the exception of those associated with cardiovascular and neurological forms of the disease. It can occur about four years after an untreated primary infection. Several body locations, tissues, and organs may be involved, including the skin, bone, mouth, face, nose, portions of the upper respiratory tract, stomach, liver, and testes. A soft tumorlike swelling, known as a **gumma,** may develop in a number of internal organs such as the brain, heart, and liver. Gummas in these critical organs would be fatal.

FIGURE 5.7

One of the signs of congenital syphilis, Hutchinson's teeth. Poor development of the teeth, especially the permanent upper central incisors (arrows) develop a barrel-shaped and notched appearance.

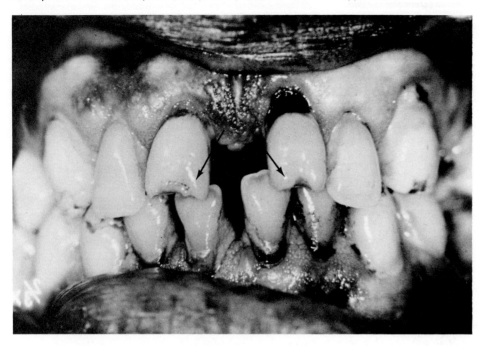

Cardiovascular syphilis tends to begin fifteen to twenty years after the primary infection. In its simplest form, the infected individual experiences a symptomless inflammation of the ascending aorta. The condition can progress to a weakening of this blood vessel until it expands to the point of rupturing. Constriction of the aorta also is possible. This condition may lead to an enlargement of the left ventricle of the heart and eventually to congestive heart failure.

Neurosyphilis develops in about 6 to 7 percent of untreated cases. It is the result of central nervous system invasion by *Treponema pallidum* during the early course of the infection. Symptoms can begin to appear two years after the primary infection. Meningitis, (an inflammation of the coverings of the brain), partial or complete paralysis, and psychological changes are but a few of the consequences associated with this form of late syphilis.

Untreated, about one-third of infected individuals will develop some form of late syphilis.

CONGENITAL SYPHILIS

Treponema pallidum is among a select few microorganisms capable of passing through the placenta to infect the fetus during pregnancy. This form of syphilis causes fetal or perinatal death in at least 40 percent of affected infants. Congenital syphilis was described in the fifteenth century and has been recognized as a distinct condition in which the source of *Treponema pallidum* is the infected mother. If the infection does not kill the fetus, the newborn will have congenital syphilis and exhibit any number of typical signs and symptoms (fig. 5.7). The skin, bone, heart, blood vessels, and blood-forming tissues may be attacked during the early or later stages of the disease. Central nervous system involvement in the fetus can often be avoided by the appropriate treatment of an infected mother early in her pregnancy.

Infected newborns generally are treated with some form of penicillin. In case of penicillin sensitivity or allergy, other antibiotics are used. Treatment is coordinated with the results of laboratory tests such as those briefly described in the next section.

DIAGNOSIS

The management of syphilis is closely linked to the results of diagnostic laboratory tests. Present-day diagnosis of all stages of the disease depends on the results of serologic tests used to detect and measure the concentrations of immunoglobulins (antibodies). Two general types of serologic tests are in use: **treponemal** (trep'-ō-NĒ-mal) **tests** that measure immunoglobulins directed against *Treponema pallidum* itself, and **nontreponemal tests** that measure immunoglobulins formed by the infected individual in response to products of injured tissues. Nontreponemal immunoglobulins are sometimes called **reaginic** (RĒ-a-jin-ik). Examples of treponemal tests include the fluorescent treponemal antibody absorption (FTA-ABS) test and the microhemagglutination *Treponema pallidum* (MHA-TP) test. Examples of nontreponemal tests include the venereal disease research laboratory (VDRL) test, and the rapid plasma reagin (RPR) test.

In untreated syphilis, the degree of reactivity in serologic tests depends on the stage of the disease. Immunoglobulins appear one to three weeks after the chancre appears. A reactive VDRL test is generally found in 65 to 70 percent of individuals with primary syphilis, 90 to 100 percent of secondary syphilis, and 75 percent of late, latent, and tertiary syphilis cases. These immunoglobulins disappear about six to twelve months after treatment of primary syphilis and within twenty-four months of treatment of secondary syphilis.

Whenever possible, direct microscopic examinations of materials from moist sores (lesions) are used to diagnose primary and secondary stages of syphilis. However, when appropriate microscopes or specimens are not available, serologic tests are used. In the case of congenital syphilis, placental tissue and the umbilical cord are excellent sources of material for microscopic examination.

Serologic tests are the major diagnostic tools in all stages of syphilis, including periods of latency. Follow-up testing also is appropriate to determine the effectiveness of treatment.

TREATMENT

The treatment of choice for primary, secondary, and early latent syphilis is some form of penicillin. The antibiotic is given intramuscularly. Symptoms in patients treated for a first attack of the disease usually disappear promptly, and a negative blood test usually is obtained within twenty-four months. Cases of neurosyphilis require high doses of penicillin.

Unfortunately, following antibiotic treatment some individuals experience a side effect known as the **Jarisch-Herxheimer reaction.** This condition results from the antibiotic's massive destruction of *Treponema pallidum.* Typical symptoms of this reaction include rapid heartbeat, fever, chills, headache, muscle soreness, sore throat, and an increased redness of skin lesions if they are present. As with the treatment of any disease, an evaluation of the results of therapy must be made. Such monitoring is done, as mentioned earlier, with serologic testing.

PREVENTION

Several preventative measures can reduce the number of syphilis cases. These include following safer sex practices such as the use of barrier devices during sexual activities and limiting the number of sex partners.

The search for an effective vaccine against syphilis as a means not only to control but to eliminate the disease has been under study and development for several decades. Progress has been slow due to the unusual features of syphilis and still unknown properties of *T. pallidum.*

FIGURE 5.8

The skin involvement in gonorrhea. This type of lesion usually
contains the infectious agent.

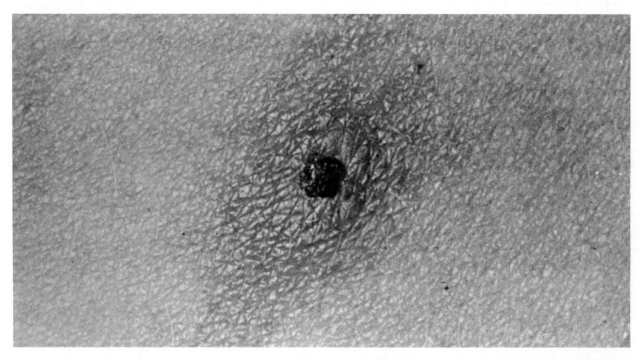

GONORRHEA
CAUSE AND TRANSMISSION

Gonorrhea (Gc) is a serious infectious disease of short
duration. It is caused by the bacterium **Neisseria
gonorrhoeae** (nī-SĒ-rē-a, gon'-Ō-rē-a), also frequently referred to as **gonococcus** (gon-ō-KOK-us).
While the disease primarily affects the male and
female mucosa (mū-KŌ-sa), the moist lining of the
genital organs, it also can involve other body areas,
such as the skin (fig. 5.8), gums, tongue, and the
throat.

Most Gc infections are acquired by sexual contact.
Infections of the rectum may occur after anal intercourse with infected persons, and infection of the
throat and other mouth parts results from orogenital sex (fig. 5.9).

The prevalence of gonorrhea in pregnant women
is variable. However, the risk of transmission from
an infected mother to her unborn is 30 to 40 percent.
The most common condition resulting from Gc
transmission and without routine application of an
antibiotic is an infection of the eyelid lining known
as conjunctivitis (kon-junk'-ti-VĪ-tis).

FIGURE 5.9

An abscess (arrow) in the mouth of a patient with gonorrhea. Such localized collections of pus in the mouth are not rare. (From D. Marini, S. Veraldi, and M. Innocenti, *Cutis* (1987) 40:363.)

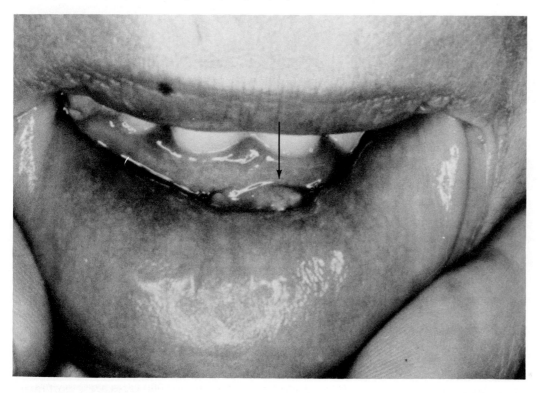

BACKGROUND

From earliest history to modern times gonorrhea has been and is a major problem causing such severe consequences as sterility, blindness, and in certain situations, death. While this disease has been recognized as a human affliction since ancient times, it remained for the well-known physician Galen, practicing in Rome during the golden age of Greek medicine, to give the disease its name. He mistakenly believed that the discharge (fig. 5.10) referred to as *Rheos,* was composed of semen, or *Gonos.* Thus, the name gonorrhea, meaning the flow of seed, was coined. One of the better known common names for this disease, "clap," was derived from the term *clappoir* used for Parisian houses of prostitution in the Middle Ages.

The history of gonorrhea is not without confusion and tragedy. As mentioned earlier, syphilis and gonorrhea were considered to be one and the same disease for almost 300 years. This confusion appears to have developed almost immediately upon the recognition of syphilis in the last years of the fifteenth century as it swept western Europe in epidemic proportions. The characteristic discharge of gonorrhea (fig. 5.10) was considered to be the first symptom of syphilis. This viewpoint is not difficult to understand, since during this period of time, the presence of more than one venereal disease in the same person was not uncommon (a situation that certainly occurs with some frequency even today). Since not all physicians of that time were convinced that the descriptions of syphilis actually were a combination of two separate and distinct diseases,

FIGURE 5.10

The typical pus-containing drip or urethral discharge (arrow) found with gonorrhea in the male. Such discharge may be cloudy yellow or greenish yellow in appearance. (Courtesy of Department of Health and Human Services, U.S. Public Health Service)

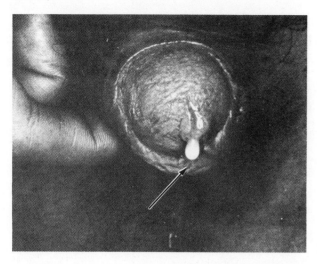

the debate continued until the tragic self-inflicted exposure by the English surgeon John Hunter in 1767. Hunter obtained pus from a patient with gonorrhea and injected himself. Unfortunately, the specimen was contaminated with the causative agent of syphilis, which added to the confused picture of gonorrhea described by the English surgeon. As would be expected, Hunter fell victim to the effects of both diseases. He subsequently developed a classic case of syphilitic heart disease and died in 1793. It is interesting to note that even though syphilis and gonorrhea were shown to be two separate diseases in the 1790s, many physicians still considered them to be the same for another fifty years.

EPIDEMIOLOGY NOTES

Even though antibiotics specifically effective against the *gonococcus* are in use, gonorrhea remains as one of the most commonly reported diseases in the United States. About 900,000 cases are reported annually. However, recent estimates suggest that there may be as many as 2.5 million affected individuals.

Gonorrhea is a difficult disease to eradicate, mainly because of its short incubation period, the presence of many asymptomatic infected carriers, the appearance of penicillin-resistant *gonococci*, and the absence of an immunity (protection) to reinfection on recovery for the disease. Several of these particular aspects of gonorrhea are described in the next sections.

A summary of the features of gonorrhea can be found in the accompanying **STD FACT FILE.**

| **STD FACT FILE** | **DISEASE**
GONORRHEA (gon-ō-RĒ-ah)
CAUSE
THE BACTERIUM NEISSERIA GONORRHOEAE (nī-SĒ-rē-ah, gon-ō-RĒ-ah) |

Source/Transmission

Infected humans; sexual intercourse and/or other activities involving direct contact with the discharge of an individual infected with gonorrhea; passage of newborn through an infected birth canal

Epidemiology

Disease is found worldwide. Some forms of *N. gonorrhea* have become resistant to penicillin thus making treatment more difficult. Several carriers of the disease are asymptomatic. Cases of oral gonorrhea are being reported.

Control

1. Injections of penicillin, or other antibiotics in cases of penicillin resistance or allergy
2. Tracing, contacting, and treating sexual partners
3. Follow-up of infected persons. Individuals should be seen three to seven days after treatment.

Prevention

Use of barrier devices such as condoms for prevention and control of the disease's spread

SIGNS AND SYMPTOMS

The particular signs of gonococcal infection differ with respect to the sex, age, and patterns of sexual practices of infected individuals. Several different groups of gonococcal infections are recognized. These include **asymptomatic genital disease, symptomatic genital disease, disseminated gonococcal infection (DGI),** and complications such as **infection of the Bartholin's glands** and **gonococcal pelvic inflammatory disease** (PID). A summary of the features of gonococcal infections is given in the accompanying **SIGNS & SYMPTOMS BOX.**

Asymptomatic Infection. Infected individuals not showing any signs or symptoms of the disease have long been recognized as a serious barrier to the control and eventual elimination of gonorrhea. More infected women (up to 75 percent) than infected men (1 to 2 percent) tend to be asymptomatic. Unfortunately, this state or condition can persist for long periods of time.

Symptomatic Gonorrhea. In men, the signs and symptoms of gonorrhea take the form of infection of the urethra, or urethritis (See chapter 3 for a description of the male reproductive system). They usually appear three to five days after sexual intercourse with an infected partner. Typical symptoms include a burning sensation on urination and the presence of a pus-like creamy white or yellow discharge from the penis (fig. 5.10).

In women, the signs and symptoms of gonorrhea usually make their appearance after an incubation period of two weeks or longer. When symptoms occur, they are frequently mild or so nonspecific and common that they are overlooked or not taken seriously. Some of the symptoms include a burning sensation on urination, the presence of an unusual vaginal discharge, backache, vaginal bleeding, and pain in the lower abdomen.

FIGURE 5.11
Localized collections of pus and the gonococcus associated with infected Bartholin's glands. These glands are situated just near the vaginal opening at the bottom of the major lips. (Also refer to chapter 3.)

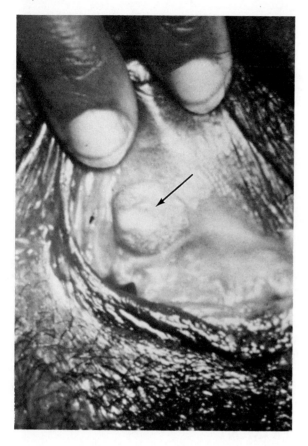

Complications. In males, two common complications of gonorrhea are infections of the prostate gland, or prostatitis, and of the urinary bladder, or cystitis. Epididymitis, an infection of the epididymis, is also a possible consequence of gonorrhea in males.

An individual with an infected prostate generally experiences fever, general discomfort, and lower abdominal pain. The condition can be detected by a physical examination similar to the one described in chapter 3.

Symptoms of a urinary bladder infection generally include painful urination, the need to urinate frequently, and the presence of blood in the urine.

In the case of epididymitis, usually the epididymis and the testes both are infected. The involved area is usually painful, hot, and swollen.

Women may experience an infection of the Bartholin's glands or **bartholinitis** (bar'-tō-lin-Ī-tis) and PID as complications of gonorrhea. Bartholinitis (fig. 5.11) causes pain and swelling of the vulva, which results in discomfort and difficulties in sitting and walking.

Gonococcal PID occurs in about 10 to 15 percent of gonorrhea cases. Lower abdominal pain, fever, and general discomfort are typical symptoms that occur during or within a week after menstruation. In untreated cases and at times after successful management of PID, women may experience pain during sexual intercourse, sterility, and **ectopic** (ek-TOP-ik) pregnancy. (In ectopic pregnancy, the fertilized egg is implanted outside of the uterus.) Gonococcal PID is a serious condition and may require hospitalization and even surgery.

Disseminated Gonococcal Infection (DGI).
Individuals with DGI generally experience fever, painful joints and bones, and a rash. In general, DGI develops in about one in 300 cases, compared to ten in 600 cases of genital gonorrhea. Moreover, it occurs six times more frequently in females than in males.

Oral Gonorrhea. Despite the common occurrence of gonorrhea, its diagnosis can present difficulties because of the various forms in which it appears. Difficult diagnoses involve the mouth and throat. Oral gonorrhea and gonococcal throat infections are not rare and mainly result from orogenital sex. Such conditions primarily occur in individuals who practice oral stimulation of the penis, or **fellatio** (fel-Ā-shē-ō). Unfortunately, in many instances, cases of throat infection are asymptomatic.

A variation of oral gonorrhea, **abscess formation,** has recently been reported (fig. 5.9). Fever, severe pain, and tenderness commonly accompany such localized accumulations of pus.

Dangers to the Newborn. The risk of gonorrhea transmission from mother to infant is 30 to 40 percent. The most common consequence is an infection

FIGURE 5.12

The appearance of a gonococcal eye infection in the newborn. The area indicated by the arrow is swollen and highly inflamed.

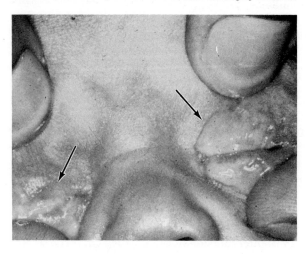

FIGURE 5.13

A microscopic view of the gonococcus (arrow), the causative agent of gonorrhea.

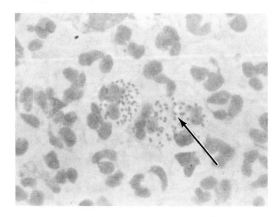

of the inner lining of the eye, known as conjunctivitis (fig. 5.12). Infections of bone and the coverings of the brain are rarer occurrences.

Newborn conjunctivitis usually appears about three to seven days after birth. There is usually a fair amount of pus and both eyes are often involved. Left untreated, permanent eye injury and blindness, referred to as **ophthalmia neonatorum** (of-THAL-mē-a, nē-ō-NA-tor-um) may result. These consequences are preventable if treatment is started within two weeks after birth.

DIAGNOSIS

In males, the diagnosis of gonococcal infection on the basis of signs and symptoms alone can be misleading, and in females it is often difficult, if not impossible. Reliable laboratory culture and appropriate tests are essential for a definitive diagnosis, as well as for situations in which legal actions for rape or divorce proceedings might develop.

A tentative identification of the *gonococcus* can be made using a staining procedure known as **Gram stain** with appropriate material obtained from infection sites, the urethra, cervix, throat, and the

rectum. In a gram-stained preparation, the *gonococcus* has a characteristic coffee-bean shape and appears both inside and outside of white blood cells (fig. 5.13).

A definitive diagnosis of gonococcal infection is achieved by isolation of *gonococci* on appropriate laboratory media and the application of sophisticated biochemical and immunological tests for the purposes of a specific identification **(color photograph 8).**

TREATMENT

As indicated earlier, gonorrhea is a difficult disease to eradicate. Increases in Gc cases caused by antibiotic-resistant gonococci, known as penicillinase-producing *Neisseria gonorrhea* (PPNG) contribute to the severity of the problem. These bacteria produce an enzyme (penicillinase) that is capable of inactivating penicillin.

Penicillin G and ampicillin are still the major antibiotics used in the treatment of gonococcal fection. With increasing gonococcal resistance to penicillin, other antibiotics have become necessary for successful treatment. Ceftriaxone (sef-TRĪ x-ōn), an antibiotic that can be given in small doses, is very effective. In cases of persons with an allergy or sensitivity to penicillin, antibiotics such as tetracycline and erythromycin may be used.

Another factor interfering with treatment effectiveness is the ability of the *gonococci* to persist without symptoms, especially in locations away from the genitalia. Most approaches for the treatment of genital infections have lower cure rates in throat and anorectal gonorrhea. Since many of these extragenital infections coexist with genital disease, an antibiotic capable of curing all infected sites is needed to prevent treatment failure or further Gc transmission. Ceftriaxone has been one antibiotic used effectively in such situations.

PREVENTION

The major preventative measures which can reduce the incidence of gonorrhea include the regular use of barrier devices such as condoms, and if applicable, limiting the number of sexual contacts. An effective vaccine against this STD could also be quite helpful in reducing the number of new gonorrhea cases. However, to date, such preparations are not available.

THE HIGHS AND LOWS OF SYPHILIS AND GONORRHEA

From earliest history until modern days, syphilis and gonorrhea have continued to be a public health problem with consequences occurring in untreated persons as serious as sterility, blindness, and in some cases, death. The incidence of these two STDs has changed in recent years. For example, the number of gonorrhea cases appears to have peaked and is now decreasing. Syphilis cases, on the other hand, have increased slowly from 1950 and 1985, and have virtually exploded in certain well-defined geographical areas and segments of the population since that time. This is especially true for syphilis in women in urban areas and, as a consequence, congenital syphilis. In New York the rate of primary or secondary syphilis in women increased slightly between 1983 and 1986; however, between 1986 and 1988 it increased almost four times. During the same two-year period the number of reported cases of congenital syphilis rose from 57 to 357. In 1989, 950 cases were expected. Similar increases are also occurring in many other urban areas. Factors responsible for this alarming state of affairs include the spread of "crack" cocaine use and prostitution, and a lack of appropriate prenatal care.

Controlling the expanding epidemic of congenital syphilis will require various strategies. These include early treatment of infected mothers, as well as children born to infected mothers, and providing good prenatal care to all pregnant women. Of course, increased public health efforts to reduce the spread of syphilis among adults, as well as increasing and improving the education programs to reduce drug addiction are extremely important. Unfortunately, infected infants are expected to continue to appear either at birth or more likely at several weeks or months after birth.

CHAPTER 6

GENITAL CHLAMYDIAL INFECTIONS AND OTHER LESSER-KNOWN BACTERIAL STDS

Don't give a dose to the one you love most.
Give her some marmalade; give her some toast.
You can give her the willies or give her the blues,
But the dose that you give her will get back to you.

—Shel Silverstein, Don't Give a Dose

Chlamydial (kla-MID-ē-al) infections, like syphilis, some forms of gonorrhea, and other more recently recognized STDs, have dramatically increased as a result of changes in sexual behavior. With an estimated 300 million cases occurring on a worldwide basis, chlamydial infections are among the most prevalent of the sexually transmitted diseases. The risk of being infected by the causative agent ***Chlamydia trachomatis*** (kla-MID-ē-a, tra-KŌ-ma-tis) has increased as a result of the rapid spread of this bacterium throughout the population, placing many sexually active men and women and their offspring in jeopardy.

The importance and features of chlamydial infections will be presented along with several other bacterial diseases that are not well known, but have a significant impact on human reproduction and fertility, and the spread of human immunodeficiency virus. These include **lymphogranuloma venereum** (lim-fō-gran-ū-LŌ-ma, ven'-ēr-Ē-um), **chancroid** (SHANG-kroyd), **nongonococcal urethritis** (non-gon-ō-KOK-al, ū-rē-THRĪ-tis), and **toxic shock syndrome.**

The Chlamydia
Basic Features

As a group the *Chlamydia* includes pathogens that cause a respiratory infection known as parrot fever in various types of birds, and a type of blindness known as **trachoma** (tra-KŌ-ma), pneumonia, and STDs in humans. Chlamydial diseases have been recognized as early as the 19th century B.C. Trachoma, for example, is described in both ancient Chinese and Egyptian writings.

Until the 1950s the *Chlamydia* were considered to be viruses, or virus-like because of their extremely small size, and their need for living cells in order to multiply. With improvements in technology and a better understanding of their properties, the *Chlamydia* are now considered to be bacteria and not viruses. The reasons for this decision include their cellular nature (viruses are not cells), and a susceptibility to antibiotics.

The *Chlamydia* are distinguished from all other types of bacteria on the basis of an unusual life cycle (fig. 6.1), in which they appear in two different forms, *initial bodies* (IBs) which are mainly concerned with increasing the chlamydial population in an infected cell, and *elementary bodies* (EBs) which represent the infectious stage of the cycle. An infection is started by an EB attaching to the surface of a susceptible host cell. Once inside, the pathogen is now protected from the defenses of the host and is free to form IBs which reproduce rapidly and eventually fill the cell.

Within twenty hours after infection the IBs reorganize and develop into infectious EBs, which are released to attack and infect nearby susceptible cells. Each infected cell may contain up to 10,000 *Chlamydia*. A complete turn of the cycle from beginning

Figure 6.1

The chlamydial life cycle. (a) The steps of the cycle. This cycle begins with the attachment of an infectious elementary body to a susceptible cell. Once inside, the elementary body is protected and continues its development. (b) An electron micrograph of a cell containing elementary bodies (EBs), initial bodies (IBs), and an intermediate form (white arrow). The specimen used was obtained from a chlamydial infection of the cervix. (From E. M. C. Dunlop, A. Garner, S. Darougar, J. D. Treharse, and R. M. Woodland, *Genitourinary Medicine* (1989) 65: 22–31.)

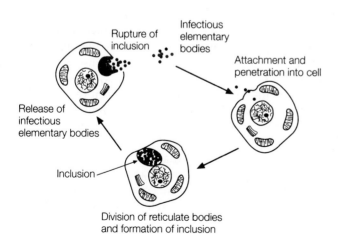

a

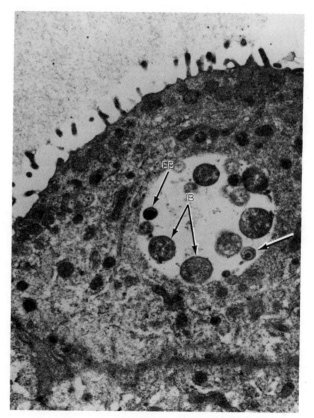

b

TABLE 6.1 | THE RANGE OF BODY PARTS INVOLVED AND TRANSMISSION PATTERNS OF CHLAMYDIA TRACHOMATIS

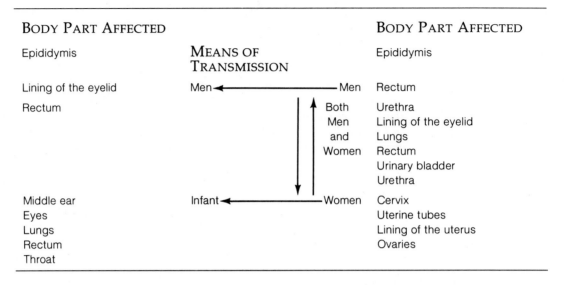

BODY PART AFFECTED	MEANS OF TRANSMISSION	BODY PART AFFECTED
Epididymis		Epididymis
Lining of the eyelid	Men ◄──────── Men	Rectum
Rectum	Both	Urethra
	Men	Lining of the eyelid
	and	Lungs
	Women	Rectum
		Urinary bladder
		Urethra
Middle ear	Infant ◄──────── Women	Cervix
Eyes		Uterine tubes
Lungs		Lining of the uterus
Rectum		Ovaries
Throat		

to end takes thirty-five to forty-eight hours. Only EBs are adapted to survive outside of host cells. Thus, they can continue to attack other cells in the same infected individual or be spread to new hosts.

CHLAMYDIA TRACHOMATIS INFECTIONS

TRANSMISSION

Chlamydia trachomatis is now well established as a significant cause of an increasing variety of major genital infections. Table 6.1 shows the broad range of infections also referred to as the *clinical spectrum* of this bacterium. It is quite obvious that not only are different age groups affected, but depending on the means of transmission different body organs are involved as well. Chlamydial infections pose a most serious health threat, especially when one considers the fact that over 3 million new cases occur per year in the United States. Moreover, many of these infections lead to infertility in more than 20,000 adolescents on a yearly basis.

Two major means of transmission are recognized for *C. trachomatis*. These are sexual and congenital. As shown in table 6.1 the pathogen can be transferred between partners and can be spread to infants born to infected mothers.

EPIDEMIOLOGY NOTES

The number of infections resulting from sexually transmitted *C. trachomatis* is difficult to determine accurately, since such cases are not reportable. Nevertheless, in the United States various studies have shown the yearly incidence of chlamydial infections to exceed those of syphilis, gonorrhea, and genital herpes combined. In many situations individuals are found to have one or more STDs in addition to a chlamydial infection. Sometimes distinguishing such infections from one another can pose problems. For example, the signs and symptoms of many chlamydial infections closely resemble those associated with gonorrhea.

Based on the isolations of *Chlamydia*, infection appears to be highest among heterosexual blacks, lower socioeconomic groups, women who have not given birth, individuals who become sexually active at relatively younger ages, and persons having a history of multiple sex partners. Explanations as to why such infections occur include the presence of asymptomatic infections, a lack of information about chlamydial infections, and avoiding the use of safer sex practices. Selected features of *Chlamydia trachomatis* infections are summarized in the accompanying **STD FACT FILE.**

SIGNS AND SYMPTOMS

This section presents only representative common infections of men, women, and newborns up to six weeks of age (**neonates**). A separate section follows describing the features of **lymphogranuloma venereum,** an STD caused by a different form of *C. trachomatis.*

It is important to note that many of the genital infections caused by *C. trachomatis* are mild, or develop without any noticeable symptoms. Unfortunately, this is especially true of chlamydial infections in women. Chlamydial infections may be discovered during a physical examination. Quite often, the first indication of a genital infection is when a sexual partner or newborn baby are found to have an inflamed eyelid known as *conjunctivitis* (kon-junk'-ti-V$\bar{I}$-tis) or another type of complication (color photograph 9). Adults acquire such problems by introducing infectious genital tract discharges into the eye either during sexual activity, or at other times by hand to eye contact. Newborns get infections by passing through an infected birth canal.

A 16-year-old female came to the emergency medicine department with a complaint of severe and sharp pain on the right side of her abdomen. The pain was continual and had started three days earlier. It increased with deep breathing, sitting up, and walking. The young patient did not have any nausea, diarrhea, pain while urinating, or vaginal discharge. Her last menstrual period began six days before her appearance at the emergency department. The patient was sexually active and used condoms. Her medical history included an episode of gonorrhea about one year earlier. The infection was treated with one dose of the antibiotic ampicillin. The patient's sex partner was also treated at that time.

The results of a physical examination revealed a marked tenderness of the upper right side of the patient's abdomen when slight pressure was applied. Her pelvic examination disclosed a normal cervix and no abnormal vaginal discharge. No unusual growths were felt on bimanual examination. (This procedure is explained in chapter 3.)

Laboratory findings included the finding of *Chlamydia* in specimens from the patient's cervix. An appropriate antibiotic was prescribed for the young patient. She was unavailable for a follow-up examination.

Various studies in recent years have shown chlamydial throat infections in both women and men practicing orogenital sex. Most such cases also are without symptoms.

Infections of Women. Although men, women, and infants all are affected in cases of genital chlamydial infection, women in particular bear a more serious burden because of the increased risk of complications. It is estimated that up to 77 percent of chlamydial infections in women are asymptomatic. These undetected and untreated cases are associated with the particular risk of upper genital tract infections such as Pelvic Inflammatory Diseases (PID). (See chapter 4 for a description of PID.)

Since *C. trachomatis* is one of the most common pathogens isolated from the cervix, it is not surprising that cervicitis is the primary infection in women (color photograph 10). While many infected women have no signs or symptoms of infection, at least one-third have signs indicating an infection. The first of these is a thick discharge consisting of mucus and pus. Other features of chlamydial cervicitis are given in the accompanying **SIGNS &** **SYMPTOMS BOX.** In most pregnant women the infection is asymptomatic and remains undetected unless tests are included in their prenatal care period.

In addition to pelvic inflammatory disease a number of other, quite harmful, complications can result from chlamydial cervicitis. These include infertility resulting from infection and damage to the uterine tubes, abnormal pregnancy, and inflammation involving the liver.

Infections of Men. *C. trachomatis* is known to cause several different infections in men. These include inflamation of the urethra of *nongonococcal urethritis* (NGU), a complication of chlamydial infections, an inflammation of the epididymis, or epididymitis (ep-i-did-i-MĪ-tis), and an inflammation of the rectum and anus known as *proctitis* (prok-TĪ-tis). A number of STD agents and other pathogens can cause infections of the rectum and anus. Infected persons experience rectal pain and an abnormal discharge or bleeding. Attention here will be given only to NGU (color photograph 10).

<table>
<tr><td rowspan="3">

**THE SIGNS
AND
SYMPTOMS
BOX**

</td><td>

DISEASE
CHLAMYDIAL CERVICITIS
(ser-vi-SĪ-tis)
INCUBATION PERIOD
7–21 DAYS

</td></tr>
</table>

First Symptoms Usually Appear: Variable, but May Appear Within 7-14 Days

Signs
1. Thick, mucus-pus (mucopurulent) discharge

Symptoms
1. Soreness in pelvic area
2. Lower back pain
3. Lower abdominal pain
4. Accompanying symptoms due to associated urethritis include:
   a. burning sensation on urinating
   b. slight fever
   c. frequent need to urinate

Complications
1. Inflammation of uterine tubes known as salpingitis (sal'-pin-JĪ-tis)
2. Infertility
3. Inflammation of the urethra, or urethritis (u-rē-THRĪ-tis)
4. Uterine bleeding
5. Inflammation of internal lining of the uterus, or endometritis (en'-dō-mē-TRĪ-tis)
6. Pregnancy complications
7. Infection of newborn
8. Inflammation involving the liver

<table>
<tr><td rowspan="3">

**THE SIGNS
AND
SYMPTOMS
BOX**

</td><td>

DISEASE
NONGONOCOCCAL
URETHRITIS (ū-rē-THRĪ-tis)
INCUBATION PERIOD
1 to 3 WEEKS

</td></tr>
</table>

First Symptoms Usually Appear: Variable, but Usually 10–21 Days

Signs
A thick discharge (usually present in the morning)

Symptoms
1. Pain or burning sensation while urinating
2. Frequent need to urinate
3. At least 25 percent of infected persons are without symptoms

Complications
1. Infection of the epididymis
2. Infertility

NGU is most frequently caused by *C. trachomatis*. The bacterium *Ureaplasma urealyticum* (ū-rē-a-PLAZ-ma, ū-rē-a-LĪT-i-kum) is another cause of NGU. This disease agent is frequently isolated from the genital tracts of both men and women. Since more than half of the men with NGU are without symptoms, or experience only a mild discomfort, medical care often is not sought. The most common symptom is the presence of a thick pus-like discharge that develops about three weeks after contact with an infected person. Left untreated, NGU may lead to an inflammation of the epididymis and sterility. A summary of the features of NGU is given in the accompanying **SIGNS & SYMPTOMS BOX.** Arthritis, an inflammation of the joints, is a common aftereffect of sexually acquired NGU. It typically develops one to four weeks after the initial infection.

Chlamydial Infections Involving the Newborn. Since *C. trachomatis* is an STD agent found in the cervix, it may be transmitted to an infant passing through the birth canal at the time of delivery. Such neonatal (nē-ō-NAT-al) infections may appear as an inflammation of the inner lining of the eyelids, or **ophthalmia neonatorum** (of-'THAL-mē-a, nē'-ō-NĀ-tor-um), pneumonia, and middle ear infections. Several studies indicate that 18 to 44 percent of infants born to infected women are likely to develop an eye infection, and 11 to 20 percent are likely to

THE SIGNS AND SYMPTOMS BOX	DISEASE OPHTHALMIA NEONATORUM (of-THAL-mē-a, nē'ō-NA-to-rum) INCUBATION PERIOD 3–9 DAYS AFTER BIRTH

First Symptoms Usually Appear: Within 3–9 Days After Birth

Signs
1. Increased redness of the inner linings of eyelids
2. Swollen eyelids due to the accumulation of excess fluid
3. Possible pus-like discharge from the involved eyes

Symptoms
Fever

Complications
1. Scarring of the inner eyelid surfaces
2. Blindness (rare)

develop pneumonia. The accompanying **SIGNS & SYMPTOMS BOX** presents the features of the neonatal infection mentioned earlier.

DIAGNOSIS

Diagnosis of chlamydial infections require properly taken specimens. Once specimens are available several different methods can be used for diagnosis. These include culture and isolation methods using tissue cultures, specifically sensitive microscopic staining techniques to show the presence of elementary bodies, and blood tests to demonstrate the presence of antibodies against *Chlamydia*.

TREATMENT

In general, once a diagnosis is made antibiotics such as the tetracyclines are used. If treatment is not successful, other options are available. With newborn infections, the antibiotic erythromycin (e-rith'-rō-MĪ-sin) is generally used.

PREVENTION AND MANAGEMENT

Prevention of sexually transmitted chlamydial infections may be achieved with the appropriate use of barrier devices such as condoms during sexual activity. In addition, since the human is the only source of the disease agent, infected persons should be treated and followed with medical visits both during and after the course of treatment. Table 6.2 lists a number of situations which require the testing of individuals for chlamydial infections.

In recent years a particular concern has been raised by the reports of high rates of asymptomatic infections among adolescent women. If such infections are not diagnosed and treated when the disease agent is confined to the lower genital tract, many young women will run the risk of complete or partial blockage of their uterine tubes. Periodic medical examinations could reduce the risk.

THE LESSER-KNOWN BACTERIAL STDS

The list of bacterial STDs has expanded beyond the limits of the original venereal diseases such as syphilis and gonorrhea. Actually most of the newer infections have been around for some time, but have been largely overlooked because of a lack of awareness of their signs and symptoms and of diagnostic tools. With improvements in detection and the dramatic increases in the number of STDs the situation has changed. Here are some examples of the not too well-known bacterial STDs.

LYMPHOGRANULOMA VENEREUM

Although it is quite likely that lymphogranuloma venereum, or **LGV,** has been known since ancient times, it was not until 1913 that it was clearly recognized as a separate venereal disease. Throughout most of its history LGV has been confused with other STDs, particularly syphilis, genital herpes, and chancroid. The introduction in 1925 of a diagnostic

TABLE 6.2 | INDIVIDUALS WHO SHOULD BE TESTED FOR CHLAMYDIA TRACHOMATIS

BOTH MEN AND WOMEN

Individuals with an STD

Individuals who have had a recent change of sex partner

Individuals with several sex partners

Individuals having problems with their reproductive and/or urinary systems

Individuals with inflamed eyelids that do not improve with treatment for chlamydial infections

MEN

Semen donor

Individuals with proctitis

WOMEN

Pregnant women with casual sex partners

Rape or sexually abused victims

Women undergoing termination of pregnancy

INFANTS

Newborns and older individual with eye infections

Newborns with pneumonia

Sexually abused victims

---

procedure known as the **Frei** (frī) skin test provided a tool with which to distinguish LGV from other diseases.

CAUSE AND TRANSMISSION

LGV is caused by specific forms or strains of *Chlamydia trachomatis*. These strains are different from those that cause trachoma and the more common forms of chlamydial STDs described earlier in this chapter. As with other chlamydial infections, LGV is almost exclusively spread through sexual contact. However, as the Signs & Symptoms section shows, the infection may involve other body sites in addition to the genitalia.

EPIDEMIOLOGY NOTES

LGV probably has a worldwide distribution. Unfortunately, accurate information as to its prevalence and incidence is not readily available. LGV is underreported and misdiagnosed because of difficulties in diagnosis linked to a general lack of awareness of the signs and symptoms of the STD. The disease appears to be more common in tropical parts of the world such as Southeast Asia, Africa, South America, and the West Indies. In the United States LGV predominately is found among African–American persons with a low economic status. This STD is also being recognized more frequently among men practicing anorectal sex. Some general features of LGV infection are given in the accompanying **STD FACT FILE**.

STD FACT FILE	**DISEASE** LYMPHOGRANULOMA VENEREUM, (lim-fō-gran-ū-LŌ-ma, ven-er-Ē-um) **CAUSE** THE BACTERIUM, CHLAMYDIA TRACHOMATIS (kla-MID-ē-ah, tra-kō-MA-tis)

Source/Transmission

Infected humans; sexual intercourse.

Epidemiology

LGV is sporadic throughout Europe, North America, Australia, and most of Asia and South America; highly common in parts of Africa, Asia, and South America. This disease may be confused with syphilis, genital herpes, and chancroid. LGV is becoming a significant infection among homosexuals where it causes an inflamed condition of the large intestine and rectum.

Control

1. Screening populations at risk and treating infected persons
2. Tracing, contacting, and treating sexual partners of those infected
3. Follow-up of infected persons after treatment

Prevention

1. Use of barrier devices such as condoms for the prevention and control of the disease's spread.

SIGNS AND SYMPTOMS

LGV has an extremely variable incubation period, ranging from three to thirty days. This range often reflects the time between the last sexual contact and the involvement of an individual's lymph nodes. The most frequent sign of LGV infection, and the main reason an infected person seeks medical attention is the increasing number of swollen lymph nodes, known as **buboes** (BOO-bows), in the groin (fig. 6.2a). Such buboes usually develop two to six weeks after infection, and because of anatomical differences are found more commonly in men than in women.

For the sake of convenience, the course of untreated LGV may be divided into three stages, the *primary stage, secondary stage,* and *tertiary stage.*

In the primary stage, the first sign lasts for only a short time and usually is painless. It may take the form of a small red spot or a shallow sore. Such primary lesions also may be found on the fingers, tongue, or around the rectum and anus. The location of lesions reflects the type of exposure and the first site of infection.

The secondary stage is marked by noticeable, enlarged, hard, and painless lymph nodes (buboes) on one side of the groin. This condition generally develops within one to three weeks after the first signs of the infection disappear. As this stage continues, the lymph nodes on both sides of the groin may become involved and give rise to a diagnostic physical feature known as the "groove sign" (fig. 6.2b). In some cases these enlarged lymph nodes may get smaller in size, break, and develop into pus-draining sores. Fever, chills, headaches, and muscular aches are typical symptoms found with this stage of LGV infection.

The tertiary stage includes a variety of serious and destructive effects resulting from the spreading of the infection (fig. 6.3 and color photograph 11). Many of these effects may be disabling as well as disfiguring, and include a narrowing of the rectum,

FIGURE 6.2

Some signs of LGV. (a) The appearance of early signs of infection including a bubo and inflamed lymph vessels (arrow) of the penis. (b) The appearance of the "groove sign," a diagnostic feature of LGV that occurs in some infected persons. (Courtesy of Centers for Disease Control)

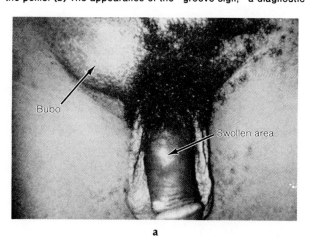

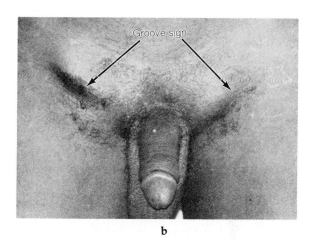

a

b

FIGURE 6.3

The destructive lesions found in lymphogranuloma venereum (LGV). (From B. Alacuque, H. Cloppet, C. Dumontel, and G. Moulin, *British Journal of Venereal Disease* (1984) 60:390–395.)

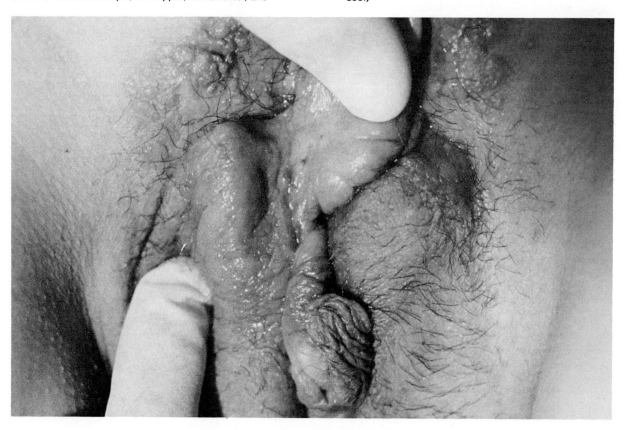

THE SIGNS AND SYMPTOMS BOX	DISEASE LYMPHOGRANULOMA VENEREUM (LGV) INCUBATION PERIOD 3–30 DAYS

First Symptoms Usually Appear: After 30 Days

Primary Stage

Signs	Symptoms
Men 1. Appearance of small, red pimples, shallow sores, or blisters on the penis, scrotum, fingers, or tongue 2. Inflammation of urethra 3. Extreme swelling of the penis so that foreskin cannot be pushed back (this is caused by an inflammation of lymph vessels)	No noticeable symptoms
Women 1. Appearance of small, red pimples, shallow sores, or blisters on the vaginal opening, fingers, or tongue 2. Inflammation of urethra and of the cervix	No noticeable symptoms

Secondary Stage

Signs	Symptoms
Both Men and Women 1. Painful and swollen lymph nodes (buboes) in the groin (inguinale area) 2. Limping caused by swollen and painful buboes 3. Buboes turn blue within 1–2 weeks 4. Rupture of buboes with the release of thick, yellow pus (may last for several weeks) 5. Appearance of swollen areas in other body areas	1. Pain in groin 2. Fever 3. Headache 4. General discomfort 5. Loss of appetite 6. Pain in abdomen and lower back (in women)

Tertiary Stage

Signs	Symptoms
Men	
1. Narrowing of the rectum	Similar to those listed in secondary stage
2. Swelling of the groin and legs caused by blockage of lymph vessels	
Women	
1. Narrowing of the rectum	Similar to those listed for the secondary stage
2. Development of tubelike connections, to the rectum known as fistulas (FIS-tū-las)	
3. Long-lasting, swollen, reddened sores involving the vulva and vagina	
4. Destruction of the urethra	

Complications

General

Painful joints, pneumonia, inflammation of the liver, and heart involvement

Men

1. Inflammation of the large intestine and anus
2. Severe swelling of groin and legs known as elephantiasis (el'-e-fan-TĪ-a-sis).

Women

1. Possible vulvar cancer
2. Elephantiasis

A CASE OF LGV

A 22-year-old woman was admitted to the hospital in May for an examination and treatment of wartlike growths on her external genitalia and in the area around the anus. These particular lesions developed two years earlier. According to the woman she had not travelled outside of Europe, and had not engaged in extramarital sexual activities.

The patient's condition started during the second month of her first pregnancy. Three or four painful pus-filled pimples appeared on the external surfaces of the labia majora. No other noticeable effects were present. Because these lesions increased in number and spread to the entire vulva area, the woman's baby had to be delivered by a cesarean (se-SAR-ē-an) operation. The newborn infant was normal and showed no signs or symptoms of infection.

Shortly after the birth, the woman's lesions enlarged, became wartlike, and spread to the area around the anus. No urinary or other symptoms were noted. However, the woman complained of pain during sexual intercourse.

A physical examination showed the presence of large wartlike growths with deep sores, and smaller red pimples covering both the healthy skin, as well as the wartlike growths (fig. 6.4). The opening to the vagina, the vagina itself, and the labia minora were not affected, although they appeared slightly swollen.

Laboratory tests showed the presence of a *Chlamydia trachomatis* strain, known to cause *lymphogranuloma venereum*. Treatment of the infection was carried out with various antibiotics. While the treatment corrected the pain experienced during sexual activities, little improvement occurred with the wartlike growths.

---

the formation of abnormal passages or tunnels between the rectum and vulva, deep sores, and severe swelling of the genitalia resulting in the condition known as **elephantiasis** (el'-e-fan-TĪ-a-sis). A general summary of LGV infection is given in the accompanying **SIGNS & SYMPTOMS BOX.** A distinction also is made between the infection as it occurs in men and women (color photographs 12 and 13).

DIAGNOSIS

Diagnosing LGV on the basis of the physical features of the disease alone is difficult because of similarities to other STDs and even certain cancers. Thus, laboratory tests serve as the major reliable means for diagnosis. A number of modern enzyme tests, microscopic staining techniques, and culture procedures are in use. Specific tests to demonstrate antibodies to the causative agent are also available.

TREATMENT

Infected individuals are treated with antibiotics such as the tetracyclines. Advanced forms of LGV may require surgery to lessen the effects of the infection or to correct any deformities resulting from the disease.

PREVENTION AND CONTROL

The use of barrier devices, such as the condom, during sexual activities may help to prevent infection. In addition, a greater awareness of LGV and early screening of individuals at risk for infection followed by adequate treatment should contribute to preventing and controlling the spread of LGV as well as the severe forms of the infection.

FIGURE 6.4

Lymphogranuloma venereum involving the vulva. Note the many large wartlike lesions (arrows). Smaller lesions and red pimples are present around the anus and neighboring areas. (Courtesy of Professor G. Moulin, Hospital de L'Antiquaille, Lyon, France)

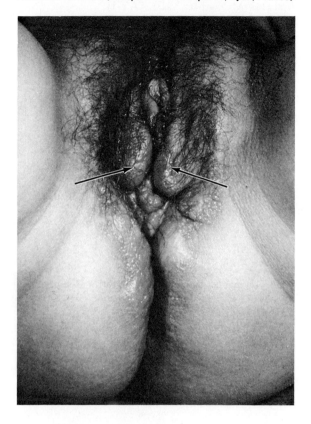

CHANCROID

Chancroid or **soft chancre** (SHANG-ker) has been recognized as a disease for centuries. It was, and often still is, confused with other STDs including syphilis. In 1852, P. Bassereau clearly showed chancroid to be different from syphilis, and seven years later A. Ducrey identified the causative agent which still bears his name.

CAUSE AND TRANSMISSION

Chancroid is a sexually transmitted infection caused by the bacterium *Haemophilus ducreyi* (hē-MOF-il-us, dū-KRĀY-i). In most reports, men have a much higher incidence of this disease than women. Moreover, chancroid is more commonly found in uncircumcised men. Several features of this STD are given in the accompanying **STD FACT FILE.**

EPIDEMIOLOGY NOTES

Chancroid is found worldwide, but appears to be most common in tropical and subtropical countries. In some third world societies, this STD ranges between endemic to epidemic levels. Endemic chancroid, whether found in these areas or Western countries, is commonly associated with prostitutes. Prostitution appears to be the source for ongoing infections in men. Historically, sailors acquired chancroid in seaports, and usually from prostitutes. Today, chancroid continues to occur sporadically among individuals who have travelled to endemic areas. In addition, this STD is believed to be an infection of individuals with relatively low standards of cleanliness.

Infections mixed with other STDs are possible with chancroid. Syphilis, genital herpes, and HIV infection are likely candidates.

SIGNS AND SYMPTOMS

The incubation period for chancroid in males varies from one to fourteen days following sexual contact. In females, this period is somewhat longer for reasons that are not clear. Typical lesions or chancroidal sores first appear at the sites of sexual contact. These lesions, which begin as small red pimples, develop into sores or ulcers within twenty-four hours. Classic chancroidal ulcers, which occur in the majority of men (fig. 6.5a), generally are painful, irregular in shape, soft, and sharply outlined (color photograph 7). A foul odor occurs with some infections.

The most common locations for such lesions in males include the internal surface of the foreskin, glans, penis, and shaft of the penis. The scrotum, anus, and thighs also may be involved. In women, lesions develop on the labia, clitoris, vestibule, and anus (fig. 6.5b). While extragenital ulcers are rare, they can occur on fingers, breasts, lips, the tongue, and more recently the ankle.

DISEASE
CHANCROID (SHANG-kroyd), OR SOFT CHANCRE (SHANG-ker)
CAUSE
THE BACTERIUM HAEMOPHILUS DUCREYI (Hē-MOF-il-us, dū-KRĀY-i)

Source/Transmission
Infected humans; sexual activities

Epidemiology
The disease is found worldwide, but occurs more commonly in tropical and subtropical areas. More men than women are infected. Prostitution appears to play a major role in disease transmission. Chancroid is more commonly found in uncircumcised men.

Control
1. Treatment of infected individuals and all sexual contacts
2. Counseling of infected individuals as to methods of prevention

Prevention
The use of barrier devices such as condoms during sexual activities.

FIGURE 6.5

Features of chancroid. (a) Chancroid (genital) ulcers can be seen on the prepuce of this male (A). In addition, a swollen bubo (B) about to break open can be seen on the thigh. (b) Chancroid infection of the female genitalia showing ulcers of the labia minora (A), and near the middle of the left thigh. Additional sites of infection can be seen at points C and D. (From G. W. Hammon, M. Slutchuk, J. Scatliff, E. Sherman, J. C. Wilt, and A. R. Ronald, *Reviews of Infectious Diseases* (1980) 2:867.)

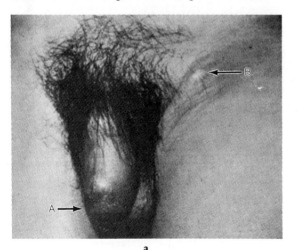

a

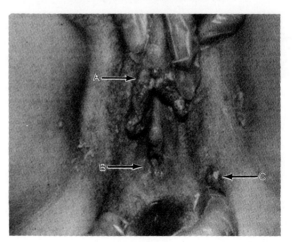

b

<table>
<tr><td rowspan="4">THE SIGNS AND SYMPTOMS BOX</td><td>DISEASE
CHANCROID</td></tr>
<tr><td>INCUBATION PERIOD
1–5 DAYS</td></tr>
</table>

First Symptoms Usually Appear: Within 1 Week After Exposure

Signs	Symptoms
Men	
1. Reddened areas in the groin	Pain and tenderness in the groin
2. Formation of one or more irregularly shaped and painful genital sores (ulcers)	
3. Sores in and around the anus	
4. Foul smelling, pus-like discharge oozing from the ulcers	
5. Swollen areas in the groin may break open and release foul smelling pus-like discharge	

Women
The signs and symptoms are similar to those described for men.

Complications
Relapses.

Within one week after an ulcer forms, the lymph nodes in the groin generally become swollen in 40 percent of men, and 25 percent of women. If left untreated, these lesions develop into deep, pus-producing sores. A general summary of chancroid is presented in the accompanying **SIGNS & SYMPTOMS BOX.**

DIAGNOSIS

The finding of genital sores during a physical examination is not sufficient for diagnosis. The isolation and identification of the causative bacterium from specimens by laboratory methods provide the basis for an accurate diagnosis.

TREATMENT

The use of appropriate antibiotics such as the tetracyclines is effective for the treatment of chancroid cases. Usually such treatment is completed within ten days. With treatment ulcers heal quickly, but often leave deep scars.

PREVENTION AND CONTROL

As is the case with several other STDs, the use of barrier devices such as the condom during sexual activities can reduce the spread of chancroid. Control of this STD can also be helped by the treatment of sexual contacts of men with genital ulcers, as well as prostitutes showing the signs and symptoms of the infection.

A MODERN-DAY CASE OF CHANCROID

A twenty-eight-year-old male was seen at the dermatology clinic of a modern health center because of painful sores on his penis and scrotum. Apparently he had had the sores and a large lump over his right groin area for two weeks. The large lump also produced a pus-like discharge. The patient admitted to having had sexual relations with a prostitute about one week before his problems began.

Physical examination showed the presence of several deep sores (ulcers) covered by a pus-like discharge at the base of his penis. A highly reddened mass, measuring about a half-an-inch was also found in his right groin. Specimens were taken from these areas and sent to the laboratory for diagnosis.

Laboratory findings revealed the presence of the bacterial agent of chancroid. The patient was treated with the antibiotic erythromycin. After seven days, the patient's condition improved dramatically, and after two weeks' time the sores and mass completely disappeared.

GRANULOMA INGUINALE

Granuloma inguinale (gran′ū-LŌ-ma, IN-gwi-nal-ē) is a long-lasting sexually transmitted disease. This infection, also known as **Donovanosis** (don-ō-VA-nō-sis) was first described in 1882 by K. Mcleod. It may be confused with other STDs such as lymphogranuloma venereum and genital warts, as well as nonsexually transmitted diseases or conditions such as penile cancers, and the side effects of certain drugs. The confusion comes from the genital growths and tumors that develop during the course of a granuloma inguinale infection.

CAUSE AND TRANSMISSION

Granuloma inguinale is believed to result from an infection with the bacterium *Calymmatobacterium granulomatis* (ka-lim′-ma-tō-bak-TĒ-rē-um, gran-ū-LŌ-ma-tis). Sexual contact is considered to be the means of disease transmission.

EPIDEMIOLOGY NOTES

Granuloma inguinale is found mainly, but not exclusively, in tropical and semitropical areas of the world. It is endemic in various parts of Africa, southeast Asia, southern India, and New Guinea. Sporadic outbreaks of this STD have occurred in southern and southeastern states of the United States. Infection occurs more frequently with men than with women. Low socioeconomic status, lack of personal hygiene, poor educational standards, and many sexual partners are factors contributing to the occurrence of this STD. Selected features of granuloma inguinale are given in the accompanying **STD FACT FILE**.

SIGNS AND SYMPTOMS

While the incubation period is not known exactly, it generally ranges from a few days to four or five months. In most cases of infection, the main lesion, a firm red pimple or papule (PAP-ūl), develops on the genitalia. Additional papules soon occur, eventually break open, and become sores of varying sizes and appearances (color photograph 14). While many such ulcers are painless, others are tender, bleed on touch, and cause disfiguring and even destruction of the genitalia (fig. 6.6). In men, for example, if left untreated, the infection may destroy the entire penis. Long-lasting infections in women may result in severe swelling of and the forming of growths on the external genitalia.

Other body sites may become involved. For example, infection of the perianal area can follow anal intercourse. In addition, the infection may spread to

DISEASE

GRANULOMA INGUINALE (gran'-ū-LŌ-ma, IN-gwi-nal-ē) OR DONOVANOSIS (don-ō-van-Ō-sis)

CAUSE

THE BACTERIUM, CALYMMATOBACTERIUM GRANULOMATIS (ka-lim'-ma-tō-bak-TĒ-rē-um, gran-ū-LŌ-ma-tis)

Source/Transmission

Infected humans; sexual contact, nonsexual transmission may be possible. The perianal area be affected following anal intercourse.

Epidemiology

The disease is found worldwide, generally in tropical areas.

Poor hygiene, educational standards and low socioeconomic status favor its occurrence and transmission. More males than females have the disease, and generally individuals in their 20s or 30s become infected.

Control

Treatment of infected persons with appropriate antibiotics such as tetracyclines

Prevention

1. Use of barrier devices such as condoms to prevent the spread of the disease
2. Use of education programs to inform individuals about the disease, and its prevention.

FIGURE 6.6

Features of granuloma inguinale. An inguinal bubo and developing sore (arrow) are shown. A site of infection also can be seen on the penis. (Courtesy of Centers for Disease Control)

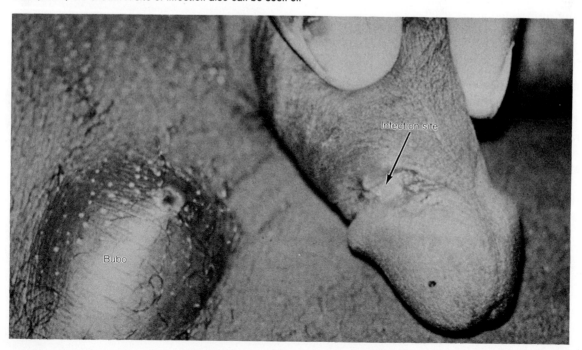

DISEASE
GRANULOMA INGUINALE (gran'-ū-LŌ-ma, IN-gwi-nal-ē), DONOVANOSIS (don-ō-VAN-Ō-sis)
INCUBATION PERIOD
VARIES, BUT GENERALLY EXTENDS FROM 2 WEEKS TO SEVERAL MONTHS

First Symptoms Usually Appear: Several Weeks After Contact With an Infected Person

Signs
1. Single or many painless sores, having beefy, red, coarse bases
2. Strong sour odor associated with sores
3. Sores spreading to other body parts such as the throat, eyelids, and chest
4. Scarring of sores

Symptoms
Some discomfort in the genital area

Complications

Men
1. Possible cause of genital cancers, primarily involving the penis and/or scrotum
2. Destruction of the penile shaft
3. Narrowing of urethral and anal openings
4. Scarring of infected areas
5. Swelling of involved areas producing an elephantiasis-like condition
6. Infection may involve bones and joints resulting in arthritis

Women
1. Narrowing of the vaginal areas
2. Scarring of infected areas
3. Involvement of uterine tubes
4. Swelling of involved areas producing an elephantiasis-like condition
5. Infection may involve bones and joints resulting in arthritis

the mouth, throat, chest, and large intestine. A summary of a granuloma inguinale infection is given in the accompanying **SIGNS & SYMPTOMS BOX.**

Complications also develop in untreated cases of this STD. In men, the most important of these conditions include possible destruction of the penile shaft and the development of a form of cancer involving the penis. In women, blockage and closure, or scarring of the uterus, uterine tubes, and ovaries may develop as complications.

DIAGNOSIS

The diagnosis of granuloma inguinale depends on both the finding of the characteristic genital lesions, and demonstrating the causative agent in specimens taken from the infected person. In the laboratory the infection is confirmed by showing the presence of Donovan (don-Ō-van) bodies. These are large, nucleated cells containing the causative bacteria.

TREATMENT

Granuloma inguinale has been a difficult infection to treat for many years. Until the early part of this century, surgery was used to remove infected tissue. Chemicals of various types, were also in use and were effective for treating the early stages. Today, treatment usually takes two to four weeks and involves the use of antibiotics such as ampicillin or the tetracyclines.

BACTERIAL VAGINOSIS

Vaginal infection can be caused by microorganisms that increase their numbers when the microbial population normally present in the vagina is thrown out of balance by some type of predisposing condition. Such conditions, which include pregnancy, menstruation, and the use of oral contraceptives, change the acid level and sugar concentration in the vagina. Several microorganisms are able to take advantage of the situation and establish an infection. One of these, the bacterium *Gardnerella vaginalis* (GARD-ner-el-la, VAJ-in-a-lis) interacts with other bacterium to cause *bacterial vaginosis* (BV). Thus, unlike other STDs, BV is not caused by a single infectious agent.

CAUSE AND TRANSMISSION

Gardnerella vaginalis currently is involved with about 50 percent of vaginosis cases. Although the exact role of this bacterium in infections is not known, it can be spread by sexual intercourse. Men occasionally get an infection of the penis after sexual contact with a woman who has vaginosis. The disease agent can be spread to newborns passing through an infected birth canal. Selected features of bacterial vaginosis are given in the accompanying **STD FACT FILE.**

SIGNS AND SYMPTOMS

The major complaint expressed by infected women is the presence of a foul-smelling, or fishy, vaginal odor. This odor may increase after sexual intercourse or menstruation. Infected men also may have discharge. A summary of the infection is given in the accompanying **SIGNS & SYMPTOMS BOX.**

DIAGNOSIS

The diagnosis of bacterial vaginosis caused by *G. vaginalis* is made on the physical finding of a foul-smelling, or fishy discharge and the microscopic examination of a vaginal discharge in the laboratory. When the chemical known as potassium hydroxide is added to vaginal secretions a distinct and intense fishy odor is produced. This so-called "sniff-test" is fairly conclusive for a diagnosis. Microscopic examination of specimens showing the surfaces of vaginal cells overrun by *G. vaginalis* also is used to confirm the diagnosis. These characteristic cells are known as **clue cells** (fig. 6.7).

TREATMENT AND PREVENTION

A variety of medications are available for treatment of infected individuals and their sex partners. Currently **metronidazole** (me-TRON-i-da-zol) is commonly prescribed. This drug eliminates the bacteria

FIGURE 6.7

A special microscopic technique is used here to show the difference between a normal cell (b) removed from the vagina and a clue cell (a). (From A. Blackwell and D. Barlow, *British Journal of Venereal Diseases* (1982) 58:387–393.)

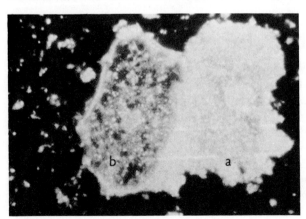

DISEASE
TOXIC SHOCK SYNDROME (TSS)
CAUSE
THE POISON KNOWN AS TOXIC SHOCK SYNDROME TOXIN 1 (TSST–1) FORMED BY
THE BACTERIUM STAPHYLOCOCCUS AUREUS.

Source/Transmission
Tampons and other materials contaminated with toxin-producing *S. aureus*. May be sexually transmitted by women with the condition.

Epidemiology
This disease has been found most frequently in menstruating women who use tampons. TSS also occurs in men, children, and nonmenstruating women, usually by exposure to the causative agent.

Control
1. Successful treatment and control involves the early recognition of TSS, and may require the removal of a tampon, draining the infected site, or surgical removal of damaged tissue.
2. Antibiotics may also be used.

Prevention
Education programs emphasizing the cause and prevention of TSS

that interact with *Gardnerella,* and allows the normal microbial population to repopulate the vagina. The use of barrier devices such as condoms during sexual intercourse may control the spread of the disease agent to others.

TOXIC SHOCK SYNDROME
CAUSE AND TRANSMISSION

Reports of a relatively new disease, closely associated with women during menstruation, began to appear in the late 1970s. In several cases of the illness the bacterium *Staphylococcus aureus* (staf'-il-ō-KOK-us, or-Ē-us) was isolated from specimens taken from the throat, vagina, or other localized sites of infection. Later investigations showed the production of a poison, or **toxin,** produced by this bacterium, caused the condition, which eventually became known as **toxic shock syndrome (TSS).** In 1980, a dramatic increase in the number of TSS cases was reported in the United States. The suddenness with which the disease struck, its tendency to single

out young women who had been previously healthy, and its severity (often with a fatal outcome) brought TSS forcefully to the public's attention. Various reports of the disease clearly linked the use of a new super-absorbent tampon with the disease. Tampons are rolls of material that are inserted into the vagina to absorb the flow of blood during menstruation. In the case of TSS, however, tampons were left in longer than usual, and caused small tears in vaginal surfaces that provided the right conditions for bacteria to grow and multiply. In recent years manufacturers have dramatically lowered the absorbency and changed the chemical composition of the tampons they sell. As a result, the tampons that are available and being used today are quite different from those used in the early 1980s.

Although infrequent changing of super absorbent tampons accounts for most TSS cases, contraceptive sponges and diaphragms also are now known to cause and increase the risk for nonmenstrual forms of the disease. Men, women, and children may acquire TSS by other means, including infections and the exposure to, or the use of materials harboring toxin-producing *S. aureus*. Some cases of TSS-causing bacteria have been sexually transmitted. Selected features of TSS are given in the accompanying **STD FACT FILE.**

SIGNS AND SYMPTOMS

A fever and a rash are the earliest signs of TSS. The fever may range between 103° to 105° F, and the rash which consists of flat, red spots, may resemble a mild sunburn. Other features of this illness are given in the accompanying **SIGNS & SYMPTOMS BOX.**

DIAGNOSIS AND TREATMENT

Diagnosis of TSS is generally based on the findings of a physical examination, and the laboratory isolation and identification of *S. aureus* from blood and urine specimens.

Successful treatment of TSS involves early recognition of the illness, and may require the removal of a contaminated tampon, draining the infected site of infection, or surgical removal of any damaged tissue. Appropriate antibiotics also may be used.

PREVENTION AND CONTROL

Women should use tampons as directed by the manufacturers of the product. In addition, male sexual partners should use barrier devices such as condoms during sexual activities.

GAPS IN KNOWLEDGE

Sexually transmitted vaginal infections are common among sexually active women. In the past ten or so years great strides have been made in the understanding of these disorders. Nevertheless, there remain large gaps in the knowledge of infectious vaginal and related diseases. Differences of opinion

---

THE SIGNS AND SYMPTOMS BOX	**DISEASE** TOXIC SHOCK SYNDROME (TSS) **INCUBATION PERIOD** VARIABLE, BUT GENERALLY WITHIN 7 DAYS

First Symptoms Usually Appear: During the Menstrual Cycle

Signs
1. Generalized rash
2. Vomiting and diarrhea
3. Inflammation of eyelids

Symptoms
1. High fever
2. Dizziness
3. Headache
4. Sore throat
5. Muscle cramps
6. General flu-like symptoms

Complications
1. Shedding of skin
2. Possible involvement of kidneys, liver, and gastrointestinal tract
3. Sometimes TSS is fatal

---

exist about various aspects of these infections. Controversy is particularly evident surrounding the "sometime disease agents" that appear to be harmless members of the vaginal microbial population, but under some conditions cause infections. Future studies and scientific developments are expected to provide a better perspective on such vaginal infections and their prevention and control.

CHAPTER 7

THE HERPES VIRUSES— SEVERAL CAUSES FOR CONCERN

Who'd go to bed with me if they thought they'd get herpes? Look, I don't want to give it to anyone else, but I don't want to ruin my whole sex life either.

—Karen B.

INTRODUCTION

Centuries ago, Tiberius placed a ban on public kissing in Rome in an effort to control an outbreak of **herpes labialis** (HER-pēz, LĀ-bē-al-is), or herpetic infections of the lips, mouth, and face (fig. 7.1). Today there is still a need to control these infections as well as the cases of herpes genitalis (HER-pēz, jen-i-TAL-is), or genital herpes, which have reached seriously high levels. An estimated 300,000 to 500,000 new cases occur each year in the United States alone. Estimates of recurring infections appear to be in the millions.

Five major herpes viruses are capable of infecting humans. These include herpes simplex virus (HSV) type 1, and herpes simplex virus type 2. HSV-1 usually is found above the waist and causes most cold sores or fever blisters, while HSV-2 seems to prefer regions below the waist and is responsible for about 80 percent of genital herpes (color photograph 17a). It is also possible for either virus to take the other's place. Type 2 can cause cold sores, and type 1, which is not usually connected with sex, can also infect the genitalia. Each virus can be passed from one body location to another during oral-genital sex, for example.

The other herpes viruses are **varicella-zoster virus** (var′-i-SEL-a, ZOS-ter) which causes both chicken pox (varicella) and an infection

FIGURE 7.1

A typical case of primary herpes simplex virus type 1 infection of the mouth. This well-known condition generally includes the formation of blisters (arrows), open sores or ulcers, and fever.

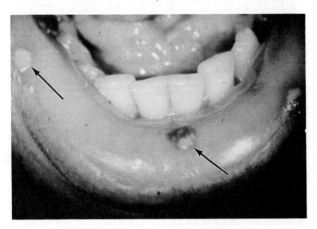

of nerves called shingles (zoster); **cytomegalovirus** (sī'-tō-meg'-a-lō-VĪ-rus) which is responsible for a variety of infections of the eye, respiratory system, and the gastrointestinal tract; and **Epstein-Barr** (EP-stēn-BAR) virus known for its ability to cause a **mononucleosis** (mon-ō-nū-klē-Ō-sis)-like illness, in which an infected person develops fever, sore throat, and swollen lymph nodes. Both the varicella-zoster and Epstein-Barr viruses are usually not spread by sexual contact. Kissing and sharing contaminated forks and spoons are linked to Epstein-Barr infections. These viral disease agents as well as the other herpes viruses are commonly found in persons with HSV infections and poorly functioning immune systems.

In most individuals, herpes virus infections are mild, and in several instances ignored. Unfortunately, in other situations, infections can be devastating. Through the years, herpes infections have also raised several causes for concern. For example, fear of getting or spreading the infection as well as recurring episodes of genital herpes can strain social, sexual, and marital relations. Some persons find it very difficult to work, socialize and otherwise carry on a normal life because of their herpes infection. Still others are greatly concerned over the associations found to exist in certain cases between Epstein-Barr virus, cytomegalovirus, the herpes simplex viruses, and cancer.

This chapter will concentrate on the features and effects of the sexually transmitted herpes viruses.

THE HERPES SIMPLEX VIRUSES

The herpes simplex viruses are large deoxyribonucleic acid (DNA)-containing disease agents that have a remarkable ability to infect the surface (mucosal) linings of various body passages and cavities such as the mouth and vagina (fig. 7.2).

Two distinct herpes simplex viruses exist and are known as types 1 and 2. While these disease agents share certain genetic and immunologic properties, they can be identified by specific laboratory tests. From a practical point of view, the herpes simplex viruses are distinguished from one another on the bases of the conditions each causes. As mentioned earlier, type 1 virus is found in most infections above the waist, while type 2 virus is associated with conditions below the waist.

The herpes simplex viruses, as well as other herpes viruses, do not survive well outside the human body. They can be readily inactivated by ultraviolet light (sunlight), and a variety of chemicals such as those found in common disinfectants.

COLD SORES OR FEVER BLISTERS (HERPES SIMPLEX TYPE 1 INFECTION)
CAUSE AND TRANSMISSION

The term *herpes*, from the Greek "to creep" has been in medical use for at least twenty-five centuries. The condition known as *cold sore*, or *herpes febralis*, was first described around 100 A.D. While the mouth is the most common site for HSV type 1 (HSV-1) infection, other body locations can be involved. These include the breast, the surface of the eye, the fingers (color photograph 15), the anus, or the rectum. Rectal herpes is commonly due to HSV-1, either because of finger or oral contact. Infected individuals can infect the eye by rubbing or scratching a cold sore and then carrying the virus to the area of the eye on contaminated fingers. The fingers of individuals whose hands come into contact with secretions from the mouth also may become infected. HSV-1 also causes genital herpes. The virus in such cases is spread by

FIGURE 7.2

A number of herpes simplex viruses attached to a susceptible cell. The nucleic acid part of the viruses (arrows) can be seen easily. (E. Lycke, B. Hamark, M. Johansson, A. Krotochwil, J. Lycke, and B. Jvennerholm, *Archives of Virology* (1988) 101:87–104.)

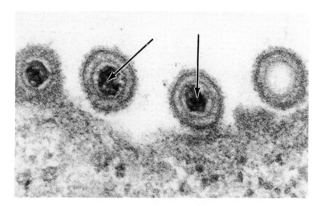

fingers or oral contact. Selected features of HSV-1 infection are given in the accompanying **STD FACT FILE.**

In general, HSV-1 is spread through kissing an infected person, or physical contact with contaminated eating utensils, drinking glasses, or toothbrushes. In addition, the virus can be spread by persons without symptoms.

SIGNS AND SYMPTOMS

The primary or initial infection with HSV-1 commonly occurs during early childhood usually between the ages of six months and five years, and is nonsexually acquired. About three to seven days following contact with the virus, painful blisters appear on and below the tongue and other mouth parts (fig. 7.1). These blisters, which may run together, eventually break, forming open, oozing sores or ulcers. Within a few days lesions also appear on the lips and about the chin, and may spread to the throat and tonsils. Crusts eventually form over the ulcers as the infection episode comes to an end and healing begins. The entire sequence from blisters to crusts and the shedding of virus which begins early in the infection, lasts about twelve to fourteen days. Healing of the sores may take another few days or so. Symptoms in many children may be mild or absent. Adults also may have asymptomatic or mild infections. However, the primary infection in some children and adults can be severe and accompanied by intense pain, difficulty in swallowing, and even weight loss.

Recurrences. Following the primary infection, the virus goes into an inactive, or latent, phase where it remains for the lifetime of the individual. This type of hibernating situation develops early in the infection when the virus travels from the infected area along nerves to nerve tissue outside the brain and spinal cord. Here the virus remains until it is awakened to cause new attacks. Reactivation of HSV-1, known as a *recurrence*, may occur at any time by mechanisms that are not completely understood. Several diverse and general factors have been shown to play a role in viral reactivation. These include high fever, stress, excessive exposure to the sun and wind, severe bacterial infections, colds, and menstruation.

During reactivation viral multiplication occurs in nerve tissue. This event is followed by the new viruses travelling along nerves to mucosal or skin surfaces where they cause a new infection. With each recurrence the body's immune system organizes a fierce and usually effective attack on the activated viruses. Unfortunately, some viruses are able to escape this attack and hide in body cells, thus being protected from the immune system and medical researchers. This is one reason why a permanent cure has not yet been found.

Recurrences develop more frequently and tend to last longer in individuals with some form of immune system defect. Complications occasionally occur and involve the eyes and the central nervous system. HSV-1 is one of the causes of blindness in the United States. Additional features of HSV-1 infection are given in the accompanying **SIGNS & SYMPTOMS BOX.**

DIAGNOSIS

Cold sores can often be diagnosed by the typical appearance of the condition. However the signs and symptoms may not always be clear-cut, and may resemble those of other diseases. Thus, laboratory tests often are needed. Laboratory diagnosis of HSV-1 infections include microscopic examination, virus cultivation, and the direct identification of viral parts known as *antigens*. All of these approaches require specimens from the lesions of the infected individual. In addition, blood tests to detect antibodies to HSV-1 also can be used.

MANAGEMENT AND TREATMENT

Following the diagnosis of HSV infection, the infected person should be told about the nature of the infection, its signs and symptoms, the likelihood of recurrence, contributing factors to recurrences, and the potential for infecting others. While most cases of infection do not require treatment, it is important to keep infected surfaces clean and dry when possible. Since some lesions may be painful, medical attention may be needed. Antiviral drugs also may be beneficial. Treatment of HSV infections is still in its infancy and no particular drug is considered to be a cure.

GENITAL HERPES

Genital herpes has been known since 1736, when the French physician Jean Astruc first described the condition. The disease soon became well recognized, and by the nineteenth century a number of reports of genital herpes began to appear. One of these reports, made in 1886, drew attention to the observation that genital herpes often appeared after a venereal infection such as syphilis, chancroid, or gonorrhea.

CAUSES AND TRANSMISSION

Because genital herpes is not a reportable disease, it is difficult to make an accurate estimate of its occurrence. Nevertheless, 300,000 to 500,000 new cases are believed to occur each year in the United States alone. Statistics of this kind clearly emphasize that herpes simplex virus, type 2 (HSV-2) infection is a common STD in modern society.

HSV-2 infection is acquired from a person shedding the virus at the time of sexual intercourse or contact with genital secretions. The practice of anal intercourse has resulted in an increasing number of cases of primary herpes proctitis (prok'TĪ-tis), an inflammation of the rectum and anus.

STD FACT FILE

DISEASE
GENITAL HERPES
CAUSE
HERPES SIMPLEX VIRUS (HSV) TYPES 1 AND 2

Source/Transmission
Infected humans; sexual activities with infected persons

Epidemiology
Herpes infections are found worldwide. HSV-2 is the most common cause of genital ulcers in the female genital tract. The majority of primary genital infections are found in sexually active persons. The mortality rate among neonates is extremely high and may approach 50 percent. Recurrent HSV-2 infections may reach 50–80 percent. Rectal herpes, often seen in homosexual males, is commonly caused by HSV-1.

Control
1. There is no drug cure for HSV infections
2. Treatment is directed toward shortening the time and lessening the discomfort of the signs and symptoms
3. Acyclovir (a-SĪ-klō-vir) is commonly used in treatment
4. Counseling of infected individuals and sex partners as to prevention and the cycle of the infection

Prevention
1. Condoms and spermicidal jellies should be used to prevent spreading of the infection
2. Avoidance of sexual activities during outbreak or presence of blisters
3. Washing of the genital area after sexual activity

The presence of HSV-2 infection during pregnancy carries with it an increased risk of spontaneous abortion and premature birth, and the possibility of acquiring a life-threatening neonatal infection at time of birth. Since most cases of neonatal infection appear to result from contact with the virus-infected vaginal tract at the time of birth, a cesarean (se-SĀR-e-an) delivery is advisable. In this procedure the baby is surgically removed from the uterus usually by way of the abdomen.

Transmission of HSV-2 to a newborn infant occurs mainly during the times when maternal symptoms are not obvious or present. Thus expectant, infected mothers should be tested before labor. Factors involved in determining whether or not an exposed infant becomes infected are not fully known, but include the amount of virus present and the defenses of the newborn to prevent infection. Selected features of genital herpes are given in the accompanying **STD FACT FILE**.

EPIDEMIOLOGY NOTES

Genital herpes is found throughout the world. The human is the only known natural source of HSV-2. Most adult cases of infection are found in sexually active persons, and are frequently accompanied by other STDs. The incidence of HSV-2 infection increases as sexual activity increases, and is uncommon before puberty.

Neonatal HSV-2 infection is a major complication of maternal genital infection. Approximately 1 case in 7,500 live births occur per year in the United States. The **mortality rate** ranges from 60 to 80 percent, with at least half of the survivors having permanent nervous system injury.

FIGURE 7.3

The sequence of signs in genital herpes with a special look at the formation of blisters, ulcers, and crusts, and viral shedding.

(a) The events of primary infection. (b) The events in a recurrent infection.

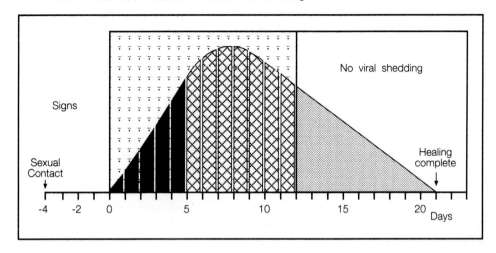

a. **Primary infection**

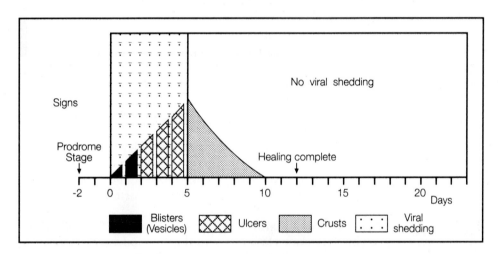

b. **Recurrent infection**

SIGNS AND SYMPTOMS

A primary or initial HSV-2 infection usually begins with local symptoms such as itching and soreness of the genitalia. Many infected individuals also experience enlarged and tender lymph nodes in the groin and surrounding areas, fever, headache, and general discomfort. The presence of these symptoms generally is followed by the development of red spots or **macules** (MAK-ūls), blisters or **vesicles,** and **ulcers.** The ulcers eventually come to contain pus.

Crusting, scab formation, and finally healing occurs (fig. 7.3). In men, lesions concentrate on the glans, prepuce and penile shaft (fig. 7.4a). Scattered lesions may also develop on the scrotum, thigh, and buttocks (color photograph 16). In women, vesicles and other lesions occur on the labia (fig. 7.4b) and spread to the inner thigh surfaces. Women also have a vaginal discharge, an inflammation of the cervix, or cervicitis, and experience more painful lesions in general.

FIGURE 7.4

The appearances of primary or initial genital herpes (arrows).
(a) In the male. (b) In the female. Refer to the **SIGNS AND
SYMPTOMS BOX** for additional features of this disease.

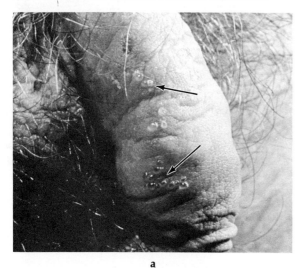

a

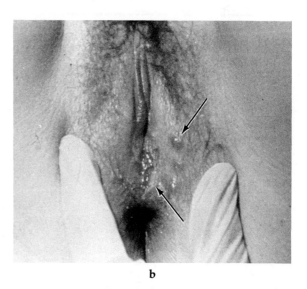

b

A summary of genital herpes is given in the accompanying **SIGNS & SYMPTOMS BOX.**

Recurrences. As is the case with HSV-1 infections, recurrences occur with HSV-2. About 50 to 80 percent of infected individuals experience recurrences in one year. Both the severity of the initial infection and the ability of the immune system to defend the body against HSV-2 influence recurrences. The symptoms, signs, and body sites of infection remain limited to the genital region. Compared to primary infections, recurrent episodes are usually shorter and milder in relation to symptoms and virus shedding (fig. 7.3b). The actual lesions are fewer, heal more quickly (fig. 7.5), and occur mostly on the penile shaft and the labia. Painful lesions appear to be more commonly experienced by infected women.

Recurrences last from eight to twelve days. In addition, such episodes may be asymptomatic in both men and women.

About 60 percent of HSV-2 infected persons experience a **prodrome** (pro-DRŌM) **stage** before exhibiting the typical genital lesions. This prodromal period refers to the time between the earliest symptoms and the appearance of the actual infection. It can develop within a few days after sexual contact. Itching, burning, and tingling or numbness in the genital area generally are experienced in the prodrome thirty minutes to forty-eight hours before the appearance of lesions.

Several factors have been identified as possible triggers for recurrences. These include menstruation, sexual intercourse, stress, and even the rubbing or friction produced by wearing tight clothing.

Neonatal Herpes Simplex Virus Type 2 Infection. Having a primary genital herpes infection during pregnancy carries the risk of transmitting the causative virus to the unborn child. This risk is much greater with the primary disease than with recurrent infection. The major source of HSV-2 to the newborn is through contact with the infected mother's genital tract at the time of delivery. Transmission of the virus from mother to infant occurs mainly during asymptomatic episodes of maternal infection. Newborn infections appear to develop more

THE SIGNS AND SYMPTOMS BOX	**DISEASE**
	GENITAL HERPES (HSV-2)
	INCUBATION PERIOD
	3–5 DAYS

First Symptoms Usually Appear: May Appear Within 1 Week After Exposure, but Symptoms are Highly Variable

Signs

Men

1. Swollen lymph nodes in the groin
2. Many small, painful blisters or vesicles in and around the genitalia
3. Healing of involved area occurs within 2 weeks

Women

Similar to those listed for men

Symptoms

1. Tenderness in groin
2. Fever
3. Pain on urination
4. Pain in area of blisters

Similar to those listed for men with the exception of pain on urination

Complications

General

Recurrence of blisters

Women

1. Abnormal growths of cervical tissue (tumors)
2. Cervical cancer

Newborn

Complications that may occur with infants infected during birth include

1. Severe central nervous system injury
2. Death

FIGURE 7.5

The less extensive involvement of recurrent genital herpes. (a) In the male (arrow). (b) In the female (circled area).

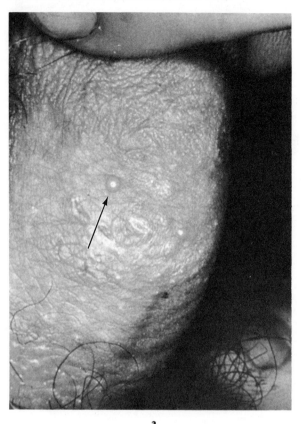

a

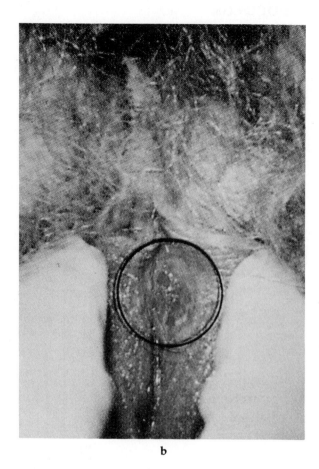

b

frequently with mothers having primary infections than with those with recurrent ones.

The appearance of symptoms usually occurs within one week after birth. However, evidence may not become obvious until three to four weeks later. Neonatal infection can range from a localized skin infection to central nervous system involvement and a spreading of the disease to several organs such as the liver and adrenal (a-DRĒ-nal) glands. The associated symptoms can include irritability, fever, vomiting, diarrhea, poor feeding, and breathing difficulties. Skin lesions are found in about half the cases. Central nervous system infection carries with it the possible danger of severe brain injury and other consequences (fig. 7.7). Because of the wide range of symptoms and effects, neonatal herpes disease is a possible consideration with infants that become ill during the first weeks after birth.

Unfortunately, maternal genital infections are asymptomatic and often unrecognizable in physical examinations. Expectant women with a history of infection, or women whose sexual partners have such a history, should be checked with appropriate laboratory tests during the last weeks of pregnancy. This approach is also of value to identify potentially exposed newborns.

A CASE OF GENITAL HERPES

What can a person experience with genital herpes? How bad can the condition become? Well, here is an example. A 37-year-old male was first seen in an STD clinic complaining of pain in his penis and groin, burning during urination, and the presence of a slight discharge. These symptoms developed after sexual intercourse with an unknown companion. A preliminary examination showed a blood-stained urethral discharge and an abnormal amount of blood in the urethral opening. On the basis of a laboratory examination of the discharge, a preliminary diagnosis of a nonspecific urethritis was made. The patient was given an appropriate antibiotic and asked to return four days later.

On his return the patient said that he felt much worse, and complained of difficulty in breathing, dizziness, and being generally confused. Without any delay the patient was admitted to a hospital ward.

On examination, a blackened area of skin surrounding the urethral opening, together with a number of flattened, pus-containing blisters (fig. 7.6a) were noted. Other findings included swollen glans, prepuce, and penis shaft, a reddened and hot shaft, and different sized pus-filled blisters widespread over the patient's skin surfaces (fig. 7.6b). The patient also was found to have a slight fever and continual drowsiness.

Several specimens were taken and tests performed to find the cause of the patient's genital infection. Tests for gonorrhea, syphilis, and human immunodeficiency virus were negative. Viral cultures were positive for herpes simplex virus type 2. Based on these findings an appropriate medication was selected and applied to the skin and penile lesions. The patient's condition improved rapidly, but recurrences developed at various skin locations six to seven months later.

PREVENTION

To decrease the risk of neonatal infection cesarean delivery is recommended for expectant mothers with obvious lesions and those actively shedding virus as shown by laboratory tests. If herpetic lesions or other problems are not present during labor, delivery should be normal and uneventful.

As mentioned earlier, HSV infection in early pregnancy may cause spontaneous abortion. However, infection of the fetus during pregnancy is not common. Thus, therapeutic abortion is generally not recommended for pregnancies complicated by HSV infection.

Another item of concern is the risk of infected infants transmitting disease to others. Generally, such infants are placed into isolation, separated from others in a newborn nursery, and closely observed for several weeks for any evidence of infection. When handling her newborn infant in the hospital, the mother wears a gown and washes her hands before and after contact. Infants born by cesarean delivery or by normal (vaginal) delivery to women with no evidence of recent HSV infection usually are not placed into isolation. In general, most hospitals handle the contact between newborn and mother on an individual basis.

DIAGNOSIS

Genital herpes often can be diagnosed on the basis of the lesions found on physical examination (figs. 7.4 and 7.5, and color photograph 17). However, because such signs and symptoms may resemble those

FIGURE 7.6

A case of herpes simplex virus type 2 infection. (a) The penile lesion. (b) An example of the pus-filled blisters found on the patient's skin surfaces. (From J. F. Peatherer, I. W. Smith, and D. H. H. Robertson, *British Journal of Venereal Diseases* (1979) 55:48–51.)

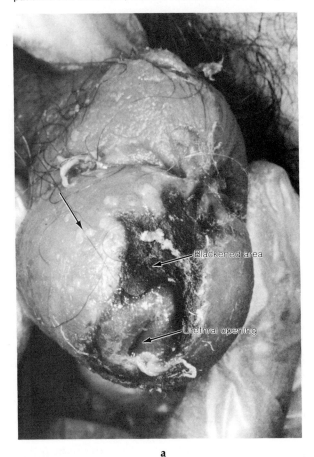

Blackened area

Urethral opening

a

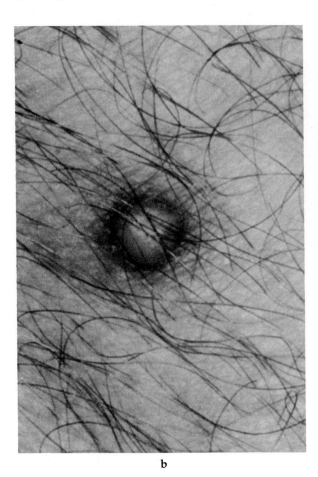

b

found with other diseases, laboratory identification is needed. Laboratory approaches include the use of scrapings or other specimens taken from genital sores for microscopic examination to show the presence of multinucleated giant cells (fig. 7.8), special staining, and enzyme techniques to demonstrate viral parts, and the isolation of virus in tissue cultures. The Pap smear, mentioned in chapter 4, is of particular value in diagnosing HSV-2 infection.

TREATMENT

The treatment of genital herpes has several goals. Among these are: shortening the duration of symptoms; reducing the possibilities of complications; and preventing the spread of HSV and the development of latent or hidden infections, and recurrences. Decreasing virus transmission and eliminating established latent infections are important to approaches for the treatment and prevention of genital herpes.

FIGURE 7.7

A newborn (neonate) infant with herpes simplex virus infection. The virus-containing blister or vesicles (arrows) can be seen on the trunk of the body. About 90 percent of neonatal herpes cases result from contact with the infectious genital secretions of the mother.

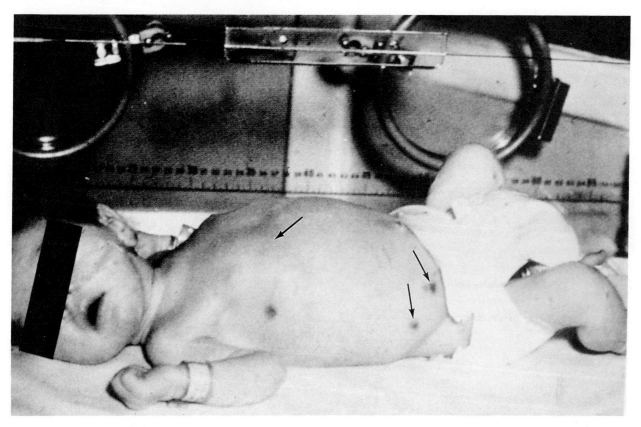

While a number of drugs are under study, the major form of treatment revolves around the antiviral drug **acyclovir** (a-SĪ-klō-vir). While treatment with this medication dramatically shortens the course of the infection, no major effect on the reduction of recurrences has been observed. Thus, HSV-2 infected individuals still need counseling about the signs, symptoms, and contributing factors of recurrent infections.

THE IMPORTANCE OF COUNSELING

Genital herpes is an emotional disease, particularly since it is recurrent, may interfere with sexual intercourse, and may be of potential importance in the development of cervical cancer. Infected persons often need a great deal of advice and emotional support, especially since their condition is incurable at the present time. When counseled such individuals should be warned that they are infectious when blisters, sores, or crusts are present. They should abstain from sexual intercourse once such lesions are noted, or sooner if prodromal symptoms are present (fig. 7.3b). It should also be pointed out that other forms of intimacy are safer. Some persons with HSV-2 infection may also find it useful to talk with fellow sufferers.

FIGURE 7.8

The results of a stained Pap smear showing HSV–2 infected giant cells (arrows) from a patient's cervix. These cells typically contain many nuclei.

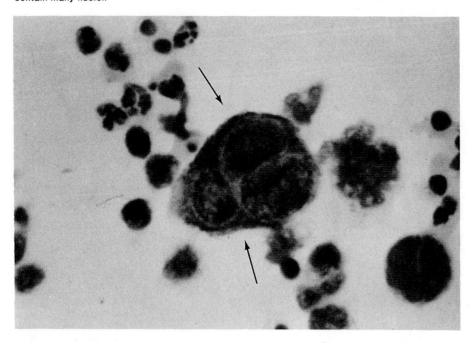

PREVENTION

Generally speaking, no proven effective means to prevent HSV-2 infection is known. While the use of barrier devices such as condoms may reduce the possibility of transmission in asymptomatic cases, the disease may still be spread if blisters and other lesions are present on the genitalia and neighboring body areas.

CYTOMEGALOVIRUS – A CAUSE OF SEXUALLY TRANSMITTED AND CONGENITAL INFECTIONS

Cytomegaloviruses (sī-tō-meg'-a-lō-VĪ-rus-ez), as mentioned earlier, belong to the herpes virus family. They are widely distributed in nature, especially in human populations in all areas of the world. A cytomegalovirus (CMV) infection typically causes an enlargement of infected cells with the development of distinctive structures, called *inclusion bodies,* in their nuclear and cytoplasmic regions (fig. 7.9). The term "cytomegalia" was adopted to emphasize the unusual size of infected cells.

Early evidence that CMV might be an STD was provided by the results of studies in 1972 in which the virus was isolated from cervical secretions and semen. Since then the virus has been found in asymptomatic homosexual men living in the same geographical area. CMV also is often isolated from body fluids such as blood, semen, and urine of homosexual men with AIDS.

Cytomegaloviruses currently are the major cause of birth defects, hearing loss, and mental retardation in congenitally infected infants. CMV infection has also been found in persons with transplanted kidneys and bone marrow.

CAUSE AND TRANSMISSION

Maternal infection plays an important role in the transmission of CMV to newborns. Congenital infections may follow initial, reactivated, or recurrent

FIGURE 7.9

The cytomegalovirus. (a) The presence of large intranuclear (arrows) and many small cytoplasmic (arrow heads) inclusions in an infected cell. (b) An enlarged view taken through an electron microscope showing the individual CMVs. (From M. T. Brady and Associates, *Pediatric Pathology* (1988) 8:205–214.)

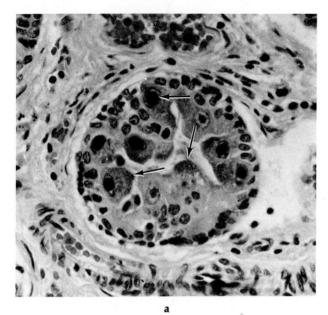

a

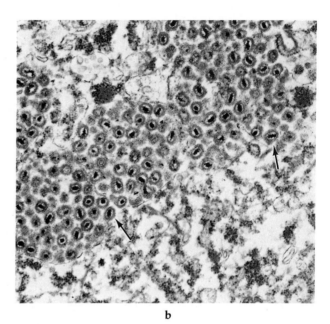

b

maternal infections. More severe outcomes of infection generally develop if expectant mothers become infected during the first three months of their pregnancy. About 1 percent of all babies are born infected. Infection results from exposure to CMV as the baby passes through an infected cervix during the birth process. Breast milk of infected mothers also has been implicated as a source of the virus.

Childhood infections also occur and are common in crowded living environments. CMV is spread largely by contaminated breast milk and close personal contact with infected individuals.

CMV also is transmitted sexually. However, it can also be spread among adults by close personal contact, contaminated blood, and organ transplants.

EPIDEMIOLOGY NOTES

CMV infections are widely distributed, and in most situations do not produce obvious symptoms. While the age at which an individual becomes infected is not always the same, the prevalence of CMV infections is related to socioeconomic status, and to geographic location in certain situations. Individuals living or playing under crowded conditions are more likely to have CMV infection early in life. This has been observed in day-care centers and nursery schools. CMV transmission among preschool children in these environments is quite high. Additional features of CMV infection are given in the accompanying **STD FACT FILE.**

Depending on the age and resistance (immunity) level of the infected individual, CMV can cause a range of disease conditions. In normal hosts (children and adults with normal functioning immune systems), a mononucleosis-like illness is commonly found. This condition is similar to infectious mononucleosis generally caused by another herpes virus, the *Epstein-Barr virus.* Typical symptoms include fever, muscle pains, headache, sluggishness, and a slight yellowing of the skin and eyes known as jaundice (JAWN-dis).

In congenitally infected newborns, CMV infections may produce symptoms ranging from fever to severe brain damage and neurological abnormalities. Other effects that may occur include enlarged liver, spleen, inflammation of the eye, and small purplish, blood-filled spots on the skin.

Individuals with abnormal or poorly functioning immune systems, **(immunocompromised hosts)** which include recipients of organ transplants, and HIV-infected persons, exhibit a variety of unfavorable effects. Individuals who receive infected organs may develop the mononucleosis-like illness described earlier, inflammation and destruction of the light sensitive portion of the eye (the *retina*) (color photograph 18), a lung infection, and painful sores along the gastrointestinal tract. The risk of rejecting transplanted organs also is increased with CMV infection. HIV-infected persons may experience similar conditions, but may also develop additional damaging effects involving the brain and its coverings. A general summary of CMV infections is presented in the accompanying **SIGNS & SYMPTOMS BOX.**

DIAGNOSIS

Diagnosis of CMV infection is generally dependent on laboratory tests. These include virus isolation, electron microscopy and related techniques, blood tests for specific antibodies, and special biochemical procedures to detect viral nucleic acid.

TREATMENT AND PREVENTION

At the present time, there is no effective treatment for CMV infections. Ganciclovir (gan-CĒ-klō-vir), a relatively new drug has been licensed for treatment of sight-threatening CMV infections. A number of other preparations are under study. Drugs are available, however, to reduce the symptoms and severity of the infection.

Prevention of CMV infections also is of major importance. The major approach currently being considered is the development of a vaccine.

THE SIGNS AND SYMPTOMS BOX	**DISEASE** CYTOMEGALIC INCLUSION (sī-tō-meg-A-LIK, in KLŪ-zhun) DISEASE (CID), OR CYTOMEGALOVIRUS INFECTION **INCUBATION PERIOD** UNKNOWN

First Symptoms Usually Appear: Variable for Adults. Newborns May Show Symptoms Within 3 Months

Signs

Adults
1. Swollen lymph nodes
2. Mild yellowing of tissues (jaundice)

Children (Newborns)
1. Yellowing of body tissues (jaundice)
2. Enlarged spleen and liver
3. Small bleeding spots in the skin
4. Smaller than normal head size
5. Indications of mental retardation
6. Difficulty in controlling body movement and coordination

Complications

Newborns
1. Pneumonia
2. Enlargement of body organs
3. Central nervous system damage

Symptoms

1. Fever
2. Headache
3. Low energy level
4. Muscle pain
5. Other symptoms listed for mononucleosis in the text

1. Fever
2. Muscle pain
3. Low energy level

THE HERPES VIRUSES—A CANCER CONNECTION

The herpes viruses, primarily those spread through sexual contact, are a major public health problem affecting millions of people annually throughout the world. The consequences of infection range from being annoying and troublesome to being life threatening. Serious diseases of the newborn can be a complication of genital infection since infected women can actively shed virus at the time of delivery.

Another particular area of concern is the possible relationship of HSV-2 infection to cervical cancer. The possibility of such an association has been the subject of controversy for nearly 20 years. Even though the relationship is not fully established or proven, women with recurrent genital herpes should have regular, yearly Pap smear examinations (see chapter 3). Any noticeable changes detected in such smears would be early ones, and should be curable. Cervical cancer occurs in only a small number of women with genital herpes; however, it is a curable condition if detected early.

CHAPTER | 8

GENITAL WARTS, MOLLUSCUM CONTAGIOSUM, AND HEPATITIS B INFECTION

I have at present a person who had long been liable to piles, who some time ago was attacked with condylomatous excrescences (surface growths) from a venereal taint; to these succeeded a common abscess (infection) from inflammation and last of all the parts have become cancerous.

—*Benjamin Bell, 1793.*

INTRODUCTION

On a global basis cervical cancer is an extremely important preventable disease. It is estimated that approximately 400,000 women worldwide develop cervical cancer yearly. This disease ranks second only to breast cancer as a documented cause of death from cancer in women. Although declining in incidence and mortality as a result of early detection programs in many developed countries, cervical cancer still remains the most important cancer in many parts of the developing countries.

For more than a century there has been the suspicion that sexually transmitted agents may contribute to the cause of cervical cancer. Furthermore, during the past twenty-five to fifty years much attention has focused on the role of viruses such as the herpes viruses and the **papilloma** (pap-i-LŌ-ma) **viruses** (HPVs) in the cause of anorectal cancers involving the vaginal, vulvar, and perianal areas.

A major portion of this chapter will deal with the human papilloma viruses as STD agents and the cause of genital warts. Attention will also be given to two other viruses that can be transmitted sexually to cause **molluscum contagiosum** (mō-LUS-kum, kon-TĀ-jē-ō-sum) and **hepatitis B infections.**

Condylomata Acuminata (Genital Warts)

Although the subject of genital warts has been of increasing interest and concern in recent years, the disease has been known and evidently observed quite commonly in the ancient world. Physicians in the ancient world referred to the growths or tumors (fig. 8.1) associated with the skin as "figs" or **condylomas** (kon'-di-LŌ-mas). Since then they have been called **venereal warts** and **condylomata acuminata** (kon'-di-LŌ-ma-ta, a-KUM-i-na-ta). The last term, which means "pointed wartlike growths," is currently used for the condition.

For many years after syphilis made its appearance in Europe in the fifteenth century, genital warts were thought to be a particular feature of this STD. While this belief eventually was discarded it was replaced by other viewpoints suggesting that the disease resulted from gonorrhea or from an irritation caused by contact with genital secretions. Several studies beginning in the late nineteenth century and continuing for fifty years showed that condylomata acuminata, also referred to as **anogenital** (a-nō-GEN-i-tal) warts, were caused by a human papilloma virus. These viruses were actually seen in 1949 by electron microscopy in specimens from common skin warts (fig. 8.2). Some nineteen years later, virus particles of a similar appearance were observed in genital wart specimens. It is now known that there are a number of human papilloma viruses (HPVs) capable of attacking several different body sites (color photograph 19).

The Virus

Papilloma viruses are a group of small deoxyribonucleic acid (DNA) viruses, which cause a class of harmless, or **benign** (bē-NĪN) tumors of the skin or mucous membranes referred to as *papillomas*. Such tumors include warts and condylomas. Many warts are generally harmless, local growths, which shrink and disappear after a time. Their initial formation is probably caused by some injury to the skin surface which allows the HPV to invade the deeper-lying skin-producing layers. The viral infection stimulates cell growth and reproduction and the eventual formation of a wart.

Figure 8.1

The appearance of warts. (From T. Shiohara and Associates, *Journal of American Academy of Dermatology* (1989) 21:307–391.)

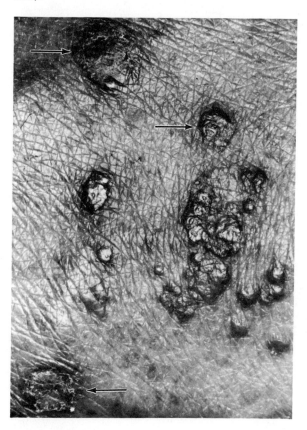

Figure 8.2

An electron micrograph showing the virus particles obtained from a case of skin warts.

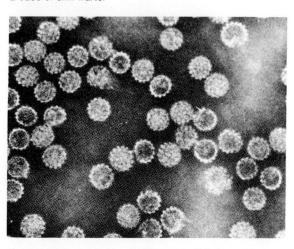

FIGURE 8.3

Two examples of oral condyloma acuminata (arrows), an increasingly common sexually transmitted condition. (Photo on right from S. Butler, J. A. Molinari, A. Plezia, P. Chandrasekar, and H. Venkat, *Reviews of Infectious Diseases* (1988) 10:544.)

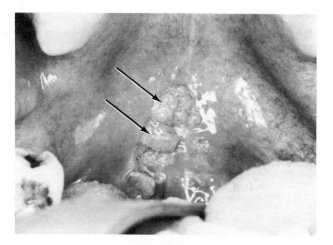
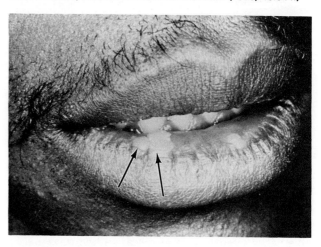

Modern biochemical and related techniques, among them **recombinant DNA technology,** have shown the existence of at least fifty different types of HPVs. The different virus types are distinguished from one another on the basis of their DNA properties. Only a small number of the HPVs are generally associated with genital warts.

CAUSE AND TRANSMISSION

HPV infections are spread through scratches of the skin, by sexual contact and a baby's passage through an infected birth canal. HPVs also have been transmitted by oral sex (fig. 8.3). Such oral infections may be caused by several genital tract HPV types and by other HPV types which infect the mouth exclusively.

Genital warts or condylomata acuminata are generally associated with HPV types 6, 11, 16, 18 and 31, as described in the accompanying **STD FACT FILE.**

Like other STD causative agents, human papilloma viruses may be spread from an infected mother to her offspring. Transmission most likely occurs as the fetus passes through an infected birth canal. A small proportion of infants born to infected mothers develop benign tumors in the mouth, throat, or other parts of the breathing passages. Adults infected through oral-genital exposure to HPV can develop a similar condition. HPV types 6 and 11 account for most such infections. A summary of selected features of genital warts is given in the accompanying **STD FACT FILE.**

Whether or not genital warts can be transmitted by contaminated, inanimate objects or materials is not known.

EPIDEMIOLOGY NOTES

In the mid-1970s it was recognized that the cervix was frequently infected with HPVs and that precancerous conditions of the cervix could not be distinguished from HPV infections occurring in the same sites. During the last ten years or so evidence has been accumulating which implicates specific HPV types as causes of certain genital cancers. This includes the finding of the nucleic acid of HPVs in cervical cancer cells and the presence of such HPV nucleic acid integrated into the genetic material of normal host cells.

A significant number of cervical cancers have been found to contain HPV types 16 and 18. These two viral types also have been reported to be present in cancers of the vulva, vagina, and penis. In addition, a number of possible sexually and nonsexually related risk factors also have been identified. The sexually related risk factors for cervical cancer include an early age for first sexual intercourse, multiple sexual partners, and a history of STDs.

STD FACT FILE

DISEASE
CONDYLOMATA ACUMINATA (kon'-di-LŌ-ma-ta, a-KUM-in-a-ta), GENITAL OR VENEREAL WARTS
CAUSE
HUMAN PAPILLOMA VIRUSES (HPV) TYPES 6, 11, 16, 18, AND 31

Source/Transmission
Sexual activities with infected individuals, including anal intercourse. Children may develop condyloma as a result of sexual abuse by an infected adult.

Epidemiology
Disease is found worldwide. Genital warts are found among sexually active adults.

Control
1. The use of liquid nitrogen or cryotherapy, electrosurgery, laser applications, or medications such as podophyllin (pod-ō-FIL-in) to remove lesions
2. Avoiding sexual activity with multiple sex partners
3. Counseling of infected persons as to features of the disease
4. Use of barrier devices such as the condom during sexual activities

Prevention
1. Use of condoms to prevent spread of the infection
2. Examination and treatment of infected sex partners

Among the nonsexually related risk factors, smoking, the use of oral contraceptives, and diet are considered to be possible contributing influences. Smoking appears to have a significant association with cervical abnormalities. The risk of cervical cancer, as well as genital warts, is apparently increased in women who are long-term smokers, heavy smokers, and users of nonfilter cigarettes. The relationship between oral contraceptive use and cervical cancer has been examined in several studies. While the results have not been conclusive, it appears that long-term users of such contraceptives are at highest risk. A possible explanation for these associations is their effect on an individual's immunity or resistance which is known to be affected negatively by cigarette smoking and high levels of hormones similar to those found in oral contraceptives. The possible role of diet in the development of cervical cancer is just beginning to be considered. Several studies have shown an association between a low dietary intake of either vitamin A or vitamin C, and a high risk for cervical cancer.

The mechanisms by which HPV infection and behavioral and other risk factors interact in the possible development of cervical, or other anogenital cancers, are not clear. It is obvious from various studies that these factors play a role, but how remains to be determined.

SIGNS AND SYMPTOMS

Genital warts occur in genital and perianal areas and are seen most often in young sexually active adults. The incubation period varies from several weeks to twenty months. In some cases an infection may be a short one without any major noticeable symptoms, or it may persist for years and include the formation of single or many flat, or soft, fleshy growths that run together to form large masses (fig. 8.5).

In men, genital warts vary in appearance. Some may be flat, while others may take on the appearance of small "cauliflowers." Generally they are soft, fleshy, and contain small blood vessels, and may first develop on the glans, prepuce, penile shaft, the corona, or other related areas which are open to

GENITAL WARTS OF THE VULVA AND CERVICAL CANCER IN A YOUNG WOMAN

A twenty-six-year-old white woman was admitted to the gynecology service of a major medical center. She complained of having sharp groin and vaginal pain for at least four months. The woman also indicated that she had had vaginal and vulvar warts for about eight years without any form of treatment.

The personal history of the patient revealed that she was a drug abuser and that she had had sexual relations with a number of partners. Her first experience was at eight years of age, when she was sexually abused by her stepfather and foster parents. She had been a transient since the age of fifteen, riding throughout the United States with truckers.

On physical examination, the vulva was found to be covered with large flat warts and a number of smaller, pointed, condylomata acuminata. One lesion had a number of open sores (fig. 8.4). Many flat, cancerous-appearing growths were found between the various types of warts. The uterus and neighboring regions were found to be fairly normal.

Laboratory findings showed the presence of *Gardnerella*, one of the causative agents of *bacterial vaginitis* and *Trichomonas* infection. Blood tests were positive for *Chylamydia*.

Treatment of the patient included the surgical removal of all abnormal growths and lymph nodes from the surrounding region. Laboratory study of the diseased tissues showed the presence of HPV.

injury or irritation during intercourse (fig. 8.6). Injury during intercourse allows the entry of HPV. Genital warts are more common in uncircumcised men, and appear beneath the prepuce. The scrotum is not commonly involved.

In the case of anal warts, the growths in men first develop on the perianal area, and can also appear internally. These warts can become quite large. Internal warts are found in over 50 percent of individuals with surface condylomas.

In women, genital warts are quite similar to those seen with men. They are frequently found at the vaginal entrance and on the labia, the urethra, and the cervix. Involvement of the perianal and surrounding regions may also occur (fig. 8.4). A general summary of this disease is given in the accompanying **SIGNS & SYMPTOMS BOX.**

Newborns infected during the time of birth may develop the condition known as **juvenile-onset respiratory papillomatosis** (pap-i-lō-ma-TO-sis). In this infection, growths or papillomas develop in the throat, and may cause hoarseness or may interfere with normal breathing. The condition may appear within a few months, or ten or more years after birth. Removal of the growths is necessary to keep the airway of the infected newborn clear.

DIAGNOSIS

The diagnosis of genital warts includes distinguishing it from other conditions involving the genitalia. These include harmless growths, warts that may develop in secondary syphilis, and cancerous tumors. A **colposcope** (KOL-pō-skōp), which is a magnifying optical instrument, is of value in detecting HPV infection in women (color photograph 2). The Pap smear also is of major importance in such cases.

A more specific diagnosis of HPV infection can be made with the detection and study of viral nucleic acid in specimens from infected individuals.

TREATMENT

Anogenital HPV-caused warts may be either uncomplicated or associated with a form of potential cancerous growth in the same or other parts of the

FIGURE 8.4

The vulva with various warts and cancerous growths. An open sore (arrow) of the cancerous growth near the anus is also shown. (From T. V. Dinh, L. C. Powell, Jr., E. V. Hannigan, H. L. Yang, D. R. Wirt, and R. B. Yandell, *Journal of Reproductive Medicine* (1988) 33:510.)

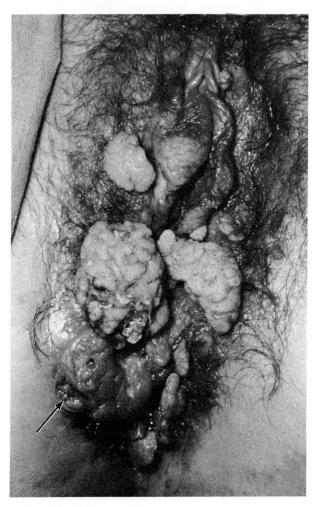

FIGURE 8.5

A case of anogenital warts in a 3½–year–old child. This child also was found to have AIDS-related complex (acquired immune deficiency syndrome-related complex). (From D. Laraque, *New England Journal of Medicine* (1989) 320:1220.)

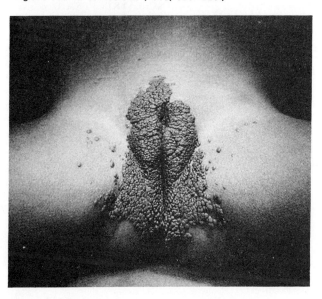

FIGURE 8.6

A severe case of condyloma acuminata (arrows) in a male. (Courtesy of H. Zachariae, Professor of Dermatology, Marselisberg Hospital, Arhus, Denmark)

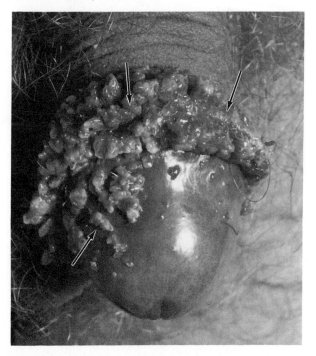

DISEASE
GENITAL (VENEREAL) WARTS OR CONDYLOMATA ACUMINATA
(kon'-di-LŌ-ma-ta, a-KUM-i-na-ta)
INCUBATION PERIOD
1 to 3 MONTHS

First Symptoms Usually Appear: Within Incubation Period or Up to Several Years

Signs

Men
1. Single or many soft cauliflower-like growths around the genitalia
2. Anal and perianal growths common among persons practicing anal sex

Women
Growths and other signs are similar to those described for men

Complications

Women
1. Cervical cancer
2. Severe itching or irritation
3. Burning sensation on urination
4. Sores and bacterial infections

Men
1. Penile cancer
2. Large, painful and perianal lesions that may cause blood in stools and/or difficult bowel movements
3. Sores and secondary bacterial infections
4. Burning sensation on urination

Symptoms

1. Generally no pain
2. Some burning or irritation in the involved areas
3. Most cases are without symptoms

Most cases are without symptoms

---

genital tract. The general aim of treatment for uncomplicated cases is to cure an unpleasantly appearing infectious condition (fig. 8.4), while the approaches associated with potential cancerous lesions is to prevent an invasive cancer from developing. Currently available techniques are either **invasive** (destructive) or **noninvasive.** Invasive techniques include **cautery** (KAW-ter-ē), a means of destroying tissue by freezing, heat, corrosive chemicals, or electrical current; **cryosurgery** (krī-o-SER-jer-ē), the exposure of tissue to extreme cold; **diathermy** (DĪ-a-ther'-mē), the application of high temperatures; general surgery; and carbon dioxide laser (LĀ-zer). The noninvasive techniques include the use of tissue-destroying chemicals such as **trichloroacetic** (trī-klor-ō-a-SĒ-tik) **acid,** agents that interfere with tissue reproduction such as **podophyllin** (pod-ō-FIL-in) and related materials (fig. 8.7), and antiviral substances such as the **interferons** (in-ter-FĒR-ons).

FIGURE 8.7
The commercial product Warticon used to treat genital warts. The applicator, which can be used for several warts as well as for single ones, also is shown. (Courtesy of KABI, Middlesex, England)

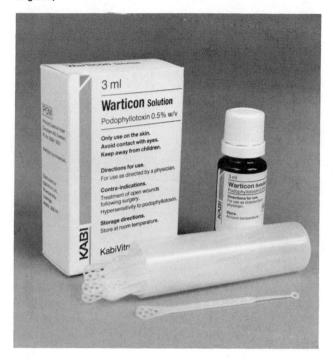

APPROACHES TO CONTROL

The general practices described in chapter 4 and elsewhere certainly apply to controlling the spread of HPV infections. Particular consideration should be given to avoiding sexual activity with multiple sex partners, the definite use of barrier devices such as condoms during sexual activities, and seeking medical services when genital warts are noticed. It must be noted that both male and female sex partners of individuals with apparently uncomplicated genital condylomas may also have growths that are potential cancerous conditions associated with the cervix, vulva anus, and penis. Thus, thorough physical examinations of sex partners are clearly needed on a regular basis especially if wartlike growths are present.

MOLLUSCUM CONTAGIOSUM

Molluscum contagiosum (mo-LUS-kum, kon-TĀ-jē-ō-sum) is a viral infection which results in the formation of soft growths or tumors on the skin and mucous membranes. This condition was first described in 1817 by Bateman, who referred to it as "molluscum," a common term then in use for growths that had little stems. Additionally he added the term "contagiosum" to emphasize the ease with which the infection could be spread from person to person. Bateman felt that the "milky fluid" which could be squeezed from the growths (fig. 8.8) was responsible for the transmission of the disease.

CAUSE AND TRANSMISSION

Molluscum contagiosum is caused by a deoxyribonucleic acid (DNA) pox-virus. The virus can be spread both sexually and nonsexually. Support for the sexual transmission is provided by the development of genital growths in sexual partners and prostitutes, and the peak ages of the disease's occurrence (20–26 years), which are similar to those of other STDs.

The nonsexual form of the disease appears to be found primarily among children. It is spread by direct contact with the skin of infected persons and/or articles contaminated by such individuals, such as gymnastic equipment and towels. The general features of this viral disease are given in the accompanying **STD FACT FILE.**

SIGNS AND SYMPTOMS

The general tumor-like growths which range in color from a pearly white to a light pink, mainly develop on the genitalia, face, and hands of the infected individual within two to seven weeks of exposure. A whitish paste easily can be squeezed from a central depression in these tumors. While the number of the growths vary from person to person, individuals with lowered resistance can have as many as 1,000. A summary of this disease and its features are listed in the accompanying **SIGNS & SYMPTOMS BOX.**

FIGURE 8.8
Molluscum contagiosum. (a) The back of an infected individual showing the large number of the pearl-like growths. (b) A closer view of the pearl-like growths or blisters characteristic of this viral infection.

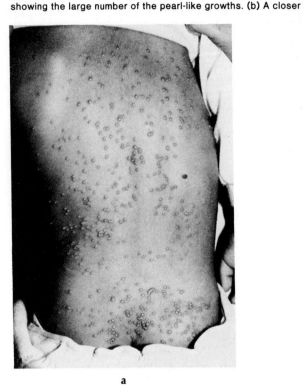

a

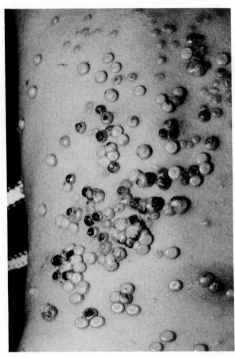

b

STD FACT FILE	**DISEASE** MOLLUSCUM CONTAGIOSUM (mo-LUS-kum, kon-TĀ-jē-ō-sum) **CAUSE** MOLLUSCUM CONTAGIOSUM VIRUS (A POX-VIRUS)

Source/Transmission
Infected humans. Virus may be spread by sexual contact, as well as by direct or close contact with blisters or their contents.

Epidemiology
The disease is found worldwide. It most commonly affects children and sexually active adults. Infection has been found among users of public baths and swimming pools.

Control
1. Removal of growths by appropriate methods, such as cryotherapy
2. Disinfecting contaminated articles used by infected individuals

Prevention
1. Use of protective barrier devices such as condoms during sexual intercourse
2. Avoiding direct contact with contaminated articles

THE SIGNS AND SYMPTOMS BOX

DISEASE
MOLLUSCUM CONTAGIOSUM (mo-LUS-kum, kon-TĀ-jē-ō-sum)
INCUBATION PERIOD
2–7 WEEKS

First Symptoms Usually Appear: Within 2–7 Weeks

Signs
1. Painless pearly white to flesh colored blisters with central depressions
2. Blisters or growths commonly found on the trunk, and anogenital regions

Symptoms
Generally painless and without symptoms

Complications
1. Bacterial infections resulting from scratching
2. Pus and scar formation
3. Infection of the eyelids

DIAGNOSIS

The diagnosis of molluscum contagiosum usually is made on the finding of the pearly white growths on the face, trunk, legs, and genitalia. However, microscopic examination of specimens obtained from infected persons may be necessary to show the presence of the virus or evidence of infection.

TREATMENT

Treatment of this disease is necessary, not only to relieve the discomfort experienced by some individuals, but also to prevent further spread. Treatment generally involves the removal of the growths by chemicals or by localized freezing.

HEPATITIS B VIRUS (HBV) INFECTION

Although viral hepatitis is unquestionably an ancient disease, it is currently one of the world's major public health problems. In 1988, it was the third most common infectious disease (just behind chicken pox and gonorrhea) reported in the United States. Most of the common hepatitis-causing infectious agents can be spread by sexual and/or **parenteral** (par-EN-ter-al) routes which includes the use of contaminated needles or syringes, blood transfusions, and perinatal transmission from an infected mother to her fetus. At least four different hepatitis viruses are recognized. These are hepatitis A, B, C, and D (Delta) viruses, respectively.

Hepatitis A virus generally is acquired by the ingestion of contaminated food or water. This viral disease agent also can be sexually transmitted through oral-anal contact. Hepatitis B virus (HBV), as a later section will indicate, is transmitted by contaminated blood or blood products and contaminated syringes and needles. It also can be spread sexually and from an infected mother to her fetus. Hepatitis C virus is spread by contaminated food and water, while hepatitis D virus transmission is associated with contaminated blood or blood products.

THE VIRUS

A great deal of current interest has come to focus on HBV. Three reasons can account for such interest. First, the infectious agent follows the same routes of transmission as the human immunodeficiency viruses, and is found in over 90 percent of persons with AIDS. Second, HBV has been shown to interact with hepatitis D virus and to change normal liver cells into cancerous ones. Hepatitis B virus is being increasingly recognized as an important cause of long-lasting or chronic liver disease and liver cancer. With viral interactions of this type actual working, questions are being raised as to whether or not a similar relationship can develop with human immunodeficiency viruses. Finally, HBV can infect lymphocytes (white blood cells), remain in this type of cellular environment, and produce a stable, long-lasting infection that does not destroy the infected cells. In this protected arrangement the immune system of the infected individual is powerless in dealing with disease agents.

Virus Organization. HBV is a complex, deoxyribonucleic acid (DNA) containing an infectious agent

FIGURE 8.9

Hepatitis B virus (HBV). (a) An electon microscopic view of the virus. (Courtesy of C. R. Howard). (b) The various parts of HBV.

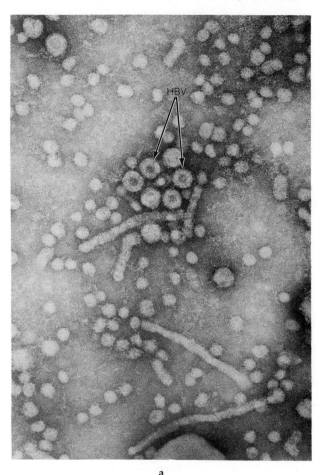

a

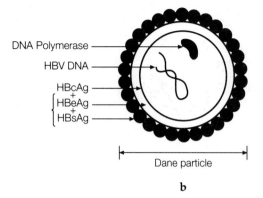

DNA Polymerase

HBV DNA

HBcAg
+
HBeAg
+
HBsAg

Dane particle

b

referred to as the *Dane particle* (fig. 8.9). It contains an outer shell known as the hepatitis B surface antigen (*HBsAg*), and an inner shell known as the hepatitis B core antigen (*HBcAg*), which holds the viral DNA. A sub-unit of the core antigen known as the hepatitis "Be" antigen (*HBeAg*) is of value as an indicator of an active infection. Many of these viral parts are of importance to diagnosis, determining recovery from infection, and vaccine production.

TRANSMISSION

The likely routes of transmission for HBV are similar to those found with human immunodeficiency viruses (HIVs). Principally, they include homosexual or heterosexual sexual activities, exposure to virus-contaminated blood or blood products, sharing of virus-contaminated injection materials by intravenous drug users, and viral transmission from an infected mother to her fetus or newborn. In addition, health care professionals such as dentists, surgeons, and medical laboratory workers are at an increased risk to HBV infection because of possible exposure to contaminated blood during the performance of their respective jobs.

EPIDEMIOLOGY NOTES

HIV and hepatitis B infections occur with increased frequency in sexually active homosexual men, intravenous drug abusers, recipients of contaminated blood or blood products, infants born to infected mothers, and heterosexual contacts of infected persons. Since both viruses are found in body fluids such as blood, semen, and saliva, their routes of transmission are recognized as being similar.

Infection is more frequently found in individuals who practice anogenital and oral-anal forms of intercourse and rectal douching before or after intercourse. (Douching refers to directing a stream of hot

STD FACT FILE	**DISEASE** HEPATITIS B **CAUSE** HEPATITIS B VIRUS (HBV)

Source/Transmission

Infected humans: sexual activities; rectal intercourse; use of virus-contaminated needles and syringes; contaminated blood and/or blood products. Infected mothers may infect their unborn.

Epidemiology

Disease is found worldwide. Hepatitis B infection is a common problem among homosexual males. Disease may be acquired by nonsexual means including sharing of contaminated needles, injection of virus-contaminated blood or blood products and tattoos made with contaminated needles.

Control

1. Use of condoms during sexual activities
2. Injection of gamma globulin and/or specific antibodies against hepatitis B virus (hepatitis B immunoglobulin)

Prevention

1. Immunization with currently available vaccine
2. Avoidance of anal sexual practices
3. Avoidance of the use of unsterile needles and syringes

or cold water onto or into a body part). The common feature of these practices appears to be injury to the rectum and the probable loss of a small amount of virus-contaminated blood.

Several factors have been shown to predict the outcome of HBV transmission in adults and children. These include the age and resistance (immune status) of the newly infected individual, and the site and route of virus transmission. A summary of the general features of HBV infection are given in the accompanying **STD FACT FILE.**

SIGNS AND SYMPTOMS

Only about 50 percent of hepatitis B virus infections present evidence of disease. The first signs and symptoms of such infections generally appear after an incubation period of 45 to 160 days. They are typical of most viral hepatitis conditions and include weakness, jaundice (a yellowing of the skin and eyes), fever, loss of appetite, abdominal pain, liver tenderness, nausea, vomiting, constipation, and general discomfort. Infected individuals usually pass dark-yellow-to-orange colored urine, and light-colored stools.

The short term of acute infection generally will run its course in three to four weeks. Some symptoms, however, may last for as long as six months.

Infections persisting for more than six months are referred to as the chronic form of the disease. Complications of various kinds can develop with the chronic state. They include liver failure, a breakdown of liver structure known as **cirrhosis** (si-RŌ-sis), and cancer.

Newborns infected by their mothers may be without symptoms. However, if the infection does result in symptoms, they generally include weakness, appetite loss, nausea, abdominal pain, jaundice, and weight loss. Once infected these infants

<table>
<tr>
<td>

THE SIGNS AND SYMPTOMS BOX

</td>
<td>

DISEASE
HEPATITIS B
INCUBATION PERIOD
45–60 DAYS

</td>
</tr>
</table>

First Symptoms Usually Appear: Around 45–60 Days After Exposure, Variable

Signs
1. Yellowing or jaundice
2. Dark orange urine
3. Gray or clay-colored stools
4. Fever

Symptoms
1. Pain in upper, right portion of the body
2. Constipation may or may not occur
3. General weakness
4. Loss of appetite

Complications
1. Inflammation of the liver with moderate enlargement and tenderness
2. Chronic liver disease
3. Liver cancer

may continue to harbor HBV for a long time, and eventually develop the complications mentioned earlier. The features of HBV infection are given in the accompanying **SIGNS & SYMPTOMS BOX**.

DIAGNOSIS

The physical diagnosis of hepatitis in general can be made on such findings as jaundice, dark orange urine, and an enlarged and tender liver. Specific laboratory confirmation of HBV infection is provided by blood tests showing injury to the liver and establishing the presence of specific parts of the virus such as *HBsA* and antibody for the hepatitis B core antigen (*HBcAg*). (Refer to figure 8.9 for an explanation of viral parts.)

TREATMENT

In general, there is no specific medical treatment for any viral hepatitis condition. However, the use of human interferon has shown some promise in chronic cases of the disease. Recovery depends on: the general health of the infected individual, following a routine of adequate rest, and good nutrition.

PREVENTION

Preventing HBV infection in contacts of infected persons may possibly be achieved with the injection of specific HBV antibodies known as **hepatitis B immune globulin** within forty-eight hours after exposure.

A major advance has been made recently in the area of infection prevention. A commercial vaccine (fig. 8.10) is available for use by the general public and health care professionals. It is recommended for a number of individuals, including sexual and household contacts of hepatitis B virus carriers, as well as homosexual males, health care workers with routine exposure to blood, heterosexually active persons with multiple partners, and intravenous drug users.

The vaccine is safe and free from any major side effects. It is a genetically engineered product containing a highly purified form of virus-free HBsAg. Further details of vaccine production and the types of resistance that can be acquired through their use are presented in chapter 15.

INCREASING PRIMARY HEALTH CONCERNS

After years of apathy and neglect, STDs such as genital warts and HBV infection are finally becoming recognized for the magnitude of illnesses they cause and the intensity of human suffering they can generate. Despite the advances being made in the areas of diagnosis, treatment, and vaccine production, avoiding high-risk behavior still remains the most logical way to prevent the STDs described in this and other chapters.

FIGURE 8.10
Examples of successful vaccines available to prevent hepatitis B.
(Courtesy of Smith, Kline and French)

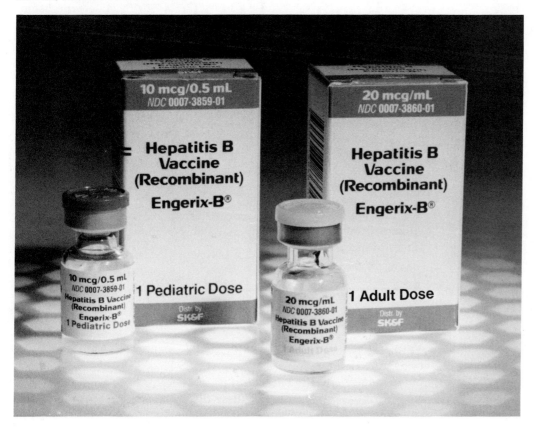

CHAPTER 9

YEASTS, PROTOZOA, AND ECTOPARASITES AS STD AGENTS

It seems logical that the aches or itches which distract ordinary citizens from business or love affairs may become, in chiefs of state, forces of history.

—Arno Karlen, Napoleon's Glands

INTRODUCTION

With increasing knowledge of disease agents that can be sexually transmitted, a number of infections have been found to be common but generally ignored because of the absence or mild nature of symptoms. Unfortunately, some of these disease agents may still cause serious injury to the reproductive system and certainly can be spread to sexual partners. This chapter will pay particular attention to the yeast infection **candidiasis** (kan'-di-DĪ-a-sis), the protozoan disease **trichomoniasis** (trik-ō-mo-NĪ-a-sis) and the infestations caused by the itch or **scabies** (SKĀ-bēz) mite and the pubic or crab louse.

Genital Candidiasis

Genital or vulvovaginal candidiasis (VVC) is found throughout the world and results from infections by the yeast, **Candida albicans** (KAN-di-da, AL-bi-kans) and related yeastlike microorganisms (fig. 9.1). Generally a yeast infection is a minor condition in both sexes, but its high incidence and frequent recurrences, especially in women, along with the accompanying discomfort makes the disease of special concern. In many countries VVC remains the commonest form of vaginal infection, especially in the warmer climates. It is estimated that about 75 percent of all women will experience at least one episode of this disease.

Cause and Transmission

Yeasts favor moist skin surfaces and mucous membranes. They are frequently isolated from the mouth, throat, large intestine, and vagina of normal, healthy individuals. *C. albicans* has been identified as the cause of several diseases, of which candidal vaginitis and vulvovaginitis in women, and inflammation of the glans penis, known as **balanitis** (bal-a-NĪ-tis), in men, may be sexually acquired. In the United States, candidal vaginitis is second only to the bacterial form of the disease (chapter 6) and three times more frequent than *Trichomonas* vaginitis described in the next major section of this chapter. Vaginal candidiasis also occurs in sexually inactive women.

Women acquiring *vaginal candidiasis* through sexual intercourse is probably infrequent. However, men contract infection with the yeast from women with vaginal candidiasis. A relationship between oral sex and genital candidiasis has also been reported.

Infants born to vaginally infected mothers are at risk of developing *Candida* infection of the mouth known as *oral thrush* (fig. 9.2).

Epidemiology Notes

Several factors are known to predispose individuals to or trigger genital and other forms of candidiasis. These include pregnancy, cancer, overweight, use of oral birth control pills, diabetes, and a breakdown

Figure 9.1

The appearance of the yeast *Candida albicans* (From M. D. Steinmetz, J. Moulin-Traffort, and P. Régli, *Mycoses* (1987) 31:40–51.)

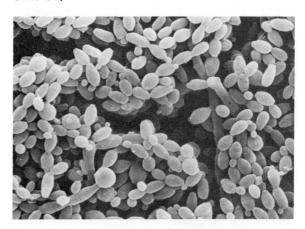

of the immune system. Pregnancy and menstruation seem to aggravate yeast infections, as does the long and continued use of certain antibiotics, steroids, or drugs that interfere with the functions of the immune system. Although the influence of some oral contraceptives is not entirely clear, their continued use does increase the risk of genital yeast infections. The increased warmth and moisture produced by the wearing of tight-fitting clothing such as jeans, and nylon or synthetic fiber undergarments also are contributing factors. Selected features of genital candidiasis are given in the accompanying **STD FACT FILE.**

Signs and Symptoms

About 30 percent of infected women may not show symptoms. Others experience mild to severe symptoms. The common complaints reported by symptomatic women include intense itching and, at times, soreness of the vulva and the area around the anus, a burning sensation both during and after intercourse, and pain or burning if urine comes into contact with an irritated vulva. On physical examination, a reddened and swollen vulva, and the presence of a thick, cottage-cheese-like discharge in the vagina (fig. 9.3a) are commonly found. The discharge, which may stick to vaginal walls in the form

FIGURE 9.2
A case of a yeast infection of the mouth.

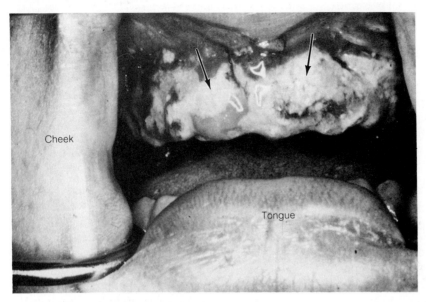

Cheek

Tongue

STD FACT
FILE

DISEASE
GENITAL THRUSH, OR CANDIDIASIS (kan'-di-DĪ-a-sis)
CAUSE
THE YEAST, CANDIDA ALBICANS (KAN-di-da, AL-bi-kans)

Source/Transmission
Infected humans. Infections are sexually transmitted in about 40 percent of cases. Transmission of *C. albicans* by oral sex acts has been reported.

Epidemiology
Disease is worldwide. Currently, *C. albicans* is the most common potential pathogen in the female genital tract. Several factors may predispose to candidiasis: cancer, diabetes, pregnancy, menstruation, and possible side effects of certain antibiotics.

Control
Prompt diagnosis and treatment with appropriate antifungal agents

Prevention
Not wearing tight-fitting jeans and nylon or synthetic fiber undergarments may help to prevent recurrences.

FIGURE 9.3

Genital yeast infection candidiasis. (a) The involvement of the vagina. A white, cottage-cheese-like discharge (arrows) generally sticking to the sides of the vagina and cervix is a common finding. (b) A case of male candidiasis. Here the patches of the yeast can be seen on the glans of the penis. (Courtesy of Centers for Disease Control)

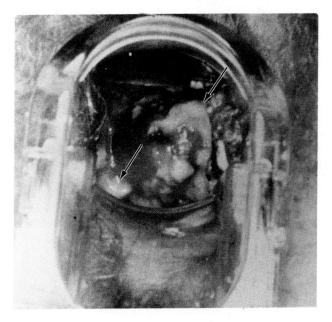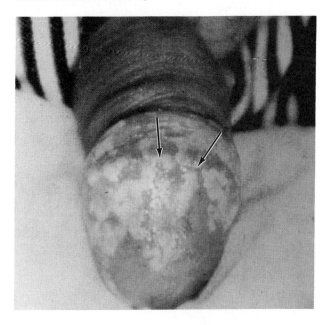

of white patches, appears to be more common in pregnant women.

Men with genital candidiasis may have few or no symptoms. Penile itching, irritation, and burning are among the common complaints of infected persons. The signs of infection range from small red spots and blisters to the appearance of white patches on the glans (fig. 9.3a) and other parts of the male genitalia.

A general summary of the features of genital candidiasis is given in the accompanying **SIGNS & SYMPTOMS BOX.**

DIAGNOSIS

Quite commonly the diagnosis of a genital yeast infection is based on physical examination and laboratory findings. In the laboratory simple microscopic examinations of specimens are used to exclude the presence of other possible causes such as the protozoan **Trichomonas vaginalis** (trik-ō-MŌ-nas, VAJ-in-a-lis), and the various bacterial disease agents described in chapter 6. Unfortunately, yeast infections

FIGURE 9.4

The creamy, white growth of the yeast *Candida albicans* obtained from a specimen taken from an individual with genital candidiasis. Growing the yeast in the laboratory is the most reliable method for identification.

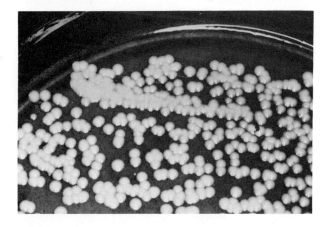

can be missed if diagnosis depends only on such examinations. Thus, the culture of specimens is used as a reliable method of identification for both symptomatic and asymptomatic cases (fig. 9.4).

DISEASE
CANDIDIASIS (kan-di-DĪ-a-sis)
INCUBATION PERIOD
VARIABLE

First Symptoms Usually Appear: Variable

Signs

Men
1. White discharge from penis
2. Itching patches on the penis and scrotum

Symptoms
1. Generally no symptoms are present
2. When symptoms are noticeable they can include:
   a. Itching areas on penis and scrotum
   b. Redness and soreness around anus

Women
1. Thick cheesy vaginal discharge

1. Intense itching of genitalia
2. Burning sensation on urination

Complications

Women
Secondary bacterial infections of genitalia and reproductive system

Newborn
Mouth and throat infections resulting from passing through an infected birth canal

TREATMENT

A number of antifungal products such as nystatin (NIS-ta-tin) and miconazole (mī-KON-a-zōl) are available for the treatment of genital candidiasis. These include creams, lotions, aerosol sprays, and vaginal tablets. Usually the first step in the local or surface treatment requires a gentle cleansing of the infected area. This is then followed by applying an antifungal cream or other product. Oral medications also are available.

TRICHOMONIASIS OR TRICHOMONAS INFECTION

The symptoms of **vulvovaginitis** (vul'-vō-vaj'-i-NĪ-tis), which include an abnormal vaginal discharge, local itching and/or irritation, and a noticeable odor, cause a substantial number of individuals to seek treatment for a possible STD. The most common causes of the condition include the yeast *C. albicans* (described earlier in this chapter), the bacterium *Gardnerella vaginalis* (described in chapter 6), and the protozoan *Trichomonas vaginalis*. Of these diseases agents, *Trichomonas* has been most traditionally linked with sexual transmission. Selected features of this disease are given in the accompanying **STD FACT FILE.**

A CASE OF VVC

A twenty-one-year-old woman went to a local STD clinic because of a persistent sharp pain in her lower back and severe vaginal itching and burning. She also was experiencing some discomfort and pain during sexual intercourse.

In obtaining her personal history, it was learned that the young lady was a waitress for several years at a well-known coffee shop. She was required to wear a tight fitting uniform which included black nylon pantyhose. The job was quite demanding and quite often the patient went directly to bed in her work clothes. About two weeks earlier, she had begun to notice a slight cream-colored cheesy vaginal discharge. Soon thereafter the vaginal itching and burning sensation began.

On physical examination, the vulva and the folds of skin between the vulva and the legs were fiery red in color. The redness extended to the anus. Crack-like sores in these areas, and a whitish cheesy vaginal discharge also were noted. Specimens for laboratory study were taken.

On the basis of the various physical examination findings, an antifungal topical cream was prescribed and the patient was told to apply the medication twice daily and to return to the clinic in a week. She was also asked to refer her sexual partners to the clinic.

The laboratory findings showed the presence of *Candida albicans* in all the specimens studied.

The patient did not return to the clinic. In addition, the sexual partners did not appear.

DISEASE
TRICHOMONIASIS (trik-o-mō-NI-a-sis), ALSO KNOWN AS TRICH AND TV
CAUSE
THE PROTOZOAN, TRICHOMONAS VAGINALIS (trik'-Ō-MŌ-nas, VAJ-in-a-lis)

Source/Transmission
Infected individuals; sexually transmitted. Very few infections may result from direct contact with contaminated examination instruments, or bath or toilet articles.

Epidemiology
The disease is worldwide. Trichomoniasis is highest in women between the ages of 16 to 35. Infection is common in sexual partners of women having the higher incidence of the condition.

Control
Treatment of infected individual

Prevention
Treatment of all sex partners, whether having symptoms or not

CAUSE AND TRANSMISSION

The role of *T. vaginalis* as a major disease agent in human urogenital infections was established in the first half of this century. A significant percentage of volunteer women and men inoculated with the microorganism developed typical signs and symptoms of trichomoniasis.

Several lines of evidence also have established the importance of sexual contact in the transmission of *T. vaginalis*. This disease agent accounts for up to 25 percent of all symptomatic vaginal infections in the United States. About 180 million new cases occur each year on a worldwide basis. The highest incidence of infection occurs between the ages of sixteen to thirty-five. Among the consistently described risk factors associated with transmission are increased levels of sexual activity and multiple sex partners. Infection is common among prostitutes and uncommon in virgins.

Trichomoniasis is most prevalent among the sex partners of infected persons. About 30 to 40 percent of male sex partners are found to harbor the causative agent.

Nonsexual transmission of *T. vaginalis* in adults is relatively infrequent. Newborns may acquire the disease agent by passing through the birth canal to an infected mother. Such infections occur in about 5 percent of female babies born to infected mothers.

Finding the disease agent in young, premenstrual girls can indicate some form of sexual abuse.

SIGNS AND SYMPTOMS

Incubation periods for trichomoniasis vary from three to twenty-eight days. Among the usual signs found with the infection in women is the presence of a bubbly, yellow-green and foul-smelling vaginal discharge. Itching and local irritation of the vulvogenital area may also be experienced by some infected women (color photograph 20). Symptoms appear to be more intense during menstruation. Many women may be asymptomatic. The presence of gonorrhea is about three times higher in women with trichomoniasis than among women without this infection.

The majority of infected men are without symptoms. Many seek treatment because their sexual partners show symptoms. Approximately 20 percent of men with gonorrhea harbor *Trichomonas*. This finding emphasizes the importance of a thorough examination of individuals for other STDs.

Female babies born to infected mothers exhibit a vaginal discharge. Some may even have a fever and show signs of a urinary infection. A summary of the features of trichomoniasis is given in the accompanying SIGNS & SYMPTOMS BOX.

DIAGNOSIS

While a physical examination of an infected woman may reveal a reddening and general swelling of the involved genital area, actual diagnosis is dependent on the basis of microscopic examination of the vaginal discharge. Pap smears described in chapter 4 also may show evidence of an infection. Urine, genital secretions, or urethral specimens are used for diagnosis in the case of an infected male. Finding the disease agent in such specimens (fig. 9.5) is generally sufficient for diagnosis. Special staining and culture techniques also are used.

TREATMENT

Treatment for trichomoniasis was inadequate until the early 1960s. It is now available and relatively straightforward. Metronidazole generally is the drug used.

SEXUALLY TRANSMITTED ECTOPARASITES

Certain forms of disease-causing agents are able to live on or in the skin of their hosts. Such forms of life are called **ectoparasites** and the relationship is referred to as an **infestation** (in-fes-TA-shun). Scabies and **phthiriasis** (thir-Ī-a-sis), or the crabs, are two examples of sexually transmitted diseases that fall into the category of infestations.

SCABIES—THE "ITCH"
CAUSE AND TRANSMISSION

Scabies is an infestation caused by the mite **Sarcoptes scabies,** variety **hominis** (sar-KOP-tēz, SKA-bēz, variety HOM-i-nis). This mite (fig. 9.6b), which

FIGURE 9.5

A microscopic view of a specimen taken from a patient with *Trichomonas*–caused vaginitis. Large numbers of the protozoan are shown. (Courtesy of Centers for Disease Control)

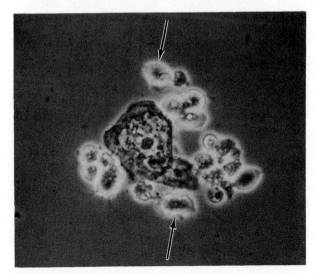

can barely be seen by the naked eye, is spread only through close contact. The ectoparasite can barely survive being off the human body for more than a few minutes.

Scabies is one of the few sexually transmitted diseases which is also often spread nonsexually in households and other areas. It may be transmitted by close contact with infected persons such as bedfellows, family members, or patients in a variety of health care facilities. Cases of scabies can occur where children exchange clothing or spend the night at one another's homes. Infested dogs also may be a source of mites.

In sexually active young adults, sexual transmission is likely. Moreover, scabies is more readily transmitted when partners spend the night together, rather than by brief sexual contact as in the cases of syphilis and gonorrhea. In recent years, mite

FIGURE 9.6

Scabies in an AIDS patient. (a) The involvement of the hands by the scabies mite. (b) The scabies mite obtained from a skin scraping. The original magnification is 40X. (From J. C. Hall, J. H. Brewer, and B. A. Appl, *Cutis* (1989) 43:325.)

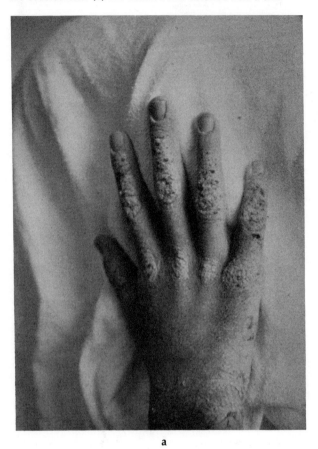

a

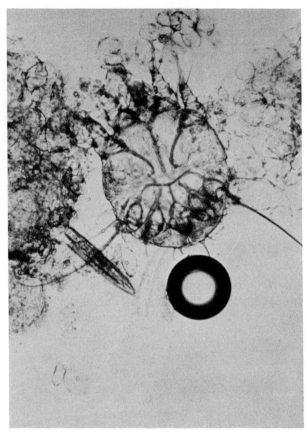

b

infestation is frequently seen in sexually active homosexuals.

BACKGROUND

The itch mite was discovered in 1687, and marked scabies as the first human disease with a known cause. The general features of the disease are given in the accompanying **STD FACT FILE.**

The adult female itch mite has a round body and four pairs of legs, which allow it to walk rapidly on skin surfaces. After finding a suitable location, the female mite digs or burrows into the top skin layers. Within a few hours, she begins to lay two or three eggs per day. These hatch and eventually develop into adult mites in about ten days. It is not unusual to find ten or more mites on one infested person. The greater the mite load in an individual, the greater is the likelihood of transmission.

SIGNS AND SYMPTOMS

The first signs of scabies appear within four weeks after contact with an infected person. This time is needed by the mite to develop from the egg to the adult stage. Normally, all parts of the body except the face may be infested by the scabies mite. Infants and individuals with immune system defects, or so-called **immunocompromised persons,** may have face involvement.

The characteristic feature of the disease is the **skin burrow** or irregular dirty-appearing line formed by the movement of a pregnant female mite. At times, reddened blisters formed near the end of the burrow indicate an allergic reaction. Infested individuals generally experience intense itching at night in involved areas. Since the mite favors the cooler parts of the body, burrows and blisters often are located on the penis, scrotum (color photograph 21) and breast. Fingers often are the first areas involved (fig. 9.6a). Other body parts frequently infected include the waist, buttocks, ankles, abdomen, and the area around the armpits. The general features of scabies are given in the accompanying **SIGNS & SYMPTOMS BOX.**

A rare form of this infestation, known as *crusted* or *Norwegian scabies,* may develop in mentally retarded, physically disabled, or immunocompromised individuals. The condition is highly contagious because of the large number of mites present in the crusts that develop on the skin. Whereas the usual number of female mites is about ten to fifty per person in a typical scabies case, an individual with the Norwegian form of the infestation may have hundreds.

Diagnosis

Scabies is generally diagnosed by finding any stage of the mite or its typical black fecal pellets, known as **scybala** (SIB-a-la), in lesions. Skin specimens may be obtained by vigorous scraping with an oiled sterile scalpel over the involved area to remove the tops of several burrows. This material is transferred to a glass slide and examined microscopically.

Another approach used is the **burrow ink tests** or **BIT.** Here a burrow is rubbed with the underside of an inexpensive pen so as to cover it with ink. An alcohol-soaked pad then is used to remove the excess ink from the surface. The remaining ink flows into the mite burrow forming a characteristic dark, zigzag line extending across and away from the entrance to the burrow.

Treatment and Control

Several **miticides** (MĪ-ti-sīds) or **scabicides** (SKĀ-bi-sīds) are available for treatment of infested individuals. These include lindane (LIN-dan), and crotamiton (krō'-ta-MĪ-ton) creams. All materials should be applied as directed. Sexual contacts and family members of an infested person also should be treated. In addition, mite-containing articles such as clothing, pajamas, and bedding should be washed in hot water, and laundered accordingly.

Since some individuals with scabies may experience extreme itching, medication may be needed to provide relief. Another problem that may develop is a bacterial infection due to the scratching and contamination of the mite burrows. In such cases antibiotics usually are used to control the problem.

Norwegian Scabies and AIDS — Pubic Lice or the "Crabs"

For many years, the louse, a wingless insect, was confused with the scabies mite. However, since the mid-1800s the true nature of lice was recognized. Today, three different types of lice are known to afflict humans. These are the **body louse, head louse** and the **pubic** or **crab louse.** Since the head louse is usually a problem for children only, and the body louse usually lives on or in clothing rather than on the human, the following discussion will be limited only to the crab louse.

Cause and Transmission

Phthiriasis (thir-Ī-a-sis), or crab louse infestation, is easily spread by sexual contact, the major means of transmission. The crab louse, or **Pthirus pubis** (THIR-us, PŪ-bis), favors the pubic region, where it resides and feeds. However, these lice can find a home elsewhere on the body, wherever there is hair. Such sites include the armpits, eyebrows, and eyelashes.

Infestations can also result from contact with lice-containing bath towels, bedding, and toilet seats.

Background

The crab louse is broader than it is long (fig. 9.7). Its second and third pairs of legs have crablike claws, which help the louse to firmly attach to pubic hairs. The life cycle of this ectoparasite, egg to egg is about twenty-five to thirty days. It can live away from the body of a host for only a few days since the louse must have a blood meal on a regular basis for survival.

Epidemiology Notes

Sharp increases in the number of crab louse infestations have occurred in the United States and western Europe. These increases are believed to be related to the so-called recent sexual revolution, especially in young unmarried individuals. About one-third of crab louse cases also have other STDs, including gonorrhea, chlamydial infection, and trichomoniasis. Among fifteen-to-nineteen-year-old's, the infestation is more common in females than in males. However, it is more common in males than in females over twenty years of age. The general features of pubic louse infestation are given in the accompanying **STD FACT FILE.**

Signs and Symptoms

The most common area affected in a case of crabs is the pubic region. Intense itching is the most obvious symptom of the infestation. Other areas that

NORWEGIAN SCABIES AND AIDS

A thirty-year-old man was first seen by his family physician in April 1989. He appeared extremely tired, and exhibited swollen lymph glands in his neck. The man complained of a severe headache, blocked sinuses, and a chest cold. Laboratory blood tests suggested the possibility of a developing human immunodeficiency virus (HIV) infection. Antibiotics and other appropriate medications were given to the patient to control his various symptoms.

Some eight months later, the patient noted a growing loss of appetite, sudden weight loss, regularly occurring night sweating, and periodic bouts of fever and chills. He went back to the family physician because he also noticed a skin rash on his legs, buttocks, and genitalia. On the basis of the rash's appearance the patient was given an ointment to apply to the involved areas. After two weeks' use of the ointment the rash disappeared only to reappear some three months later. The rash itched terribly and involved most surfaces of the body. Skin scrapings were taken and sent to the laboratory. The specimens showed the presence of scabies mites.

A similar medication was given to the patient with the same general directions for applying it, and told to come back in one week. Unfortunately, the condition became worse over the week, and a bacterial infection developed in addition, due to the scratching of the blisters. The patient was hospitalized. He was given antibiotics for the bacterial infection, and treated with cool water baths and medications for the scabies. The entire body, with the exception of the eyelids, was treated for the scabies eruption. This time the approach used was effective. The patient was asked to refer his sexual partners for an examination and possible treatment.

DISEASE
PHTHIRIASIS (thir-Ī-a-sis), ALSO KNOWN AS "CRABS"
CAUSE
PTHIRUS PUBIS (THIR-us, PŪ-bis), THE CRAB LOUSE

Source/Transmission
Infested humans; sexual contact. Crabs also can be spread nonsexually by contact with lice-infested bath towels, bedding, and toilet seats.

Epidemiology
Disease is found worldwide. At least one-third of infested individuals have additional STDs such as gonorrhea, chlamydial infections, or trichomoniasis. Crabs are found more commonly in females than in males aged 15 to 19, and more in males than females over 20 years of age.

Control
Prompt treatment of infested individuals

Prevention
1. Treatment of all sexual contacts
2. Appropriate tests should be made for the detection of other STDs

FIGURE 9.7
(a) A microscopic view of the pubic louse. (Courtesy of the Reed and Carnrick Pharmaceutical Company). (b) An egg (nit) at the base of a hair. Nits usually hatch within seven days.

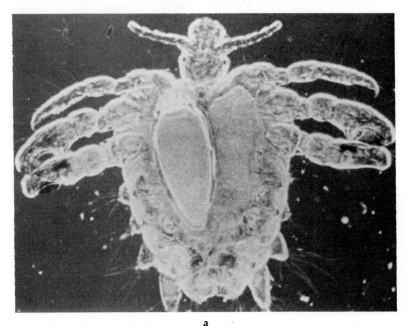

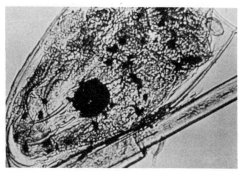

a   b

may be involved include the thighs, the trunk of the body, and hairy regions such as eyelashes, eyebrows, mustache, and beard.

At times characteristic sky-blue spots may develop on the thigh and trunk (fig. 9.8). These lesions generally fade within a short time. See the accompanying **SIGNS & SYMPTOMS BOX** for other features of this STD.

DIAGNOSIS

Interestingly, the diagnosis of crabs frequently is made by the infested host. Most commonly, the diagnosis is made by finding and identifying adult lice and/or their numerous eggs, or *nits,* on or near pubic hairs (fig. 9.7b). Pubic lice infestation is one of the few STDs that can be diagnosed by physical examination alone.

THE SIGNS AND SYMPTOMS BOX

DISEASE
PHTHIRIASIS (thir-Ī-a-sis), ALSO KNOWN AS "CRABS"

INCUBATION PERIOD
4–5 WEEKS

First Symptoms Usually Appear: Within 4 Weeks

Signs
1. The development of sky-blue spots on the thigh or trunk of the body. (These spots fade after a short time.)

Symptoms
1. Itching in and around the groin and other involved areas

Complications
Bacterial infections caused by scratching

FIGURE 9.8

One form of skin eruption found in a patient with a pubic louse infestation. (From S. Brenner and I. Yust, *Cutis* (1988) 41:281.)

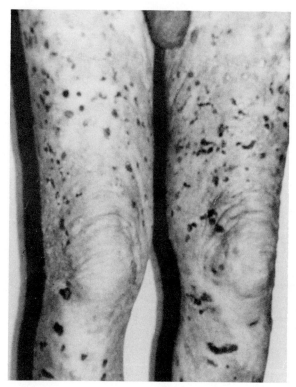

TREATMENT

Several different medications are available for treatment. Medications such as lindane are applied to the infested hairy and surrounding areas, with specific attention to the pubic area and perianal region. All sexual partners also should undergo treatment to prevent reinfestation. Possible infested underclothes, sheets, and pajamas should be washed and cleaned by machine. A hot cycle is necessary to insure that all lice and their eggs or nits have been destroyed.

THE WORLD'S HEALTH AND STDs

The broad range and general features of sexually transmitted diseases have been described in the chapters of part 2. Even though STDs are preventable for the most part, large numbers of individuals still fall victim to one or more of them. On a worldwide basis, the World Health Organization reports that one out of every twenty young adults contracts such diseases each year. The current STD epidemic is clearly more than a medical problem. Its control will depend on education and behavioral change, prompt diagnosis and treatment, and the cooperation of the infected and his or her sexual contacts.

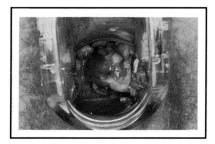

1. Vaginal discharge (Courtesy of Centers for Disease Control, CDC)

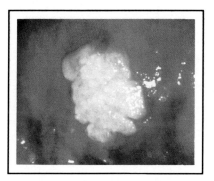

2. A cervix infected with the genital wart virus (From Dunlop, T.M.C., A. Garner, S. Darougar, J.D. Treharne, and R.M. Woodland. *Genitourinary Medicine.* **65**:22–31, (1989).)

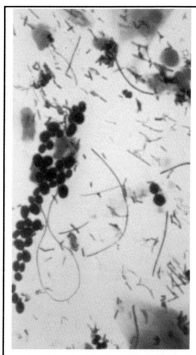

3. Microscopic view of a vaginal infection caused by the oval yeast cells shown.

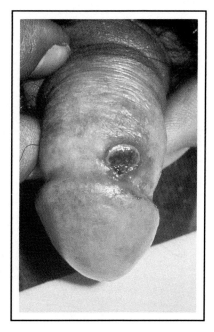

4. Chancroid (From McCarley, M. E., P. D. Cruz, and R. D. Sontheimer, *Journal of American Academy of Dermatology.* **19**:330–337, (1989).)

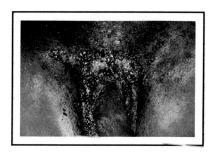

5. The sores of a chronic genital herpes infection involving the scrotum (From Alessi, E., M. Casini. and Z. Zerboni. *Journal of American Academy of Dermatology.* **19**:290–297 (1988).)

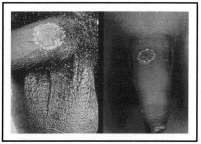

6. The hard chancre of syphilis (Courtesy CDC)

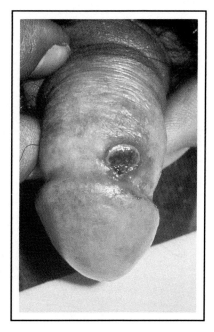

7. The soft chancre of chancroid (Courtesy CDC)

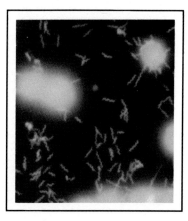

8. A microscopic view of syphilis spirochetes stained green with a fluorescent dye. (Courtesy CDC)

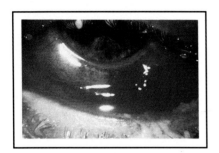

9. The appearance of an infected inner eyelid. (Courtesy CDC)

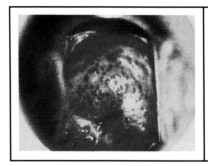

10. Chlamydial STDs. Cervicitis (left). Urethritis (right). (Courtesy Syva Company)

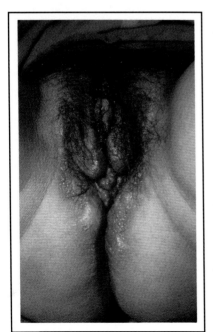

11. Elephantiasis (Courtesy CDC)

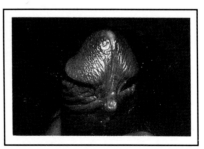

12. LGV in the male (Courtesy CDC)

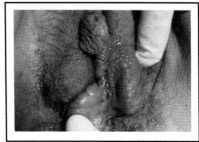

13. LGV in the female (Courtesy CDC)

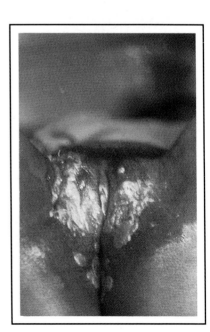

14. Granuloma inguinale (Courtesy CDC)

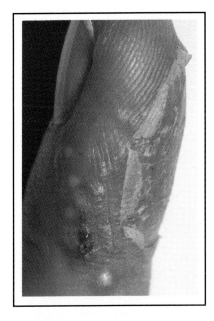

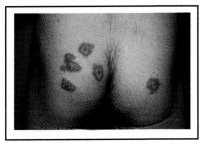

16a. Primary herpes infection of the buttocks (From Greenhouse, P.R.D.H., and R.N. Thin. *British Journal of Venereal Diseases*. **60**:346–348 (1984).)

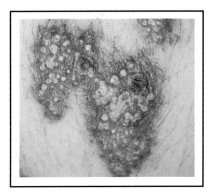

16b. A close-up view of blisters, and crusts (From Greenhouse, P.R.D.H., and R.N. Thin. *British Journal of Venereal Diseases*. **60**:346–348. (1984).)

15. Herpes infection of the finger.

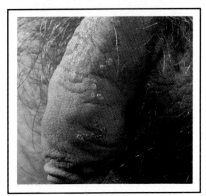

17a. Primary genital herpes

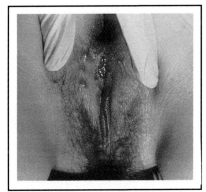

17b. Primary genital herpes of the vulva (Courtesy CDC)

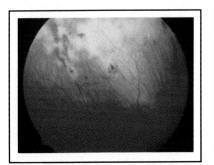

18. CMV destruction of the lining (retina) of the eye (yellow area). (From Palestine, A.G. *Revs. of Infectious Diseases*. **10**:5515, (1988).)

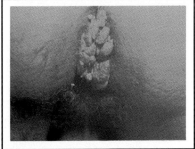

19. Anal warts (Courtesy CDC)

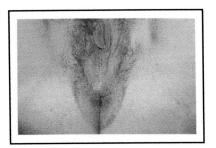

20. *Trichomonas* infection. (From Blackwell, A. *The Practitioner*. **229**:987–995. (1985).)

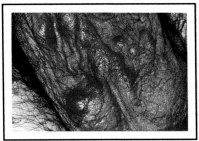

21. Scabies on a scrotum.

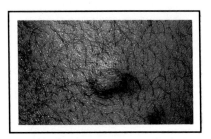

22. Kaposi's sarcoma on the skin (Courtesy CDC)

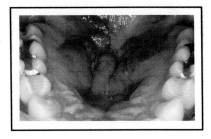

23. The purple growths of Kaposi's sarcoma in the mouth (Courtesy CDC)

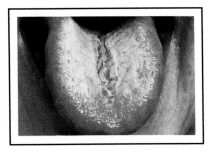

24. Yeast infection of the tongue (From Cohen, P. R. and Kurzrock, R. *Cutis*. **40**:406–409 (1981).)

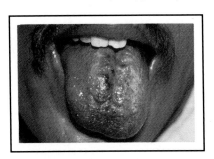

25. Opportunists at work, HSV and bacterial infections of the tongue (From Cohen, P.R. and R. Kurzruck. *Cutis*. **40**:406–409, (1987).)

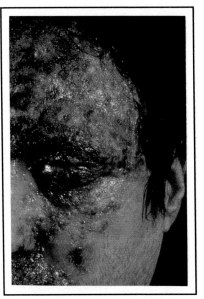

26. Severe form of shingles in an HIV infection. (From Alessi, E., M. Cusini, and R. Zerboni. *Journal American Academy of Dermatology* **19**:290–297, (1988).)

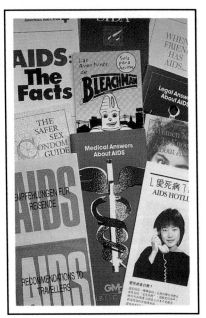

27. Example of the range of brochures dealing with AIDS

PART 3 | THE HUMAN IMMUNODEFICIENCY VIRUS (HIV) SPECTRUM

Numbers from the World Health Organization make it quite clear that acquired immune deficiency syndrome (AIDS) will remain a global health problem for many years to come. Because reporting of disease cases is not totally complete, the 1989–1990 worldwide estimates place the number of individuals infected with the human immunodeficiency virus to be about five to ten million.

Since the first reported cases of AIDS in 1981, research efforts against this disease have yielded an enormous amount of information. Unfortunately, however, it is unlikely that science will conquer HIV infection any time soon. Continued efforts to educate people on the nature of the disease and how to avoid HIV infection currently appears to be humanity's best hope against AIDS.

The AIDS epidemic continues to reveal a great deal of previously unknown facts concerning the interrelationships between social behavior, sexually transmitted diseases, opportunistic infections, cancer, and individual resistance or immunity. The chapters in part 3 provide basic knowledge and a general understanding of these and related topics.

Before going on to the chapters in part 3, test your general knowledge of HIV infection and AIDS by taking **THE 12 QUESTION AIDS CHALLENGE.**

THE 12 QUESTION AIDS CHALLENGE

Test your general knowledge of HIV infection and AIDS by answering the following questions. Indicate your responses by checking either the *true* or *false* box provided next to each question number. The answers and brief comments are given at the end of the test.

RESPONSE COLUMNS

TRUE   FALSE

QUESTION COLUMN

TRUE	FALSE	
☐	☐	1. HIV transmission has been found to occur mainly by blood, semen, cervical secretions, and (rarely) human breast milk of infected individuals.
☐	☐	2. HIV may be spread by insects.
☐	☐	3. HIV may be spread during physical contact sports such as football, boxing, or wrestling.
☐	☐	4. The use of condoms is an effective, but not a foolproof way to prevent the spread of HIV.
☐	☐	5. The risk of HIV infection to health care workers such as nurses and doctors who are taking care of HIV-infected or AIDS patients is low.
☐	☐	6. The human immunodeficiency virus can be quickly inactivated by common germicides such as ordinary household bleach.
☐	☐	7. HIV is spread by three main ways: a) having sex, vaginal, oral, or anal, with an infected person; b) sharing drug needles and syringes with an infected user; and c) an infected mother transmitting the virus to the baby before or during birth.
☐	☐	8. HIV infection can result from contact with the saliva, sweat, tears, or urine of a person with AIDS.
☐	☐	9. Recently, HIV-infected persons do not exhibit any symptoms.
☐	☐	10. HIV infection in persons practicing high-risk behavior may develop long before antibodies to the virus may be detected by blood tests.
☐	☐	11. HIV-infected children who are old enough to attend school can be admitted freely to all activities to the extent their own health permits.
☐	☐	12. Symptoms alone cannot be used to make a diagnosis of AIDS.

THE ANSWERS

1. **TRUE.** Even though the human immunodeficiency virus has been found in other body fluids, such as tears, saliva, and urine, infection has not been reported by contact with these materials.
2. **FALSE.** No reports of HIV transmission by mosquitoes or other insects have been verified.
3. **FALSE.** No studies or reports have shown HIV transmission by any form of athletic activity.
4. **TRUE.** To be effective condoms should be put on either before or during foreplay. This point also applies to oral and anal sex.
5. **TRUE.** The number of HIV infections among health care workers is low in proportion to the number employed by this industry. Most infections developed from one or more exposures to infectious body fluids and a needle stick injury.
6. **TRUE.** HIV is quite sensitive to a 1:10 dilution of ordinary bleach and water.
7. **TRUE.** These are the major ways for HIV transmission. Donated sperm from sperm banks used for artificial insemination (fertilization) and infected bones used for transplantation, while rare in occurrence, also have been reported to result in HIV infections.
8. **FALSE.** There are no reports of infection with these materials, because the HIV concentration is very low in these fluids.
9. **TRUE.** The appearance of symptoms of AIDS in an HIV-infected adult generally will take a substantial period of time. While the average incubation period for the disease is about six to seven years, indications of AIDS may appear within four to five years after incubation.
10. **TRUE.** Recent studies have demonstrated the presence of the virus at least two years before blood tests became positive for HIV infection.
11. **TRUE.** No studies or reports exist showing the transmission of HIV by HIV-infected children to others in day-care or school settings.
12. **TRUE.** The symptoms of AIDS are similar to many of those found with individuals experiencing other types of diseases affecting the immune system. Specific laboratory tests are needed to confirm AIDS.

10 THE IMMUNE SYSTEM

The development of immunity (resistance) in its broadest sense is a process by which the body learns from experience of past infections to deal more efficiently with subsequent ones.

—Sir Macfarlane Burnet

INTRODUCTION

Humans are protected in varying degrees from disease-causing microorganisms and cancers by various body cells and organs, which collectively form an **immune system.** Together, the different parts of this system provide protection, or **immunity,** by establishing barriers to invasion by infectious microorganisms or other disease agents, or by selectively neutralizing or eliminating materials recognized by the immune system as being foreign and life threatening. Used in a general way immunity refers to the ability of a host to recognize and to protect against disease. **Susceptibility,** on the other hand, is the opposite of immunity and refers to the vulnerability of a host to injury by a disease agent and/or its products.

The human body has several general defenses against disease, regardless of the type of invading pathogen involved. The immunity provided by such defenses, which include the skin and the antimicrobial substances in saliva, are considered **nonspecific.** Nonspecific defenses serve as the body's first line of defense and operate to prevent disease agents from entering the body, or if they do, to destroy them before any injury occurs.

The body is also able to respond directly to the disease agent. Such immunological responses are considered to be specific since they are provoked by and tailored to defend against particular foreign substances known as **antigens.** Specific defenses form the body's second line of defense. Both types of host's defenses serve two major functions: *1) defense against invasion by microorganisms;* and *2) surveillance for or recognition of abnormal cell types and their destruction.*

In a time when the health concerns of the public are heightened or in many cases caused by AIDS and other STDs that have firmly established themselves in the mainstream of society, there is a particular need for an understanding of the potential benefits and limitations of the body's immune system. This chapter deals with the various means and mechanisms by which the body normally combats infectious disease agents. We shall see what happens when such protection fails and what factors and conditions lower an individual's resistance.

BLOOD AND ITS FUNCTIONS

Various means and mechanisms are used by the body to normally combat infectious disease agents and other factors recognized by the body's unique defensive immune system as being **foreign.** To understand this system and how certain pathogens such as HIV can cause infection some background information about blood and its role in health and disease states is needed.

The circulatory system consists of the **heart, blood vessels,** and the **blood.** This system supplies oxygen and nutrients to all parts of the body and removes carbon dioxide and other wastes from them. Blood leaving the heart circulates through a closed system of blood vessels and subsequently returns to the heart. Its flow is regulated so that all cells receive nutrients and get rid of wastes according to their needs.

BLOOD—AN OVERVIEW

Blood participates in the removal and, in certain situations, the destruction of foreign substances and invading microorganisms. It can also play an important role in the transmission, development, diagnosis, cure, and prevention of many diseases caused by microorganisms and other agents.

The cells and other components of blood have important functions in preventing infections and protecting the body from disease. Brief descriptions of their respective functions and related properties are described here to provide a basis with which to understand selected aspects of the immune system.

THE COMPONENTS

Sixty percent of blood consists of a liquid called **plasma,** and 40 percent of **formed elements,** which are cells and cell fragments (fig. 10.1). Plasma is mainly water, and contains proteins such as **albumins** (al-BŪ-mins) **globulins,** and **fibrinogen** (fī-BRIN-ō-jen). Albumins play important roles in maintaining adequate levels of cellular nutrition and a stable internal environment in the body. Certain globulins are important in defending the body against infection. Most protective proteins, called **antibodies** or **immunoglobulins** (im'-ū-nō-GLOB-ū-lins), are found in the **gamma globulin** portion of plasma. Fibrinogen is important in the blood clotting process. In contrast to plasma, **serum,** a yellowish fluid remains after blood clots. It also contains albumins and globulins.

The formed elements of the blood include red blood cells, or **erythrocytes** (e-RITH-rō-sīts), white blood cells, or **leukocytes** (LOO-kō-sīts), and **platelets.** Red blood cells are the most plentiful of the formed elements. They account for 40 to 45 percent of the total volume of blood. Their presence and quantity are important to the oxygen-carrying capacity of the blood because red blood cells contain the oxygen-binding protein **hemoglobin.** If the body does not produce sufficient numbers of these cells or produces hemoglobin-deficient cells a condition known as **anemia** (a-NĒ-mē-a) develops.

Leukocytes contribute to various nonspecific and specific defenses of the body. They are divided into two groups based on certain cellular features. These are: 1) the **granulocytes** (GRAN-ū-lō-sīts), which have little cytoplasmic masses or granules, and oddly

FIGURE 10.1

The relationship of blood components to one another. Both plasma (liquid portion) and the formed elements are shown. The buffy coat contains platelets and various types of white blood cells.

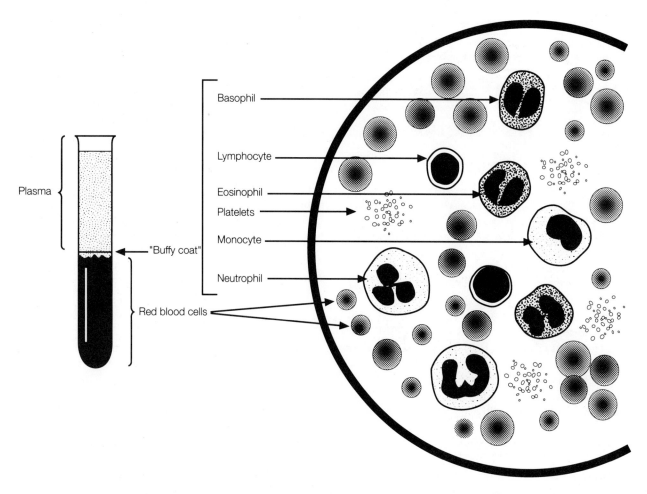

Plasma

"Buffy coat"

Red blood cells

Basophil

Lymphocyte

Eosinophil

Platelets

Monocyte

Neutrophil

shaped nuclei; and 2) the **agranulocytes** (a-GRAN-ū-lō-sīts), which lack granules, and have somewhat rounded nuclei. Based on staining reactions in the laboratory three types of granulocytes are recognized: **neutrophils** (NŪ-tro-fils), **eosinophils** (ē'-ō-SIN-ō-fils), and **basophils** (BA-so-fils). Agranulocytes include **monocytes** and **lymphocytes.** Platelets, fragments of large cells called **megakaryocytes** (meg'-a-KAR-ē-ō-sīts), are important participants in blood clotting.

LEUKOCYTES AND BODY DEFENSES

When a disease agent gains entrance to the blood, several defense mechanisms come into play. For example, through the process of **phagocytosis** (fag-ō-sī-TO-sis), many invaders are engulfed and destroyed before they can penetrate other areas of the body (fig. 10.2). In other situations involving pathogens for which the body has developed immunity,

FIGURE 10.2

Phagocytosis. (a) Selected stages or events in phagocytosis; (1) ingestion of a microorganism or other particle; and (2) digestion and eventual destruction of the ingested material.

(b) Two bacterial cells phagocytized by a neutrophil. Note the position of the bacterial cells within the cell (arrows). (From T. A. Betram et al., *Infection and Immunity* (1982) 37:1241–1247.)

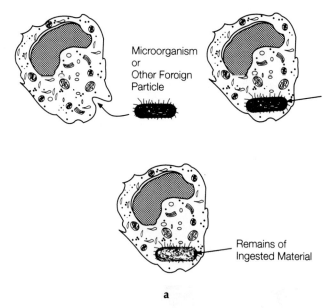

Microorganism or Other Foreign Particle

Remains of Ingested Material

a

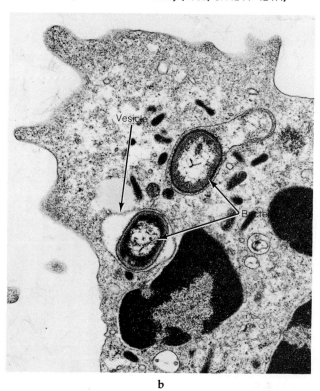

b

specific antibodies are available to attack and inactivate the disease agents before they can cause disease. Antibody production, a specific aspect of immunity, is described later in this chapter.

Neutrophils, the most abundant of leukocytes, are eager phagocytes, cells that literally eat foreign particles and substances. During an infection these cells are released from blood-forming areas of the body and ushered into the blood. Many neutrophils leave the blood and enter tissues, where they protect the skin and mucous membranes against invading pathogens and foreign substances. Eosinophils are released in large numbers in response to allergy attacks. These cells also serve as phagocytes and may neutralize poisonous substances. Basophils move into tissues, where they are referred to as **mast cells,** and release chemicals such as **histamine** (HIS-ta-mēn) and **heparin** (HEP-a-rin). Histamine starts the

body's response to tissue damage from injury or infection known as inflammation, and heparin prevents blood clotting.

Monocytes are the largest of the leukocytes and also function as phagocytes. They enter tissues and either remain stationary or wander through the body looking for, not only foreign microorganisms, but also dead cells and their remains. In tissues these large hungry phagocytes are called **macrophages** (fig. 10.3). Unfortunately, in certain situations blood cells such as macrophages can harbor STD agents such as the herpes viruses, HIV, and the gonococcus, and thereby not only protect them from the body's defenses, but also serve as sites for their growth and reproduction.

Lymphocytes are usually the second most numerous type of leukocyte in the body. They circulate in the blood and are found in large numbers of

FIGURE 10.3

The various types of blood cells in the blood and in tissues.

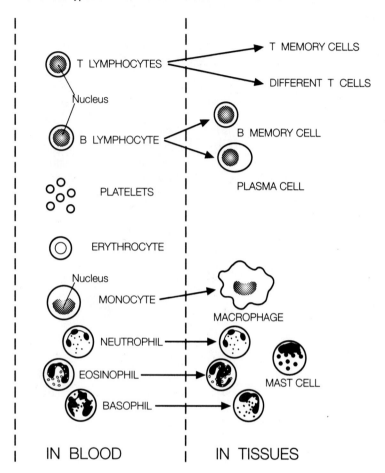

IN BLOOD | IN TISSUES

specific lymphoid tissues such as lymph nodes, spleen, and the tonsils, where they contribute to the specific immunity of the host. Lymphocytes are processed by different tissues into **B** and **T lymphocytes.** B lymphocytes give rise to smaller antibody-producing cells known as **plasma cells,** while various forms of T cells contribute to an individual's resistance by participating in antibody production and the destruction of foreign cells (fig. 10.3). Additional features of these cell types are given later in this chapter. Figure 10.3 shows the various leukocytes as they appear in other body tissues.

THE LYMPHATIC SYSTEM

The lymphatic system (fig. 10.4) is closely associated with the cardiovascular system. It consists of a network of vessels which extend throughout the body, lymph fluid, lymph nodes, and other forms of lymphatic tissues such as the tonsils, spleen, and thymus gland. The components of this system perform functions important to nonspecific and specific host defenses.

Lymph nodes are small, oval bodies that are widely distributed throughout the body, but are most numerous in the chest, neck, armpits, and

FIGURE 10.4

The blood and lymphatic systems in the human. (a) An overall view of the lymphatic system showing major locations of lymph nodes (the parts known to remove bacteria and foreign particles and cells). Note the positions of major body organs in relation to the lymph nodes. Several STDs involve the lymph nodes in the groin. (b) A diagrammatic representation of the relationship between the circulatory and lymphatic systems.

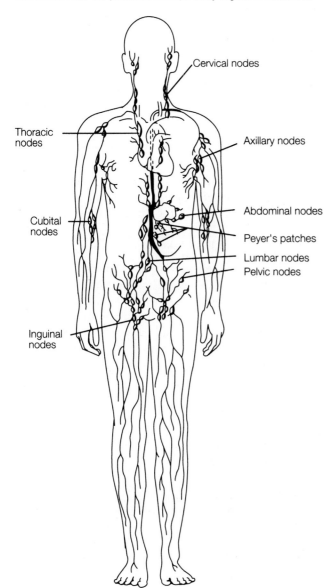

a

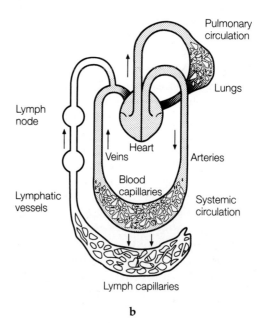

b

groin. They contain both B and T lymphocytes. Lymph vessels carry lymph fluid to and from these tissues.

Lymph nodes as well as certain other lymphatic tissues also have phagocytic cells that help to remove and eliminate disease agents and other foreign substances from blood and lymph fluids. If these phagocytic cells are overcome by disease agents the lymphatic tissue then becomes the site of infection. The body's defense system failed in this case. Swollen lymph nodes are examples of such situations and serve as a common feature of several STDs including chancroid (color photograph 4), lymphogranuloma venereum, and HIV infections. (See chapters 6 and 13.)

NONSPECIFIC IMMUNITY

Defenses that operate regardless of the disease agent serve as the body's foundation for nonspecific immunity. They are quite general and, as indicated earlier, represent the first line of protection against foreign cells and harmful substances. Factors contributing to an individual's nonspecific immunity include anatomical barriers such as unbroken skin, the mucous membranes of the respiratory and genitourinary systems, phagocytosis, inflammation, and various antimicrobial products of the body. An absence of or defect in any of these factors lowers an individual's resistance and increases susceptibility to a disease agent. The effectiveness of these factors against disease can be reduced by conditions such as alcoholism, poor nutrition, and debilitating effects of aging, fatigue, prolonged exposure to extreme temperatures, and the use of drugs which interfere or suppress immune system activities.

In the event the anatomical barriers are overcome by foreign invaders the body has other important defenses available. Phagocytosis is one of these. As described earlier, it is a process whereby the ingestion and eventual digestion of foreign matter by circulating granulocytes, monocytes, and macrophages takes place (fig. 10.2). Unfortunately, some disease agents can escape this nonspecific defense mechanism.

Inflammation is yet another of the body's defenses against infection. It can be triggered by infectious disease agents and by irritating factors such as chemicals, heat, and mechanical injury. Do you remember one of the times you either cut, burned, or scratched yourself? If the injury was not too serious, the bleeding soon stopped, and you could easily clean and bandage the wound. Many people notice in such cases that within a few hours the injured area begins to swell, hurt, turn red, and feel warm, even hot. Occasionally there also is a throbbing. These are the typical signs and symptoms of inflammation and they represent the body's first step in the repair of injured tissue. The single most important event in this process is the gathering of large numbers of phagocytic cells at the site of injury. Pus formation may also occur with inflammation. Pus is fluid formed by the remains of damaged tissue cells, dead phagocytes, and microorganisms.

FEVER

In addition to the defenses described thus far there are also overall body responses that go into action during an infection or injury. One of the most important of these is the increase in body temperature known as **fever,** a frequent sign of many diseases, and a part of the local inflammation reaction described earlier.

Normal body temperature is considered to be 37° Celsius or 98.6° Fahrenheit, and is controlled by a temperature-regulating center in the brain. Any increase above this normal level is a fever. it can be caused by various factors, including pathogens, certain processes associated with immunity, and nearly any type of tissue injury. Fever accompanying an infection rarely goes above 40°C; however, if it reaches 43°C, death usually results. Temperatures of 38.5°–39° C are known to be helpful to a person's recovery, since destruction of disease agents occurs more rapidly because of an increase in antibody production and more effective phagocytic activity.

CHEMICAL WARFARE

In addition to phagocytosis, inflammation, and fever, the body is capable of launching various types of chemical substances to interfere with the actions of pathogens and in some cases even to destroy them. Examples of these body bullets include the **proteins, complement** (KOM-ple-ment), and the **interferons** (in-ter-FĒR-ons).

Complement goes to work as soon as an invading disease agent is detected by the body. It is generally involved with important nonspecific defense reactions, including inflammation and phagocytosis. Complement is also capable of directly destroying certain disease agents.

Interferons are normally produced in response to infections caused by viruses and other disease agents. These proteins interfere with the formation of viruses and even certain cancer cells. Interferons have become of great commercial interest, especially in relation to treatment. They are used in cases of genital warts, HIV infections, and some types of cancers.

SPECIFIC IMMUNITY

Humans are protected in varying degrees from disease-causing microorganisms and cancers by an immune system consisting of a number of special cells and organs which work together to provide the host with **specific immunity.** Specific immunologic responses in contrast to those associated with nonspecific immunity are directed against particular disease agents. *What are these responses and how do they work?* The following section explains.

Generally, a person who recovers from an infectious disease has some degree of immunity or resistance toward the cause. Such resistance is created when a person's own immune system produces antibodies or other defenses against microorganisms, cells, or certain harmful substances that the body identifies as being foreign. Foreign cells and substances which provoke an immune response are called **antigens.** The *active* immunity caused by the specific immunological response can last for a few weeks, months, or years, depending on how long the antibodies remain. Adding to the person's immunity is a built-in immune system memory that not only can remember the antigen to which it reacted, but can trigger another specific response any time it again is invaded by the same antigen. Another form of immunity can be established by introducing ready-made antibodies into the body. This immunity is *passive* since the person's own immune system is not involved with the making of antibodies. (Chapter 15 provides other aspects of active and passive immunities and general descriptions of vaccines and their production.)

IMMUNE RESPONSES

The immune system has two major types of specific immune responses to foreign cells and substances. These are **humoral** (HŪ-mor-al) **immunity** and **cell-mediated immunity.** The presence of foreign invaders often sets both types of immune responses into action. Furthermore, both types of responses depend on lymphocytes, which originate from different body locations early in the development of the individual. These different cells are **B lymphocytes (B cells)** and **T lymphocytes (T cells).** Under the influence of the **thymus** (THĪ-mus) **gland,** T cells develop and acquire specific properties that distinguish them from B cells. During this differentiation process, a number of genetically determined T (thymus) antigen-reacting sites, or markers, develop on the surfaces of T cells. These surface markers not only enable such cells to recognize foreign antigens, but also are needed for the development and activation of different T cell types. After this differentiation process, the fully developed T cells migrate to lymphoid organs such as lymph nodes and the spleen, where they take on the responsibility to attack and eliminate foreign antigens, and serve as regulators of both *humoral* and *cell-mediated responses.*

Four functional T cell types are recognized and named according to their respective activities: (1) T helper (T_H) cells; (2) cytotoxic T (T_C) cells; (3) T suppressor (T_S) cells; and (4) T delayed hypersensitivity (T_{DH}) cells. The following discussions will include the respective roles played by T cells in specific immunity.

Humoral and cell-mediated responses also have certain distinctive properties that help to provide immunity. These include the ability to respond specifically to a wide assortment of antigens, and a *memory.* The memory in this case allows the immune system to respond rapidly to defend the body against an antigen to which it has previously reacted. Specific memory cells stand ready for years to quickly enable the immune system to respond faster to second and subsequent antigen exposures. This prompt recall by memory cells is called an **anamnestic** (an-am-NES-tik) response. Such responses are produced by vaccine booster shots and probably exposures to certain disease agents, and contribute to maintaining the immunity of an individual against various disease agents.

With this brief description of immune responses in mind we will now look at the two kinds of specific immunity in more detail.

HUMORAL IMMUNITY

Humoral immunity is the specific immune response which protects the body by antibodies (immunoglobulins) circulating in the blood. The term *humor* was used by people during medieval times to describe the fluids of the body. They believed that such humors were the main factors that determined an individual's level of health. Since antibodies were found in the body fluids, the associated immune response came to be known as **humoral immunity.**

FIGURE 10.5

The activities of B lymphocytes with the recognition of foreign particles (antigens). B cells are stimulated to reproduce and give rise to new (descendent) cells (clones) that differentiate into plasma cells and antigen-specific memory cells. Antibodies (immunoglobulins) are produced by plasma cells.

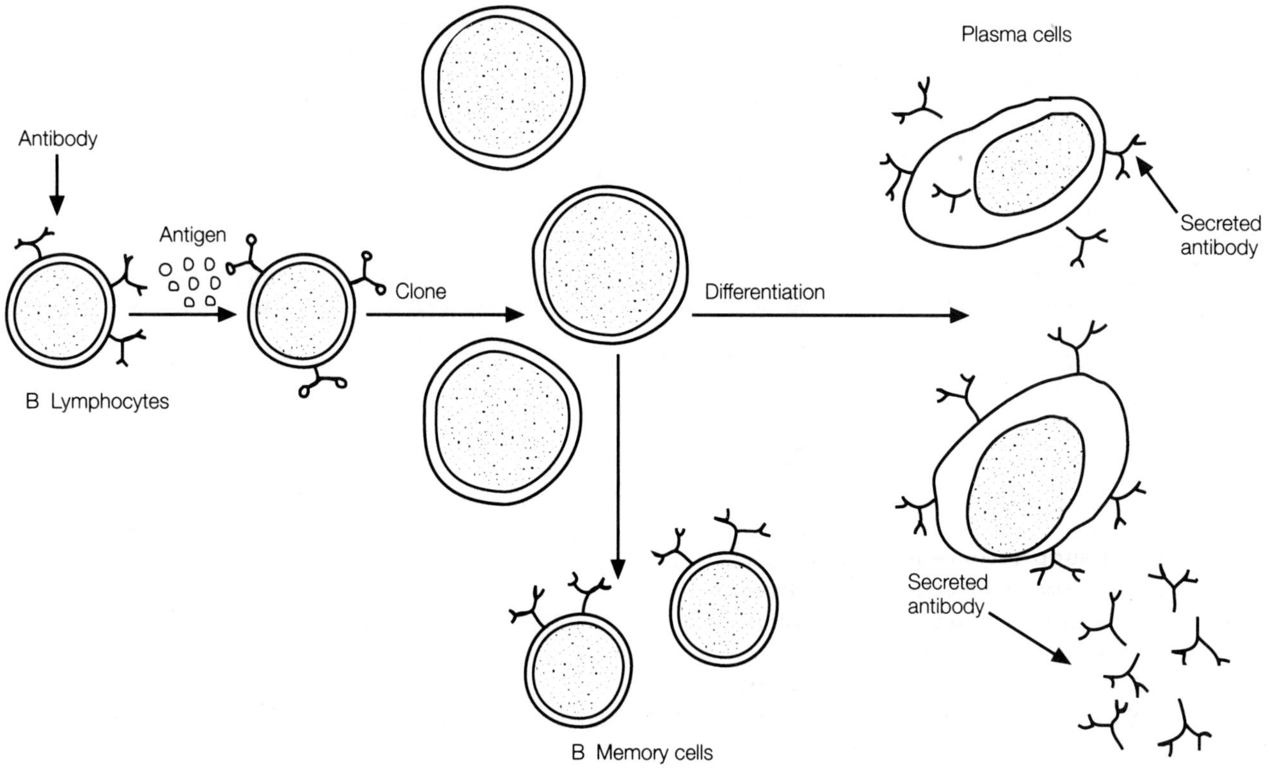

THE PRIMARY RESPONSE

The process of antibody formation is started when host B lymphocytes first recognize an antigen. In most instances, the antigens are on the surfaces of the disease agent. Each kind of B cell carries specific antibodies corresponding on its outer surface so that it can immediately attach to corresponding specific antigen. After recognizing and reacting with the antigen, B cells divide many times to form some **memory cells,** but mostly **plasma cells** (fig. 10.5). Plasma cells are large lymphocytes that produce and release antibodies. While it is active, a single plasma cell can manufacture as many as 2,000 antibodies per second.

The antibody produced in this **primary response** to the antigen (or anti-antigen) is capable of specifically attaching to the antigen. Such attachment will inactivate an antigen and may lead to the destruction of disease agents.

Memory cells do not get involved with the primary response. They simply persist in lymphoid tissue for many months to many years, and keep their ability to recognize a particular antigen ready for action.

Other Cells Involved with the Primary Response. Two types of T cells and macrophages also work with B cells. While B cells are clearly the main cells needed for antibody or immunoglobulin production, in certain cases T helper cells provide assistance by preparing antigens so that B cells can respond to them, and are thus activated. Macrophages also concentrate and prepare antigens to spark an immune response from B cells. Macrophages that have processed an antigen secrete

THE MIGHTY T HELPER CELL

The T helper cell, also known as the T_4 cell, is considered the cornerstone of an individual's immune system. In addition to cooperating with B cells to produce antibodies, these cells play several other vital roles in the host's immune responses (fig. 10.6). Without their involvement expressed in most cases through the production of lymphokines, other cells participating in immune responses would not function.

T helper cells are distinguished from other T cells by having a specific surface antigen called the **CD4 marker.** (The **CD** designation belongs to a system for the naming of lymphocyte antigens and is an abbreviation for "cluster of differentiation"). This surface feature of helper cells has become an item of special interest since the human immunodeficiency virus (HIV) is attracted to any cell that bears it. The CD4 markers act as receptors for HIV.

chemicals known as **lymphokines** (LIM-fō-kinz), which activate T helper cells. T helper cells, in turn, also secrete chemicals which activate other T cell types such as **T suppressor** cells. These cells stop the immune response once it reaches a specific point and achieves its mission in providing immunity. T suppressor cells specifically interfere with the formation of plasma cells from B cells. Both T helpers and T suppressors are considered to be **regulatory cells** since they control an individual's immune response so that it should not go on indefinitely.

What Are Antibodies? What Do They Specifically Do? Antibodies, or immunoglobulins (Igs), are Y-shaped molecules composed of four proteinlike chains—two identical light (L) chains and two identical heavy (H) chains (fig. 10.7). These chains are held together chemically, and have *constant* and *variable* regions. The variable regions of each immunoglobulin chain enable the immunoglobulin to attach to a particular antigen. Each of the millions of different immunoglobulins has its own unique pair of identical **antigen attachment,** or **binding sites,** formed from the variable regions at the ends of the L and H chains (fig. 10.7). This accounts for the ability of different immunoglobulins to attach to different antigens.

FIGURE 10.6

The importance of T_4 (helper) cells to the normal functioning of the immune system. Reducing the normal number of T_4 cells seriously cripples the immune responses and the level of host resistance.

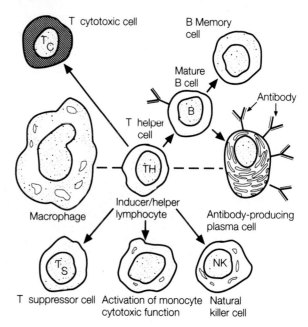

FIGURE 10.7

An immunoglobulin or antibody molecule. It consists of two identical proteinlike heavy chains and two identical light chains. The chains are linked together chemically. Each molecule has at least two sites that attach (bind) to specific parts of antigens (antigen binding sites).

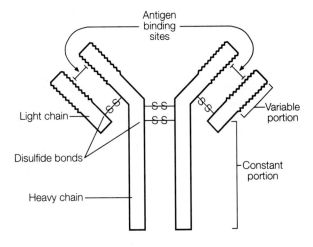

Immunoglobulins circulate in the blood and other body fluids. They are produced by the body in response to: (1) infectious disease agents; (2) preparations used for immunization (vaccines); or (3) other foreign substances such as various plant pollens which cause *allergies*. While thousands of individual immunoglobulins differing in their major structure circulate in blood, they can all be placed into one of five classes or categories: **IgG, IgA, IgM,** and **IgE**. This grouping is based on various biochemical and immunological differences. The general properties of the **Ig** classes are summarized in table 10.1.

THE SECONDARY RESPONSE

As indicated earlier, the exposure to an antigen either in the form of an actual disease agent or a vaccine usually provokes a primary response. With this exposure the antibody formation process is set into motion (fig. 10.8).

TABLE 10.1 | SELECTED FEATURES OF THE MAJOR IMMUNOGLOBULINS

TYPE	LOCATION IN THE BODY	MAJOR FUNCTION(S)
IgG	Body fluids and plasma	1. Acts against bacteria, viruses, and certain toxins (poisons) 2. Only Ig that can cross from a mother's circulation to that of her fetus and provide protection (passive immunization) 3. Contributes to increasing the effectiveness of phagocytosis
IgA	Body fluids (saliva, mucous, breast milk, urine, etc.), and respiratory tract surfaces	1. Acts against bacteria and viruses 2. Assists in phagocytosis
IgM	Plasma	1. Reacts with antigens 2. Assists with phagocytosis 3. First Ig to be secreted during early stage of primary immune response
IgD	Surfaces of most B lymphocytes	1. Aids in antigen recognition
IgE	Plasma and skin	1. Promotes allergic reactions

FIGURE 10.8

The primary and secondary antibody responses to an antigenic stimulus. Chapter 14 presents the states of immunity with which these responses are associated.

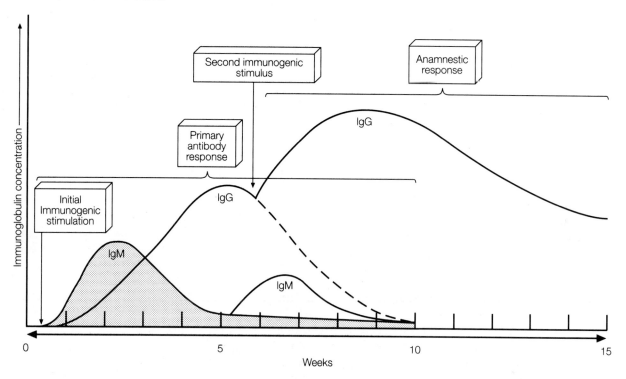

CELL-MEDIATED IMMUNITY

Certain antigens stimulate a secondary response when they enter the blood and are recognized by memory cells. The presence of these cells causes the secondary response to be faster than the primary one. Both responses are compared in figure 10.8.

High levels of immunoglobulins may remain for several months or longer, and then these levels slowly begin to move downward as the breakdown of the immunoglobulins exceeds their production. Several factors such as the type of the antigen involved, the length of exposure to the antigen, and an individual's immune system are known to influence the process. The resulting hormonal immunity is most effective in defending the body against bacteria, toxins, and viruses *before* they enter a host's cells.

Cell-mediated immunity differs from humoral immunity in that it does not require antibody formation. Early in the study of immunity, scientists found that some forms of protection against disease agents could be transferred between animals by injecting serum-containing antibodies to other animals lacking them. In short, it was possible to temporarily protect, or immunize, animals with an injection of antibodies. This form of protection as described earlier was passive. In later experiments it soon became apparent that other forms of immunity were not transferable with blood serum containing specific antibodies, but required the transfer of certain lymphocytes. These lymphocytes eventually were identified as T lymphocytes, and the type of immunity associated with them was named **cell-mediated immunity.**

Cell-mediated immunity (CMI) takes place at the cellular level, especially in cases where antigens are a part of or inside cells, and thus not open to attack by antibodies. When viruses such as the causes of genital herpes and AIDS and other foreign invaders penetrate and hide inside a cell, immunoglobulins are left powerless since they cannot pass into the invaded cells. CMI is most effective in clearing the body of virus-infected cells. It can also distinguish between cells that are normal and those changed into cancerous ones. CMI may also participate in defending the body against cancer.

THE PROCESS

The cell-mediated response begins with preparing an antigen, usually one associated with a disease agent, for T cell action. This process typically is performed by macrophages which ingest and break down the pathogen to expose its antigenic parts. Some of these parts are inserted into the macrophage's surface. T cells having the appropriate antigen receptors attach to these macrophage surface antigens. The resulting activated T cells disconnect, begin to divide, and to form different T cell types. These include the **T helper** and **T suppressor cells** (described earlier), T cytotoxic cells, and natural killer cells. At the same time these T cells are being formed, some T memory cells also are produced. **Memory cells** also help the immune system to recognize antigens to which T cells have responded previously.

Cytotoxic T cells represent the main T lymphocyte type that defends the body against virally infected cells, whereas natural killer cells act directly on cancers and possibly body cells infected by *Chlamydia*. Both kinds of cells are able to separate from cells they have attacked and damaged, and to move on and attack again.

IMMUNODEFICIENCY DISEASES — A BREAKDOWN OF THE IMMUNE SYSTEM

Immunodeficiency diseases include a wide range of disorders in which the immune system does not respond normally to an antigen because of inherited or acquired defects in B or T lymphocytes. The effects and symptoms of these conditions may be minor or may be life-threatening.

Immunodeficiency diseases develop from the lack of lymphocytes, defective lymphocytes, or the destruction of lymphocytes, and invariably lead to the weakening of an individual's humoral and/or cell-mediated immune responses. Even nonspecific lines of defense such as phagocytosis may be affected (fig. 10.9).

In recent years the **acquired** or **secondary immunodeficiency diseases** have become of great concern because of the dramatic destruction that occurs in AIDS. This group of diseases can be caused by the agents of infectious diseases such as tuberculosis and AIDS, and of cancers, or malnutrition, or drugs which suppress the immune system, and even certain antibiotics used in the treatment of various infections.

In the case of AIDS, the human immunodeficiency virus carefully selects T helper lymphocytes as its primary targets. Once the virus invades and establishes itself in these cells which play a controlling role in orchestrating the body's immune responses to infections and cancers, the stage is set for the ultimate collapse of the immune system. With the viral destruction and depletion of the body's T helper cells, the infected person thus becomes susceptible to a variety of agents waiting for the opportunity to establish infections and is unable to prevent the development of various type of cancers.

The human immune system is equipped with an abundance of weapons to combat foreign cells, substances, and various disease agents. Yet interestingly enough, despite all of these defenses, the system has an Achilles' heel, the T helper lymphocyte.

Figure 10.9

The various components of the immune system provide protection against both internal and external factors. (a) A high level of protection is in-effect in a host when exposure to disease agents, or allergy-causing substances occurs. (b) With a reduction or deficiency in one or more parts of the immune system, the more likely infections or other disease conditions such as cancers are likely to develop. Such is the case in an immunocompromised host. The more defects in the immune system the greater is the susceptibility to disease.

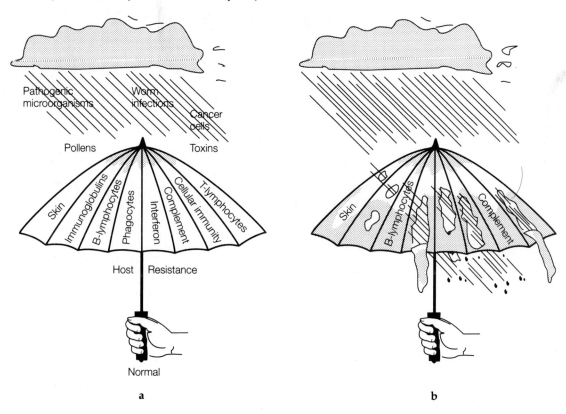

CHAPTER 11 | OPPORTUNISTIC INFECTION AND THE IMMUNOCOMPROMISED HOST

I love the doctors, they are dears.
But must they spend such years and years
investigating such a lot
of illnesses which no one's got.

Look Back and Laugh—A. P. Herbert

INTRODUCTION

"Illnesses no one's got" was the specific epidemiological clue that led to the identification of AIDS as a new disease in 1981. A rare infectious disease agent, *Pneumocystis carinii* was found in previously healthy homosexual males. Since then a wide range of disease-causing agents has been found to cause illness in persons with AIDS. Infection with human immunodeficiency virus (HIV) causes a predictable, progressive breakdown of the immune (defense) system and its associated functions. The resulting severe immune deficiency provides an opportunity for several normally harmless, as well as pathogenic, microorganisms to flourish in HIV-infected persons, and to possibly cause fatal outcomes. Such causative agents which may or may not be normal residents in or on the host are referred to as opportunists, and the conditions they cause are known as **opportunistic infections.** The individuals whose immune systems are severely injured become **immunocompromised** (im'-ū-nō-KOM-prō-mīzd) hosts, and provide the environment in which opportunists can establish themselves.

As HIV infection progresses, the infected individual passes through several stages, the last of which is AIDS (see chapter 13). The presence of an opportunistic infection is one of these stages and is used in the diagnosis of AIDS. Usually the first infections to appear are relatively harmless but annoying conditions of the skin and mucous membranes.

FIGURE 11.1

The lesions of the fungus disease sporotrichosis on the arm of an immunocompromised host.

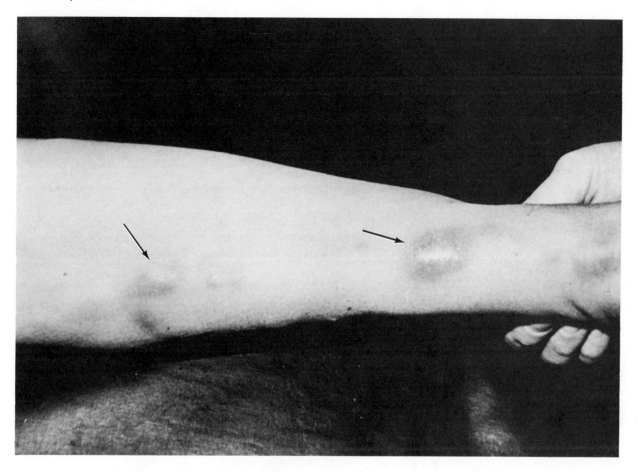

Among these may be thrush (painful sores on the inside of the mouth), shingles (infection of the nerves and skin), and an unusually severe form of athlete's foot (fig. 11.1, and color photographs 23, 24, and 25). As the resistance of the individual continues to weaken further, serious opportunistic infections usually develop.

The clinical (medical) expression of HIV infection appears increasingly complex if the effects due to opportunistic pathogens also are present. The types of opportunistic infections vary not only in populations of different geographic regions, but also according to the probable way the HIV infection was acquired. Examples of some of the most commonly occurring opportunistic infections and illnesses in AIDS patients, together with their respective causative microorganisms, are listed in table 11.1 and are described in this chapter.

TABLE 11.1 | COMMON OPPORTUNISTIC INFECTIONS IN PERSONS WITH AIDS

CAUSE	USUAL BODY SITE INVOLVED	SYMPTOMS	COMMON DIAGNOSTIC TESTS INCLUDE:
Fungi Cryptococcus neoformans	Brain	Headache, fever, confusion, behavior changes	Laboratory diagnosis includes examination of spinal fluid (lumbar puncture) and/or bone marrow. Same method is used for culture.
	Lungs	Nonspecific cough, fever, difficulty in swallowing	Chest X-rays, collection of sputum or other material for isolation and identification
	Skin	Fever blisters	Removal of blister fluid or skin for microscopic examination or culture for isolation
Candida albicans	Mouth, esophagus (the region extending from the throat to the stomach)	Difficulty in swallowing, painful sores, white thick film on surfaces of tongue and other parts	Laboratory diagnosis includes microscopic examination of film scrapings and culture for isolation and identification
Protozoa Cryptosporidium	Gastrointestinal tract	Watery diarrhea, dehydration, general weakness	Laboratory examination of stools
Isospora belli	Gastrointestinal tract	Watery diarrhea, dehydration, general weakness	Laboratory examination of stool
Pneumocystis carinii	Lungs	Dry, nonproductive cough, shortness of breath, fever, night sweats	Chest X-ray examination of respiratory system by bronchoscopy (bron-KOS-kō-pē)
Toxoplasma gondii	Brain	Headaches, sudden attack of pain, behavior changes, depression, impaired memory	Examination of brain by computerized tonography (known as CAT scan) or other methods

TABLE 11.1 | (CONTINUED)

CAUSE	USUAL BODY SITE INVOLVED	SYMPTOMS	COMMON DIAGNOSTIC TESTS INCLUDE:
Viruses Cytomegalovirus	Eyes	Loss of vision, inflammation of the retina (RET-i-na), the light-sensitive part of the eye	Laboratory diagnosis includes tests for antibody, analysis of spinal fluid, and viral isolation from various specimens
	Lungs	Cough, fever, difficulty in swallowing	
	Gastrointestinal tract	Abdominal pain, ulcers, bleeding	
	Spinal cord	Partial paralysis of legs or paralysis of both arms and legs	
Epstein-Barr virus	Tongue	White painful patches on the sides of the tongue	Laboratory tests for antibody and biopsy specimens to show virus particles
	Lungs	Cough, difficulty in swallowing, fever	
Herpes simplex virus type 1	Skin	Painful sores in clusters in and around the mouth and perianal area	Laboratory examination of tissue and culture for virus isolation and identification
	Spinal cord	Partial paralysis of legs, paralysis of both arms and legs	Analysis of spinal fluid
Varicella-zoster virus	Skin	Painful blisters, fever	Laboratory examination of tissue for virus identification
	Nerves	Severe and prolonged pain	
	Central nervous system	Headaches, vision problems, paralysis of legs	
Bacteria Mycobacterium avium-intra-cellulare	Spreads and involves various organs including liver, lungs, gastrointestinal system, and lymph nodes	Fever, heavy sweating, productive cough, weight loss, swollen lymph nodes, and diarrhea	Laboratory diagnosis includes examination and use of specimens for isolation and identification

TABLE 11.2 | EXAMPLES OF HOST DEFENSE MECHANISMS

DEFENSE MECHANISMS	GENERAL FUNCTION(S)
Physical and Chemical Barriers: Skin and mucous membranes; flushing action of urine flow, and movement of gastrointestinal contents; high acid content of gastric juices in stomach; normal microbial populations in and on the body (microbiota)	Prevent the introduction and/or penetration of foreign microorganisms from internal or external sources
Inflammatory Response: Circulating ingesting white blood cells known as phagocytes; certain cellular antimicrobial products	General ingestion and destruction of foreign microorganisms and cells, thus producing local protection
Reticuloendothelial System: (re-tik-ū-lō-en'-dō-THĒ-lē-al)	General ingestion and some destruction of foreign microorganisms and cells in tissues, thus producing both local and general body protection
Immune Response: T lymphocytes and products; B lymphocytes; plasma cells and immunoglobulins	Neutralize and/or eliminate foreign microorganisms and their products

WHAT IS A COMPROMISED HOST?

Some of the most important challenges to medicine today are associated with individuals having some form of immune system defect and the question as to how such defects predispose or affect their susceptibility to infection by microorganisms. An individual who has a lowered resistance to infection because of one or more defects in his or her host defense mechanisms is generally referred to as a **compromised** host. Table 11.2 reviews a number of these mechanisms, together with their respective functions. The development of an infectious disease in a compromised host reflects the interaction of weakened immunological and nonimmunlogical defense mechanisms with microorganisms and related disease agents. Knowing which hosts defenses are compromised is essential to developing an effective approach for prevention, early detection, and prompt treatment of the causative agents that are most likely to establish an infectious disease.

For individuals whose immunological or inflammatory defense mechanisms are compromised, the term **immunocompromised host** is perhaps more appropriate. As described in chapter 10 the major cellular members of immune responses are **T lymphocytes, B lymphocytes,** and **macrophages.** These cells are distributed throughout the body where they interact among themselves and with immunoglobulins and other components of the immune system to provide protection against various disease agents and other harmful factors.

The degree to which an individual becomes compromised or abnormally susceptible to infection depends on: 1) which immune system components or functions are affected, 2) the severity of the condition, and 3) the effect on the interactions of affected mechanisms if more than one is compromised at the same time. Thus, with individuals infected with HIV or who develop AIDS, the compromise of any of their immune system components or defense mechanisms is the major predisposing condition to life-threatening disease. As a rule, the infections of HIV-infected persons are those normally controlled by the cell-mediated responses of white blood cells such as T lymphocytes and macrophages. These cells are heavily attacked and destroyed by the HIV. In contrast, infections that are primarily eliminated by immunoglobulins, or by nonspecific defenses are normally managed fairly well, at least for a short time. The remaining portion of this chapter briefly describes several infectious diseases which develop under such conditions.

FUNGAL INFECTIONS

Destructive fungal infections have long been recognized as major complications in immunocompromised hosts following treatment for cancer or in cases of organ and bone marrow transplants. A number of fungi, including *Candida* and *Aspergillus,* account for the majority of such infections. Unfortunately, cases caused by less damaging pathogens are being found with increasing frequency. It is therefore not surprising that fungal infections should be prominent among the opportunistic infections which are so typical of AIDS. The range, and at times the severity, of fungal infections in AIDS is, however, somewhat different from that seen in cancers, or recipients of transplanted organs (table 11.1). The incidence of any fungal infection in an immunocompromised host is determined by the natural habitat (location in the environment) of the fungus and by the type of host defense mechanism involved in preventing its invasion. Thus, infections by fungi, commonly found in the environment, also depend on a compromised cell-mediated immunity for invasiveness. Since some of the fungal pathogens spread to a number of body organs, the infections they cause are referred to as **systemic.** Several examples of such infections will briefly be described.

CRYPTOCOCCOSIS

Cryptococcosis (krip'-tō-kō-KŌ-sis) ranks among the four most life-threatening infections in AIDS, along with *Pneumocystis carinii* pneumonia, cytomegalovirus, and *Mycobacterium avium-intercellulare* infections.

Cause and Transmission. The yeast *Cryptococcus neoformans* (krip-tō-KŌK-us, nē-ō-FOR-mans) is a microorganism that can cause respiratory infections and an inflammation of the coverings of the brain and spinal cord known as meningitis. In persons with AIDS the most common form of cryptococcosis is **meningitis** (me-nin-JĪ-tis). Since the yeast is commonly found in a variety of environments, including soil, pigeon droppings, and on fruits and vegetables, humans come into regular contact with it.

Signs and Symptoms. Individuals with meningitis may experience few if any symptoms. The most common symptoms include headaches, fever, nausea, vomiting, stiff neck, sensitivity to light, and personality changes.

Respiratory infection with *Cryptococcus* generally produces a cough, sputum production, and slight fever.

Infection with *Cryptococcus* also may involve other body areas, including the skin (fig. 11.2), joints, eyes, and the heart.

Diagnosis and Treatment. The feature of cryptococcosis that makes it stand out among fungal diseases is the production of a specific polysaccharide **antigen** by the disease agent. A major component of *Cryptococcus* is an outer structure known as a capsule. The capsular antigen and the yeast itself generally are found in spinal fluid specimens taken from meningitis cases (fig. 11.3). Such findings and positive cultures from specimens are sufficient for diagnosis. In skin and other noncentral nervous system infections, diagnosis is made by showing the microscopic presence of the yeast in specimens and positive cultures made from such materials.

Treatment for cryptococcosis in persons with AIDS generally involves an individualized approach in order to determine appropriate drug dosages. The combination of the two antifungal agents **amphotericin B** (am'ō-TĒR-i-sin) and **flucytosine** (flū-SĪ-tō-sēn) are commonly used.

CANDIDA INFECTIONS

Various examples of *Candida* infections have been described in earlier chapters. These conditions, the

FIGURE 11.2

AIDS-related facial lesions caused by the yeast *Cryptococcus*. (a) The facial lesions. (b) A microscopic view of a specimen taken from the facial lesion showing a large number of round yeast cells. (From S. J. Miller, *Cutis* (1988) 41:411.)

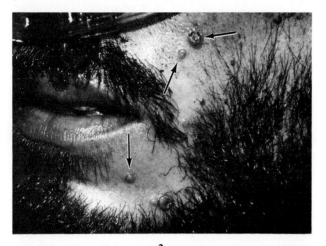

a

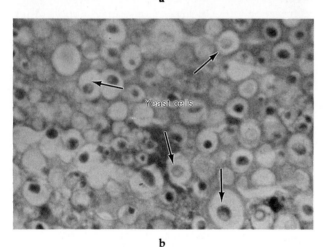

b

FIGURE 11.3

A microscopic view of material obtained from the coverings of the brain from a person with AIDS. All of the circles are the yeast cells *Cryptococcus neoformans*. (From F. Staib and M. Seibold, *Mycoses* (1988) 31:175–186.)

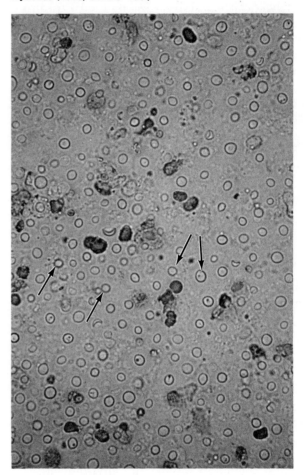

most common of which involves the throat and neighboring areas, are found during the initial stages of HIV infection. Oral candidiasis and an inflammation of the esophagus are frequently caused by yeasts such as *Candida* species.

Cause and Transmission. The various forms of *Candida* are regularly found in the human gastrointestinal and female reproductive tracts. In general, these organisms infect the mucosal membranes of

persons with AIDS, and at times may cause life-threatening conditions. The gastrointestinal tract usually serves as the major source of the yeast.

Signs and Symptoms. *Candida* infections of the mouth, throat, and esophagus are annoying to the individual. Typical symptoms, all of which may interfere with eating and nutrition, include soreness, local irritation, and difficulty in swallowing.

Diagnosis and Treatment. Oral *Candida* infections involving the mouth and related areas can be diagnosed either by the typical appearance of the condition or by microscopic examination of a smear made with material from a lesion. In the case of systemic infection, isolation and culture techniques generally are needed for diagnosis.

The treatment of infections should involve the use of topically (surface) applied antifungal drugs such as **nystatin** (NIS-ta-tin) and oral **ketoconazole** (kē-tō-KON-a-zōl). In severe forms of *Candida* infection amphotericin B is used.

ASPERGILLOSIS

The question as to whether **aspergillosis** is an opportunistic infection in persons with AIDS remains undecided. While the disease is found in HIV-infected individuals it does not occur in the same proportions as other fungus infections. The causative agent **Aspergillus** (as-per-JIL-us) is commonly found in soil, dust, and air samples throughout the world. Invasion and involvement of body organs is seen only in immunocompromised hosts.

The symptoms found with infections are similar to those described for the other fungus conditions mentioned in this section. Treatment generally may involve the use of amphotericin B.

AIDS-RELATED INFECTIONS

Some of the HIV-related infections are caused by microorganisms that are not necessarily opportunistic. The conditions they cause represent the reactivation of inactive infections that were held in check by the individual's immune system before it was attacked by HIV. These include **coccidioidomycosis** (kok-sid-ē-oyd-ō-mī-KŌ-sis), **histoplasmosis** (his'-tō-plaz-MŌ-sis), and **aspergillosis** (as'-per-jil-Ō-sis). While the causative agents of these infections can cause respiratory disease and other problems in healthy persons, they can also cause extremely destructive systemic infections involving the skin, bone, liver, and lymphatic tissues. Brief descriptions of these disease agents and their associated diseases follow.

COCCIDIOIDOMYCOSIS

Coccidioides immitis (kok-sid-ē-OYD-ēz, im-MĒ-tis), the cause of coccidioidomycosis, is a fungus common to the soil and desert sands of southwestern North America, Central America, and parts of South America. Infection usually is acquired by inhaling the disease agent.

HIV-infected persons appear to be at an increased risk for the severe form of the disease known as disseminated coccidioidomycosis. Symptoms may include a prominent cough, fever, weight loss, and a general feeling of discomfort.

Diagnosis is based on finding the causative agent by culture or in microscopically-examined tissues obtained from patients. Amphotericin B and ketoconazole are the drugs generally used for treatment. Relapses are known to occur after treatment has been discontinued.

HISTOPLASMOSIS

Histoplasma capsulatum (his'-tō-PLAZ-ma, kap-sū-LĀ-tum), the causative agent of histoplasmosis also is a soil fungus. It is found in the river valleys of North, Central, and South America. Since the fungus grows well in bird droppings, a number of outbreaks have been associated with *aerosol* exposure to such material excreted by chickens, and several types of wild birds.

Symptoms of infection are nonspecific and include fever, chills, sweats, weight loss, diarrhea, nausea, and vomiting. Such symptoms may be present for weeks to months before a diagnosis is made. In HIV-infected persons histoplasmosis has appeared years after leaving the area in which exposures occurred.

Diagnosis of histoplasmosis depends on demonstrating the presence of the causative agent by isolation and culture, or microscopically in tissues obtained from patients.

Treatment of this fungus infection involves the use of amphotericin B.

PROTOZOAN INFECTIONS

The epidemic of HIV infection has provided a clear demonstration of the the delicate balance between humans and the various protozoa in their respective microbial environments. The immunological defense mechanisms (table 1.2) mentioned earlier play the essential role in protecting the individual against a number of protozoan diseases. In persons with AIDS and other immunocompromised conditions, such antiprotozoan defenses are defective and thereby account for the high morbidity and mortality rates caused by such diseases as **pneumocystis pneumonia, toxoplasmosis** (toks-ō-plas-MŌ-sis), **cryptosporidiosis** (krip-tō-spor-id-ē-Ō-sis), and **isosporiasis** (ī-sos-pōr-Ī-a-sis).

PNEUMOCYSTIS PNEUMONIA

Pneumocystis carinii (nū-mō-SIS-tis, kar-i-NĒ) pneumonia (PCP), also known as pneumocystosis (nū'-mō-sis-TŌ-sis), remains one of the most common life-threatening opportunistic infections associated with AIDS, at least in developed countries of the world. PCP is the AIDS-defining illness in more than 60 percent of persons with AIDS in the United States at some point in their illness. An estimated 40,000 cases of pneumocystis pneumonia were expected to occur in HIV-infected persons in 1990 in the United States. Unfortunately, such cases will continue to occur despite impressive advances in preventive treatment. Thus PCP is expected to remain the most life-threatening opportunistic infection associated with AIDS for the next decade.

Cause and Transmission. PCP results from an inflammation of the lungs caused by the microorganism *Pneumocystis carinii* (fig. 11.4), which was first described in 1909 by C. Chagas. One year later the organism was rediscovered by A. Carinii, after whom it was named in 1914. Although *P. carinii* was later found in the lungs of humans and many other animals, it remained little more than a medical curiosity for some time. Its first association with human illness was reported in 1952. At this time *P. carinii* was found to cause a form of pneumonia in premature and weakened infants in central and eastern Europe following World War II.

Medical interest in *P. carinii* in the United States developed in the 1960s and 1970s when the organism emerged as an important cause of pneumonia in immunocompromised individuals. The

FIGURE 11.4

The penetration of lung tissue by *Pneumocystis*.

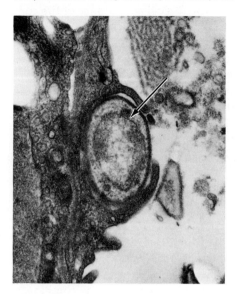

major targets were children with leukemia, persons with immunodeficiencies, and individuals receiving various immunosuppressive drugs for the treatment of cancer and the prevention of organ transplant rejection. In the 1970s, the drug trimethoprim-sulfamethoxazole (trī-METH-ō-prim, sul'-fa-meth-OKS-a-zōl) was found to be an effective treatment for PCP. Its widespread use led to a dramatic decline in the number of cases of this type of pneumonia in most major medical centers. Unfortunately, with the appearance of AIDS and HIV infections in 1981, *P. carinii* reappeared and regained medical attention (fig. 11.5).

Infection with *P. carinii* is acquired mainly by inhaling the disease agent. In various animal studies infections could not be established when soil, water, or food were used as sources of the organism.

Signs and Symptoms. PCP may appear as an infection without severe symptoms in a normal host, and as life-threatening pneumonia in an immunocompromised host. Typical symptoms of the infection include a high fever, shortness of breath, and a dry nonproductive cough (no sputum is produced). Chest pain may also be a common complaint.

FIGURE 11.5

(a) A normal chest X ray of an individual in the early stages of PCP. (b) An X ray taken four days later showing the rapid development of the disease. The white areas (arrows) show the specifically involved portions of the lungs. (From D. W. Martin, Jr., D. G. Warnock, and L. H. Smith, Jr., *Western Journal of Medicine* (1982) 13:400.)

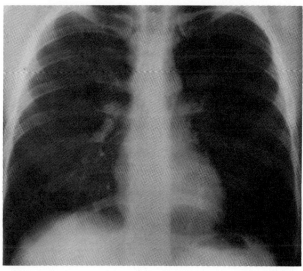

a

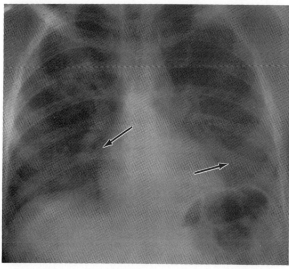

b

Diagnosis and Treatment. Chest X-rays, tests used to determine if the lungs are functioning normally, and related procedures can show abnormalities of the respiratory system. However, none of these techniques is completely sensitive to specifically pinpoint a case of PCP. Moreover, some of the procedures are expensive and take a fair amount of time to perform. Thus, establishing the presence or absence of PCP depends on demonstrating the disease agent in sputum or tissue removed during a lung examination procedure such as *bronchoscopy* (brong-KOS-kō-pē).

Over the past ten to seventeen years, two major drugs have been used to treat PCP. They are ***trimethoprin-sulfamethoxazote*** (trī-METH-ō-prin, sul-fa-meth-OX-a-zōt) (TMP-SMX) and ***pentamide isethionate*** (PENT-a-mīd, īs′-e-THĪ-ō-nāt). Both medications appear to be equally effective. While the condition in individuals receiving these drugs may become worse during the first three to four days of therapy, signs of improvement generally appear within seven to ten days.

TOXOPLASMOSIS

Toxoplasmosis (toks-ō-plas-MŌ-sis) is found throughout the world. The infection is very common in the United States. About 10 to 50 percent of the population is infected by the age of twelve years. The disease usually is mild in most humans; however, it can have serious consequences in developing fetuses, newborns, and sometimes in young children. The incidence of toxoplasmosis increases with age and does not vary between the sexes.

Cause and Transmission. Toxoplasmosis is caused by *Toxoplasma gondii* (toks-ō-PLAS-ma, GON-dē), a protozoan that infects a variety of animals. Humans usually become infected through contact with the feces of infected domestic cats that hunt for natural foods, among which are infected rats and mice. Cats not allowed to roam, and fed on canned or cooked foods, are unlikely sources of the disease agent. Fruits and vegetables exposed to flies and cockroaches, as well as unpasteurized milk and cheese, and contaminated lamb and pork also have been reported as sources of the toxoplasma. The protozoan also can be transferred across the placenta of an infected mother to her fetus, and thereby cause serious congenital defects. Such defects include blindness and mental retardation. Stillbirths and spontaneous abortions also can occur.

Toxoplasmosis found in persons with AIDS appears to result from the reactivation of an earlier acquired infection that has been inactive.

Signs and Symptoms. Immunocompetent individuals infected with toxoplasma are generally **asymptomatic.** If symptoms do appear they may last for up to one year and include swollen lymph nodes, fever, general discomfort, night sweats, muscle pain, rash, and an enlarged liver and spleen. On the other hand, the signs and symptoms of toxoplasmosis in an immunocompromised host such as a person with AIDS virtually always show evidence of an inflammation of the central nervous system (CNS), also known as an *encephalitis* (en-sef'-a-LĪ-tis). Two patterns or groups of symptoms are recognized. One group includes specific centralized abnormalities such as sudden attacks of pain, paralysis of one side of the body, seeing double, blindness, personality changes, and severe headaches that do not respond to pain-killing drugs. The other pattern consists of general symptoms including headache, weakness, muscle twitching, confusion, sluggishness, and other signs of abnormal functioning of the CNS.

Diagnosis, Treatment, and Prevention Unfortunately there are no consistent or diagnostically helpful abnormalities associated with the infection that are obvious from the history, physical examination, and routine laboratory tests. The computed tomography (tō-MOG-ra-fē) scan is the most useful procedure for detecting the infection of the CNS (fig. 11.6).

Definite diagnosis of toxoplasmosis requires demonstrating or culturing the disease agent from specimens obtained from infected persons. Treatment should be started following a specific laboratory identification.

Persons with AIDS and in whom CNS toxoplasmosis has been confirmed generally are treated with a drug combination of **pyrimethamine** (pēr'-i-METH-a-mēn) and a **sulfonamide** (sul-FON-a-mīd).

FIGURE 11.6

A view of the brain by a computerized brain scan technique. The destructive effects of toxoplasmosis are shown by the arrow. (From R. G. Ramsey and G. K. Geremia, *American Journal of Radiology* (1988) 161:449–454.)

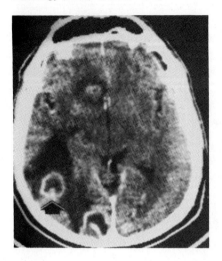

Most individuals experience an improvement within a week or two of staring the treatment (fig. 11.7). Unfortunately, relapses occur if the drug usage is stopped, thus lifelong treatment is recommended. In addition, some persons with AIDS develop an intolerance to the usual drugs, and therefore must be provided with alternatives.

Preventing toxoplasmosis requires avoiding exposure to cat fecal material and giving special attention to food and its preparation. Specific measures include cooking meats thoroughly until well done, or freezing meat at −20° C for twenty-four hours before use, washing fruits and vegetables, preventing access to food by flies, cockroaches, and related forms, and washing hands with soap and water after handling raw meat. In addition, raw eggs and unpasteurized goat's milk and cheese should not be eaten.

CRYPTOSPORIDIOSIS

Cryptosporidiosis (krip'-tō-spōr-i-dē-Ō-sis) is a relatively new addition to the list of human diseases. The disease is of particular importance in the case of AIDS since it is considered to be the most likely infection to cause a persistent, weakening or debilitating diarrhea. Cryptosporidiosis affects as many as

FIGURE 11.7

The effective treatment of toxoplasmosis shown through a brain scan. (a) A view showing many infected areas (arrows). (b) The disappearance of the infected areas shown in (a) by appropriate treatment. (From R. G. Ramsey and G. K. Geremia, *American Journal of Radiology* (1988) 161:449–454.)

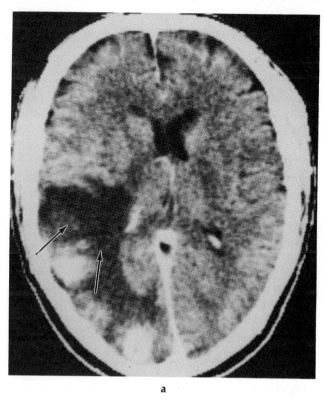

a

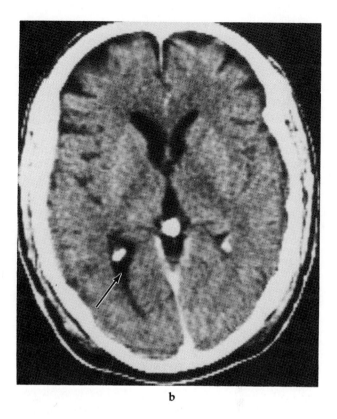

b

20 percent of persons with AIDS in the United States and up to 70 percent of AIDS patients in third world countries. Such infected individuals can develop quite extraordinary symptoms such as a severe watery diarrhea amounting to 10 to 20 liters per day. This protozoan disease is considered by many to be by far the most devastating complication of AIDS.

Cause and Transmission. Cryptosporidiosis is caused by *Cryptosporidium,* a disease agent associated with diarrheal illness in all areas of the world. Infection generally occurs from direct contact with infected persons and through the ingestion of contaminated food or water, and with men practicing oral-anal sex. Some cases also have been reported among health care workers having close contact with AIDS patients.

Signs and Symptoms. The most common observable feature of cryptosporidiosis in immunocompromised hosts is diarrhea. It is this symptom that most often leads to the diagnosis of the disease. Large volumes of fluid are lost due to this protozoan infection. Other less common symptoms include abdominal pain, nausea, vomiting, and a slight fever. At times muscle pain, headache, and a loss of appetite also are reported. Unfortunately, the diarrheal illness becomes progressively worse and may be a major factor leading to death.

Cryptosporidium infection also can extend beyond the gastrointestinal tract. It can involve the gallbladder and the respiratory system. Symptoms of respiratory infections include difficulty in swallowing, a long-lasting cough, chest pain, and soreness.

Diagnosis, Treatment, and Prevention. Diagnosis of cryptosporidiosis usually is based on laboratory examination of stool specimens which show the presence of the disease agent.

Treatment of cryptosporidiosis in a previously healthy, immunocompetent individual usually is not necessary, since after a short time the disease and its symptoms clear up spontaneously. Unfortunately, this is not the case with an immunocompromised host such as a person with AIDS. For the most part, treatment for immunocompromised hosts generally has been extremely frustrating and unsuccessful. The antibiotic **spiramycin** (spēr'-a-MĪ-sin) has been reported to be effective.

Measures to prevent infection include avoiding contact with infected hosts, proper disposal of fecal wastes, and practicing good personal hygienic habits. The latter refers to washing hands with soap and water after using bathroom facilities and before preparing food.

ISOSPORIASIS

Isosporiasis (i-SOS-pōr-ī-a-sis) has recently been recognized as an opportunistic infection in persons with AIDS. While the condition generally is seen in less than 0.2 percent of U.S. AIDS patients, it is common in infected individuals in tropical and subtropical climates. Isosporiasis is frequently found to be the initial opportunistic infection of HIV-infected persons in Haiti.

Cause and Transmission. *Isospora belli* (ī-SOS-pō-ra, bel-lē) causes isosporiasis which is a long-lasting form of diarrhea. The causative agent is acquired through the ingestion of contaminated food or water.

Signs and Symptoms Infected individuals generally experience a number of symptoms that are indistinguishable from those of cryptosporidiosis. These include diarrhea (which may last for six months), weight loss, nausea, and abdominal cramps. Fever and vomiting generally are not typical complaints.

Diagnosis and Treatment. Diagnosis of *T. belli* depends on demonstrating the causative agent in stool specimens. Its appearance is quite characteristic.

Infected individuals generally respond well and fairly quickly to treatment with trimethoprim and sulfamethoxazole.

VIRUS INFECTIONS

Various viruses also take advantage of the immunologic defects and weakened defense mechanisms of the immunocompromised host. In certain HIV-infected persons, viruses that have been inactive (latent) are activated to produce widespread (disseminated) aggressive infections. These disease agents include papilloma viruses (fig. 11.8), Epstein-Barr virus, a probable cause of hairy leukoplakia (fig. 11.9), and cytomegalovirus, by far the most common cause of a severe infection involving the retina or, the light-sensitive portion of the eye (color photograph 18). The general features of these viruses and their associated diseases have been described in earlier chapters.

SHINGLES

Other viruses, such as **herpes zoster** (HER-pēz, ZOS-ter), the herpes virus that causes chicken pox, and **shingles** (SHING-lz) are found with a high frequency among persons at risk for AIDS. The resulting herpes virus infection appears to be related to HIV infection, and causes both skin involvement and widespread disease (color photograph 26). Herpes zoster frequently occurs months to years before other opportunistic infections (table 11.1) or tumors develop. Painful and severe forms of the shingles have been associated with the development of AIDS.

A general diagnosis of zoster or shingles can be made from the appearance of skin lesions. However, confirmation is provided by laboratory tests, which include microscopic examination of material taken from skin blisters, and virus culture.

Treatment for shingles has been successful with the use of acyclovir (a-SĪ-klō-vir), a drug used with other herpes virus infections. (See chapter 7.)

FIGURE 11.8

The fingers (a) and toes (b) of a patient with AIDS and warts widely spread over the body. A human papilloma virus associated with cancer was isolated from penile warts. (From P. B. Milburn, J. L. Brandsma, C. I. Goldsman, E. D. Teplitz, and E. I. Heilman, *Journal of American Academy of Dermatology* (1989) 19:401–405.)

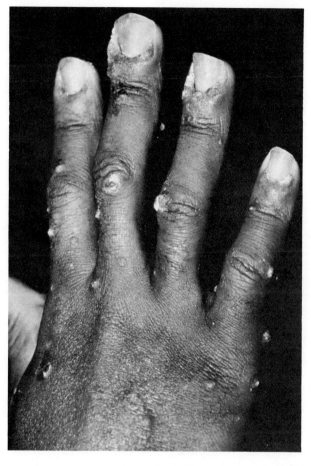

a

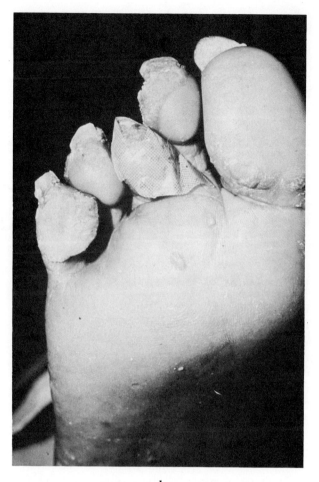

b

FIGURE 11.9

Hairy leukoplakia. (a) The appearance of the condition. (b) An electron micrograph showing virus-like particles (arrows) believed to be Epstein-Barr virus. (From E. Alessi and
Associates, *Journal of American Academy of Dermatology* (1990) 22:79–86.)

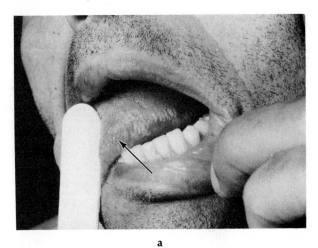

a

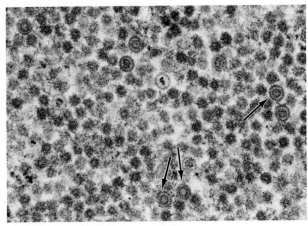

b

BACTERIAL INFECTIONS

Complications of HIV infection involve almost every organ system. Persons with advanced HIV infection have a very high incidence of respiratory-tract illness. In addition to *Pneumocystis carinii* (mentioned earlier), a variety of other microorganisms including the mycobacteria produce life-threatening situations in hosts immunocompromised by HIV. A number of studies have clearly shown that the notable decline over the past ten years in the occurrence of tuberculosis in the United States and elsewhere has been reversed by HIV infection and AIDS. Attention here will be given only to the mycobacteria and the infections they cause.

TUBERCULOSIS

Mycobacterium tuberculosis (mī′-kō-bak-TER-e-um, tū-ber′-kū-LO-sis), also known as the **tubercle** (TU-ber-kl) **bacillus,** causes tuberculosis (TB) and forms of this disease that occur in organs or body locations outside of the lungs. TB is spread by inhaling tiny airborne particles containing *tubercle bacilli* coughed up by a person with the disease. In susceptible individuals such as immunocompromised hosts, the inhaled bacteria travel into the lungs and eventually reach the air sacs of the organ where they multiply and cause tuberculosis.

While this bacterial infection can develop even in persons with normally functioning immune systems, the HIV-infected individual is more likely to develop the disease. Several studies also show that in HIV-infected persons, tuberculosis most often results from the reactivation of previously acquired but inactive infection.

Signs and Symptoms. Generally, individuals with pulmonary TB are most infectious before diagnosis and treatment. Typical symptoms in a person with TB include dry cough, fever, night sweats, weight loss and general fatigue. Many individuals also experience a tightness in the chest and breathing difficulties. Whether active tuberculosis occurs soon after exposure and infection with the *tubercle bacillus* or years later, the disease may involve several other body locations. These **extrapulmonary** (eks′-tra-PUL-mo-ne-re) forms of the disease particularly involve the lymph nodes and spread to other body parts. Symptoms experienced in such situations depend on the site affected. Tuberculosis is not any

HIV INFECTION AND TROPICAL DISEASES

The major causes of disease and death in developing parts of the world such as Africa are strikingly different from those found in technically advanced or industrialized countries. In many developing countries, poverty, ignorance, social inequities, and environmental conditions combine with inadequate health care resources to create a disease pattern having disastrous consequences. While combating endemic diseases (those normally found to a greater or lesser degree within a region) is a major problem, the rapidly spreading HIV epidemic in Africa has raised additional concerns and fears. These include the possibility of interactions between existing infectious agents and HIV, and the consequences of such interactions. While being infected with more than one disease agent is common in poor countries, individuals with such *coinfections* may experience more severe injuries or become more susceptible to other diseases. Most infants and children dying in Africa have some combination of malnutrition, malaria, respiratory infection, and intestinal worms.

The epidemiological pattern of HIV infection in Africa indicates that two major groups are at high risk. These are heterosexually active adults, and infants of HIV-infected mothers. Risk factors for the adults include multiple sex partners, other sexually transmitted diseases (especially those that lead to the formation of genital sores), sexual relations with prostitutes, and living in cities or urban areas. Diseases and/or disease conditions known to thrive in urban areas include diarrhea, respiratory infections, tuberculosis, hepatitis, and sexually transmitted diseases.

With respect to children, approximately 25 to 50 percent of infants born to HIV-infected mothers become infected with the virus. In some parts of Africa the blood transfusions given to infant-toddlers with severe malaria-caused blood loss represent another important source for HIV transmission. In 1988, a large number of children infected with malaria tragically were found to have contracted HIV infection from transfusions with virus-contaminated blood.

A number of tropical disease agents that may interact with HIV are under study. Thus far, the causative agent of tuberculosis (the *tubercle bacillus*), is the main one for which an important interaction with HIV infection has been clearly established. Hidden or inactive tuberculosis may be reactivated by the lower resistance resulting from HIV infection. In developing countries studies have found that more than 60 percent of adults have latent tuberculosis.

Other candidates that may enter into an HIV interaction include various worms, hepatitis B virus, Epstein-Barr virus, and the various causes of diarrhea. Information as to the extent and importance of these possible interactions should become available in the near future. Unfortunately, as is the case with tuberculosis, HIV tropical disease agent interactions probably will become a growing public health problem in developing countries. Such HIV coinfections may also affect the treatment and control of tropical diseases.

FIGURE 11.10

An example of a positive TB skin test. In such cases usually the involved area is swollen, reddened, and may form open sores.

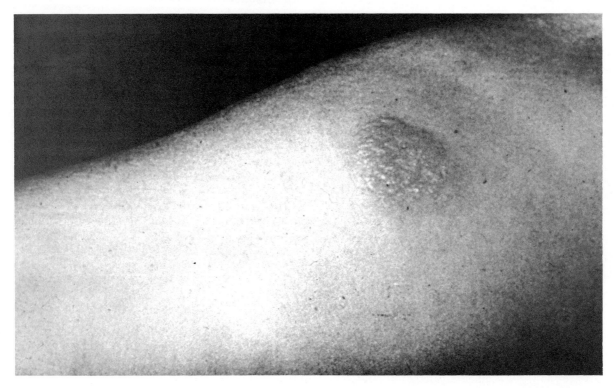

more communicable in a person with TB and HIV infection than it is in an individual with only TB.

Diagnosis. The *Mantoux* (man-TŪ) tuberculin skin test is used as a screening tool to detect both those individuals with TB and those at risk of developing the disease because of prior infection with the *tubercle bacillus*. An infection is indicated in persons without symptoms by the development of an enlarged, reddened, and sometimes ulcerating reaction in the area into which the skin testing material was injected some forty-eight hours before. (Figure 11.10)

All persons who have positive tests for HIV or who practice high-risk behaviors for HIV infection should be skin tested for TB. Unfortunately, some individuals with both HIV and TB infections may exhibit negative skin tests because of their immunocompromised condition. Chest X-rays and appropriate laboratory tests, including the staining of sputum specimens and isolation, and appropriate culture techniques for the *tubercle bacillus,* are needed for such persons. A special staining procedure known as the **acid-fast stain** is used with specimens to find evidence of a possible infection with *M. tuberculosis* and other related bacteria.

Treatment. Treatment for tuberculosis is generally based on laboratory and X-ray findings. It is especially important in cases of persons with high risk of HIV infection. Several drugs are in common use for treatment. These include **isoniazid** (ī'-so-NĪ-a-zid), **rifampin** (RIF-am-pin), **pyrazinamide** (pī'-ra-SIN-a-mīd), and **ethambutol** (e-THAM-bū-tōl). Although individuals with both active TB and HIV infection respond well to medication, treatment is necessary for a longer period of time than for persons with only TB. Generally after the first few weeks of drug treatment, most persons with TB become noninfectious.

FIGURE 11.11

A localized infection in the groin caused by the opportunistic bacterium *Mycobacterium avium–Mycobacterium intracellulare*. (a) Before treatment. (b) After treatment. (From D. J. Barbaro,

V. L. Orcutt, and B. M. Coldrion, *Reviews of Infectious Diseases* (1989) 11:625.)

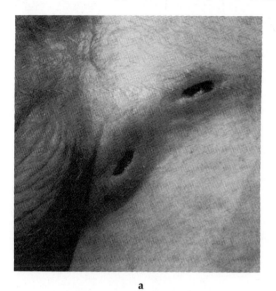

a

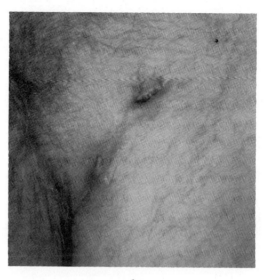

b

Control. Preventing the spread of TB is particularly important not only in the case of HIV infection but in general. Transmission of *tubercle bacilli* can be reduced by several ways, including: the early and appropriate use of anti-TB drugs, providing adequate ventilation in rooms and facilities used by persons with TB, and the covering of the nose and mouth when coughing and sneezing.

MYCOBACTERIUM AVIUM – INTRACELLULARE INFECTIONS

In the years following World War II, an increasing number of non-*tubercle bacilli* were isolated from individuals with long-standing lung disease at the Battey State Hospital in Rome, Georgia. These bacteria, often referred to as the Battey (BAT-ē) bacilli, and eventually named *Mycobacterium avium-M. intracellulare* or *M. avium* complex (MAC), are among the most frequently found opportunists in persons with AIDS (fig. 11.11).

The *M. avium* complex is commonly found in soil and water, and is known to cause tuberculosis in birds and various mammals such as pigs and cattle.

Humans with normal immune systems are relatively resistant to MAC infection.

Signs and Symptoms. Persons with AIDS and MAC infections widely distributed throughout their bodies generally exhibit nonspecific signs and symptoms. Infection in such individuals is indicated by signs such as the appearance of a high fever (often associated with drenching night sweats), diarrhea, and general weakness. Other signs of infection include swollen lymph nodes, enlarged liver and spleen, and pneumonia.

Diagnosis and Treatment. Diagnosis of MAC infection is based on laboratory findings. The fact that the causative agent can be found in several body locations is of value for obtaining specimens for special microscopic staining techniques such as the acid-fast procedure mentioned earlier for tuberculosis. Culturing of stool specimens also is used for diagnosis.

Treatment for MAC infection in immunodeficient hosts follows the recommendations of the American Thoracic Society. Antibiotics and related drugs are selected on the basis of laboratory tests used to determine the specific drug sensitivity of the disease agent. Antibiotics commonly used for treatment include **cycloserine** (sī'-KLŌ-ser-ēn) and **ethambutol.**

A WORD ABOUT WORMS AND CERTAIN GASTROINTESTINAL INFECTIONS

The sexual transmission of protozoan and worm infections by orogenital or oroanal routes has become increasingly common during the past twenty to twenty-five years, especially in young homosexual men. Most of these conditions are caused by organisms that generally are acquired through the ingestion of contaminated food or water. They include the protozoan diseases **amebic dysentery** (a-MĒ-bik, DIS-en-ter-ē), **giardiasis** (jī-ar-DĪ-a-sis), and the worm infections such as pinworm. The current situation is complicated in that many infected persons appear to be without symptoms or only slightly ill, thus making them unsuspected carriers of the disease agents. Moreover, infections may become long-lasting or chronic, and contribute to lowering the competency of the immune system, and thereby render protozoan- or worm-harboring persons more susceptible to attack by HIV.

HIV can damage organs directly. However, by progressively crippling the body's defenses, the virus also sets the stage for invasions by microorganisms and other disease agents that can reproduce wildly only because the body's immune system is defective.

CHAPTER **12** # HIV AND RELATED INFECTIONS

> The spread of HIV, the causal agent of AIDS, is a grave threat to the health of the world's population and poses a major constraint to social and economic development in many countries.
>
> *—Patrick Friel*

The human immunodeficiency virus type 1 (HIV–1) was first described by independent groups of investigators in 1983 and 1984. It was later shown to be the causative agent of the disease **acquired immune deficiency syndrome,** or **AIDS.** The original idea that AIDS might be caused by a virus developed from earlier studies involving a group of viruses known as the **retroviruses** (ret'-rō-VĪ-rus-es). These viruses cause a number of different cancers and infect a wide variety of animal species.

In the five years immediately following the initial description of AIDS, attention was focused on the isolation and description of the retroviral agent responsible for the disease and diagnostic tests for the identification of symptomatic and asymptomatic HIV-infected persons. The identification and treatment of opportunistic infectious agents also were of considerable interest and concern. This chapter mainly deals with the general features of human retroviruses, their transmission, and consideration of how HIV damages the immune and other body systems.

ENTER THE RETROVIRUSES—AN OVERVIEW

Retroviruses were so named because they reverse what seemed to be the normal flow of genetic information in a biological system such as a cell. In cells the genetic information is deoxyribonucleic acid (DNA) and is generally organized into genes. When genes are expressed, or in a sense activated, the information in the DNA is copied through a process known as **transcription** (tran-SKRIP-shun) into another chemical molecule called **messenger ribonucleic acid** (mRNA). The information in the mRNA is then read, or decoded, by another process known as **translation** (trans-LA-shun), and used as a pattern for the production of specific proteins. Thus the flow of genetic information can be shown as:

$$DNA \rightarrow MRNA \rightarrow Protein$$

RNA-containing viruses duplicate their genetic material in several different ways. For example, before the genetic information of a retrovirus can be expressed it must first be converted into a copy of itself in the form of a single strand of DNA. The enzyme performing this process is known as **reverse transcriptase** because it transcribes in a **reverse,** or retro, manner. Thus, viruses containing the enzyme are referred to as **retroviruses.** The process does not stop at this point. The newly formed DNA strand next acts as a pattern for the formation of a complementary DNA strand, and a normal double-stranded DNA is produced. This new viral DNA cannot be distinguished from the DNA in a host cell. After its formation, the viral DNA may integrate itself into the host's DNA and thereby become a permanent part of the genetic material in the host cell. Once incorporated into the host's cell genetic material, the viral DNA is referred to as a **provirus.** Here it will remain in a fairly sheltered environment until it is activated to make new RNA viral particles. Thus the flow of genetic information in retroviruses and the resulting events can be shown as:

viral RNA → single DNA strand → double DNA strand → provirus formation → NEW RNA VIRUSES

It is interesting to note that retroviruses were among the first viruses associated with specific diseases. For example, in 1904 a form of infectious blood disease known to be transmissible among horses was linked to a retroviral cause. Some years later in 1911, certain leukemias and cancers of muscle and bone in chickens were added to the list of retroviral diseases. With the development of the electron microscope in the late 1940s and early 1950s, a number of viruses responsible for many kinds of animal cancers were actually seen.

HUMAN RETROVIRUSES

It was generally believed by many scientists that retroviruses did not exist in humans. In 1970, Robert Gallo and his co-workers changed this view with the isolation and identification of a **human T cell lymphotropic** (lim-fo-TRO-pik) **virus** (fig. 12.1). Now simply referred to as **HTLV-1,** this human virus is known to cause certain types of cancers. Shortly after this discovery a related virus, HTLV-II, was identified. Infections with both of these viral agents of disease are quite common, particularly among intravenous drug users.

In 1983 and 1984, intensive investigations were carried out by a French group of scientists headed by Luc Montagnier and an American team led by Gallo. Both isolated a third human disease-causing retrovirus. The French labelled this agent **lymphoadenopathy** (lim-fad-e-NOP-a-the) **virus** or **LAV,** while the Americans designated it as **HTLV-III.** Interestingly, both groups of investigators showed that the virus could be isolated from a large number of individuals with AIDS, or with various symptoms suggestive of developing the disease. Antibodies to specific proteins of the viral agent were found in almost every case. In an effort to standardize the name of the virus, and after much debate,

FIGURE 12.1

Features of human T lymphotropic virus type I (HTLV–I). (a) An example of a lymphocyte found in individuals infected with HTLV–I. This cell is magnified 19,000 times. (Courtesy of Dr. M. T. Daniel). (b) The appearance of HTLV–I (arrows) as observed with an electron microscope. These viruses are magnified 35,000 times. (From O. Gout and Associates, *Archives of Neurology* (1989) 46:255–260.) (Courtesy of Dr. J. Lasneret)

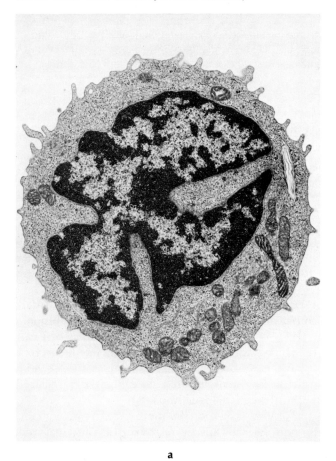

a

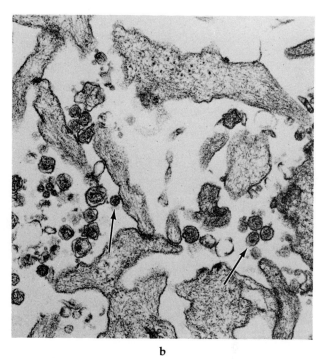

b

the agent's name was changed to **human immunodeficiency virus (HIV).** Table 12.1 summarizes several of the features associated with the various human retroviruses known to exist as of 1990.

Shared Properties of Retroviruses. While these and related viruses have distinct biochemical and genetic differences, they share a number of features. These include similar means of transmission, a particular attraction for T_4 **(helper) lymphocytes** and other cells such as macrophages and certain brain cells that carry a CD_4 protein on their surfaces, and possession of specific genes and related components important to viral replication. Many of these retroviruses are associated with host immunodeficiency, disorders of the central nervous system (CNS), and the development of several types of cancers.

Even though the retroviruses share several properties in common, they do have differences. Such differences are of value in dividing the viral group into smaller *groups.*

The Subgroups. Three different subgroups are recognized. These are **Spumivirus** (SPŪ-mē-vī-rus),

TABLE 12.1 | DISEASES CAUSED BY OR ASSOCIATED WITH HUMAN RETROVIRUSES

VIRUS	DISEASE(S) DIRECTLY OR INDIRECTLY ASSOCIATED
Human immunodeficiency virus–1 (HIV–1)[a]	Acquired immune deficiency syndrome (AIDS); AIDS-related complex (ARC); dementia (dē-MEN-shē-a), a breakdown of mental abilities; other central nervous system disorders; Kaposi's sarcoma (indirect association)
Human immunodeficency virus–2 (HIV–2)	AIDS; other immune system deficiencies
Human T cell lymphotropic virus–1 (HTLV–I)	Adult form of T cell leukemia; destruction of the spinal cord; minor immune system defects
Human T cell lymphotropic virus–2 (HTLV–II)	Hairy cell leukemia; tumors involving T helper cells; widespread lymph node disease developing from various skin disorders
Human T cell lymphotropic virus–V (HTLV–V)	Mycosis fungoides (mī-KŌ-sis, FUN-goyd-ēz). A rare form of skin cancer that eventually involves lymph nodes and internal organs; other forms of skin cancer

[a]Was first called human T cell lymphotropic virus–III (HTLV–III)

Oncovirus (ON-kō-vī-rus) and **Lentivirus** (LEN-ti-vī-rus). Their general properties briefly are as follows:

Spumiviruses are generally not associated with diseases of any kind. When they are isolated, the viruses are recognized in tissue culture preparations by the presence of clear spaces filled with fluid in infected cells.

The *oncoviruses* are animal RNA, tumor-producing or transforming agents that cause various types of leukemia and cancers in birds, cats, and other animals. Three human oncoviruses also are known: human T cell lymphotropic virus I (or HTLV-I), HTLV-II, and HTLV-V. (See Table 12.1 for the diseases currently linked to these viruses.)

HTLV-I is associated with a rare form of adult T cell leukemia and with long-lasting forms of diseases involving the spinal cord. Since its discovery in 1977, infections have been found in Japan and portions of the Caribbean on a fairly consistent level. Cases of infection also have been reported among intravenous drug abusers in the United States.

HTLV-I is primarily transmitted by sexual intercourse and transfusions with contaminated blood.

HTLV–II may be the cause of a rare form of T cell leukemia. Additional information is needed before the full extent of its disease-causing abilities can be described. Transmission of the virus is associated with intravenous drug abusers.

HTLV–V is one of the more recently discovered human disease-causing retroviruses. Certain forms of T cell leukemia are believed to result from infection with this virus. Its major means of transmission is not known.

The *lentiviruses* are known for their cell destroying abilities and slowly developing infections of animals. Several of the diseases caused by this subgroup result in paralysis, a wasting condition in which a loss of body strength and size occurs, inflammation of the nervous system, pneumonia, and painful joints and bones (arthritis). While the human immunodeficiency viruses (HIV) are lentiviruses, several other related retroviruses are known to infect and to cause immunodeficiency-like conditions.

ADULT T CELL LEUKEMIA/LYMPHOMA (ATLL)

GENERAL BACKGROUND

The occurrence or incidence of malignant lymphomas (growths in the lymphatic system), such as Hodgkin's disease in Asian countries such as Japan and China, is relatively low compared to that found in western European countries and the United States. However, in limited areas of Japan, a specific type of **lymphoid** (LIM-foyd) **malignancy** called **adult T-cell leukemia/lymphoma (ATLL),** caused by human T cell leukemia virus type 1, **HTLV-I)** is fairly common. Many healthy carriers of the virus have been found.

THE VIRUS AND TRANSMISSION

The etiologic agent HTLV–1 was discovered in 1980. It is the first human retrovirus to be clearly linked to a new growth, or neoplasm. This virus is not readily **contagious** (kon-TA-jus) under natural conditions. The natural routes of virus transmission currently recognized are: 1) from mother to child mainly through breast-feeding and 2) sexual contact.

FORMS OF THE DISEASE

Four different neoplastic conditions have been recognized since the discovery of ATLL. These are **acute, cutaneous, chronic,** and slowly developing, or **smoldering.** The acute form is the most common type of ATLL. Typical cases exhibit a form of leukemia with atypical white blood cells, lymphadenopathy, cutaneous involvement, general discomfort or **malaise** (mā-LAZ), and fatigue. ATLL patients are all adults, and appear to be more susceptible to infections by microorganisms that are normally nonpathogenic, but because of the lowered resistance of these patients are able to establish a disease process.

PREVENTION

ATLL in Japan is an important subject in the field of cancer epidemiology. Several trial intervention programs for disease prevention are under consideration. One of the most important of these is to control the vertical transmission of HTLV–1 from mother to child. Since breast feeding by a HTLV–1 carrier mother is the most conceivable route of virus transmission here, the use of artificially prepared milk is being recommended to expectant mothers who have been found to be HTLV–1 carriers.

Table 12.2 lists examples of these lentiviruses and the hosts involved.

HUMAN IMMUNODEFICIENCY VIRUS-1 (HIV-1)

HISTORICAL ASPECTS AND GEOGRAPHIC DISTRIBUTION

The human immunodeficiency virus type 1 is well established as the causative agent of the AIDS epidemic in central Africa, Europe, the United States, and most other countries of the world. The geographic origin of this virus and of the current epidemic is believed to be central Africa since descriptions of disease states typical of AIDS were reported there as early as the mid-1970s. Blood samples taken in Africa at that time and before, contained antibodies against HIV–1. The earliest antibody response to the virus dates back to 1959 and was found in stored blood samples from Zaire. Several studies suggest that HIV–1 infection began to spread epidemically in cities and towns of central

TABLE 12.2 | LENTIVIRUSES ASSOCIATED WITH IMMUNODEFICIENCY-LIKE CONDITIONS

VIRUS	HOST	DISEASE DESCRIPTION
Bovine immunodeficiency virus (BIV)	Cattle	Enlarged and infected lymph nodes
Equine infectious anemia virus	Horses	Fever, blood loss
Feline immunodeficiency virus (FIV)	Cats	Immunodeficiency
Simian immunodeficiency virus (SIV)	Monkeys	Immunodeficiency
Visna virus	Sheep	Wasting, paralysis

FOCUS ON STDs

AN AIDS-LIKE DISEASE IN CATS

A recently identified retrovirus has been shown to cause a long-lasting immunodeficiency-like condition in cats (fig. 12.2). In early reports the virus was referred to as a feline T lymphotropic lentivirus to reflect its particular attraction to a cat's T lymphocytes and its similarity to retroviruses. The name of the disease agent has been changed to feline immunodeficiency virus (FIV) to conform with international terminology for immunodeficiency-linked viruses.

FIV is infectious among cat populations and can be spread by intimate and prolonged contact. Early reports suggest that biting is an important means of transmission. Most epidemiological studies have indicated that outdoor, free-roaming male cats were at greatest risk for infection. In addition, the infection rate is two to three times higher in males versus females, and the average age of an FIV-infected cat is about five to six years of age.

The course of FIV infection generally follows a long, asymptomatic phase lasting for several months or perhaps years. During this time the virus can be isolated but symptoms are not obvious. Typical symptoms most commonly found include a running nose (increased mucous secretion), fever, swollen lymph nodes, weight loss, inflammation of the gums, diarrhea, skin sores, and opportunistic infections. Malignancies also have been found in various body organs. These conditions vary among infected cats, but generally last a fairly long time. Once symptoms appear, however, infected cats begin to shed the virus.

It is quite obvious that FIV infection resembles HIV infection in several ways. Recent studies have found additional similarities including a sensitivity to the drug AZT which is used in the treatment of AIDS. Because of the number of such similarities FIV may prove useful in drug and vaccine research studies associated with finding effective solutions to the AIDS epidemic.

FIGURE 12.2

A cat showing the effects of immunodeficiency caused by feline leukemia virus. The disease state is quite similar to human immunodeficiency syndrome caused by HIV infection. (From E. A. Hoover, *Blood* (1987) 70:1880–1892.)

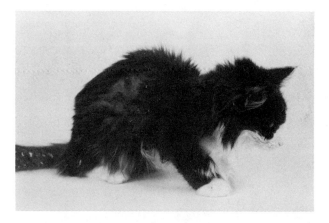

Africa during the mid- and later 1970s. Once introduced into populations where individuals were likely to have multiple sex partners, or to be exposed to blood or blood products, HIV infection spread rapidly. The rate of HIV–1 transmission is clearly related to social and economic factors.

The features of AIDS were first recognized in the United States in 1981, apparently several years after HIV–1 was introduced into the population. Blood samples collected in the United States and Europe before the mid-1970s generally showed no evidence of antibodies against HIV. It thus became apparent early on that AIDS probably originated in Africa.

In the United States, AIDS first appeared in a limited geographic area and then spread to other regions. The disease was found in socially, economically, and geographically different groups, all of which shared a tendency to be infected with similar

FOCUS ON STDs

THE TREATMENT OF HEMOPHILIA — A PAST TRAGEDY

The transmission of *bacterial pathogens* by blood or blood related products is seldom a problem in today's world. However, the transmission of other disease agents such as hepatitis B and human immunodeficiency viruses (HIV) has been and is still a cause for serious concern. This is especially the case for individuals who have abnormal bleeding difficulties such as those posed by hemophilia (hē′-mō-FIL-ē-a) and other blood clotting problems.

Hemophilia is a hereditary disease in which the blood of afflicted individuals fails to clot normally thus causing any bleeding to take a long time to stop. Effective modern treatment of such persons became available in 1965 and involved the use of commercially concentrated preparations of coagulating substances or factors needed for normal blood clotting. One of these factors, known as *Factor VIII*, may require 20,000 blood donors to obtain a sufficient quantity of it.

The enthusiasm and the hope with which the new products were greeted was slightly dampened by the early finding that all of the Factor VIII products were contaminated with hepatitis viruses. Unfortunately, about 90 percent of persons with hemophilia using the commercial products eventually showed evidence of hepatitis virus infections. Adding to this tragedy soon came the realization that the majority of persons with hemophilia or related disorders became infected with HIV–1 through the use of the commercial blood clotting factor concentrates. These preparations were manufactured before the screening of donors, and before the use of specific measures such as heat to inactivate any viruses possibly present.

Today a number of virus-inactivating measures are used to make commercial blood clotting concentrates safe and free from hepatitis viruses and HIV. In addition, newer products developed through genetic engineering technology have been found to be safe and appear to show great promise for the treatment of hemophilia.

FIGURE 12.3

An HIV-infected cell with a large number of viruses (arrows) being released.

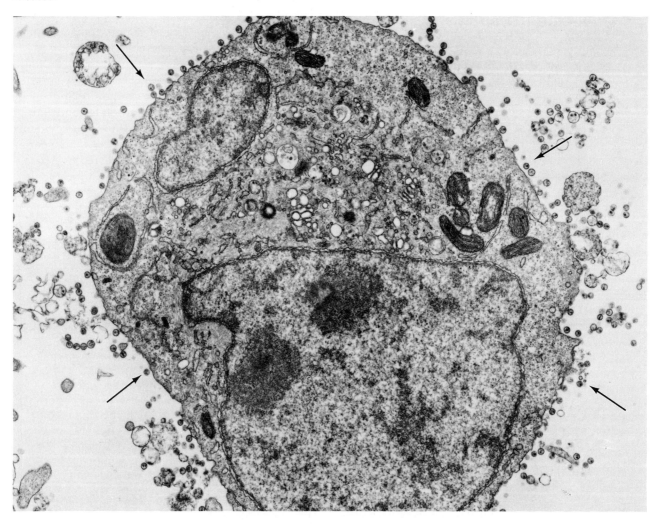

viral disease agents such as hepatitis B virus and cytomegalovirus. (See chapter 8.) Individuals within these groups who developed AIDS were found to be connected by common contacts, recipients of blood products, sexual partners, or children of affected persons.

TRANSMISSION

HIV-infected cells (fig. 12.3) and individual virus particles circulate in the bloodstream and may be present in a variety of blood products. Body fluids found to contain small amounts of HIV include tears, saliva, blood, vaginal secretions, semen, and breast milk. However, only blood, vaginal secretions, semen, and possibly breast milk of infected individuals have been associated with the spread of the virus. Transmission of HIV occurs with these sources through sexual contact, exposure to contaminated blood or blood products, or by transfer of the virus from an infected mother to her fetus, (also known as *perinatal transmission*). Table 12.3 summarizes the known routes of transmission.

TABLE 12.3 | TRANSMISSION OF HIV

KNOWN ROUTES OF TRANSMISSION

Inoculation of Blood

1. Transfusion of contaminated blood and/or blood products

2. Contaminated needle sharing among intravenous drug users

3. Needle-stick, open wound, and mucous membrane exposure to contaminated blood by health care personnel

4. Injection with unsterilized, contaminated needles

Sexual Activities

1. Anal intercourse with an HIV-infected person (includes intercourse between two men, or a male and a female)

2. Vaginal intercourse

3. Oral sex

Perinatal[a]

1. During pregnancy (intrauterine)

2. During labor and delivery

3. Shortly after birth by ingestion of HIV-infected breast milk

[a]Refers to the period beginning after the 28th week of pregnancy through 28 days following birth of a baby.

Individuals associated with various types of high-risk behavior increase the possibility of acquiring an infection. These also are listed in table 12.3 and include sexual intercourse involving infected homosexual and bisexual males, intravenous (IV) drug users, recipients of contaminated blood or blood products, and children born to mothers either with AIDS or in high-risk behavior groups. Heterosexual transmission of HIV also is possible and can occur from sexual intercourse with HIV-infected prostitutes, IV drug users, or bisexual men. Table 12.4 lists several sources and/or carriers of HIV.

HIV can also be acquired by other than sexual means. The virus can enter the body through the contamination of various types of wounds, including cuts and punctures. This potential type of danger is of concern to health care workers and others. Chapter 14 discusses the problem and measures which can be used to prevent exposure to the virus. One particular unfounded fear with blood has been in relation to *donating* blood. There is no evidence of any danger associated with blood donations (fig. 12.4), since there is no exchange of blood during the procedure.

A number of routes also have been studied and shown not to be involved in spreading HIV. For example, there is no evidence of transmission by prolonged nonsexual contact with infected individuals (fig. 12.5). In addition, infection has not been acquired through inhalation, ingestion of food or water, or by the bites of arthropods such as ticks, mosquitoes, or bedbugs. Transmission does not occur through casual contact.

Factors in HIV Transmission. *What are the chances of getting or transmitting human immunodeficiency virus during sexual activity? What factors help or interfere with spreading the virus?* These are probably two of the most commonly asked questions by individuals exposed not only to an HIV-infected person, but to all forms of STDs.

TABLE 12.4 | POSSIBLE SOURCES AND/OR CARRIERS OF HIV

ADOLESCENTS/ADULTS

Homosexual or bisexual males

Intravenous drug abusers

Hemophiliacs

Sexual partners of high-risk group members

Prostitutes

Transfusion recipients (received blood or blood products prior to 1985)

Mother practicing high-risk behavior

INFANTS/YOUNG CHILDREN

Child born to HIV-positive mother

Transfusion recipient

Hemophiliacs

Sexually and physically abused child

Various studies indicate that some persons become HIV-infected after a single or a few sexual encounters, whereas others remain uninfected despite hundreds of unprotected contacts. Situations of this type indicate that the chances of HIV infection may be greatly affected by some property of the HIV-infected partner, the virus itself, or the noninfected partner. Clearly, host or viral factors are likely to be important determiners of whether a single sexual encounter will be sufficient to transmit HIV. Specific factors such as the presence of genital sores (color photographs 4 and 6) and the type of sexual activities practiced are considered to increase the likelihood of infection. Table 12.5 lists both infectious and noninfectious causes of genital sores. The presence of uncovered genital sores (a source of HIV) during sexual intercourse and related activities increases the possibility of infection of either partner. The use of barrier devices such as a condom lowers but does not totally eliminate the risk of an infection in such situations.

As research into factors that contribute to HIV transmission continues, a clearer idea begins to emerge as to the risks involved with certain sexual practices. Figure 12.6 shows the potential risk of HIV infection for an uninfected partner or from an infected partner in relation to the type of sexual activity or practice followed.

FIGURE 12.4

AIDS is not acquired by donating blood. This poster from Brazil's Ministry of Social Assistance says exactly that: "Giving blood doesn't give AIDS." (Courtesy of World Health Organization)

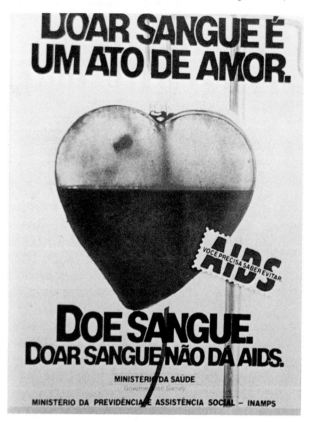

FIGURE 12.5

This poster presents a clear, simple, and direct message. You can't get AIDS by touching a person with AIDS. This is a reminder that AIDS is not transmitted by casual contact. (Courtesy of World Health Organization)

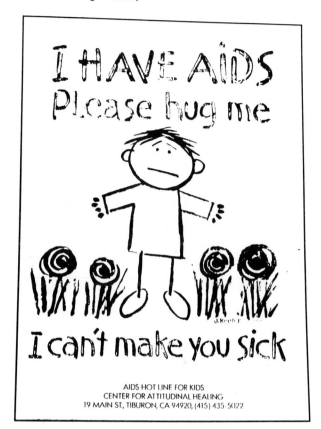

TABLE 12.5 | CAUSES OF GENITAL SORES

INFECTIOUS CAUSES

Yeast infection[a]

Chancroid[b]

Inflammation of pubic hairs

Genital herpes[c]

Granuloma inguinale[b]

Herpes zoster (shingles)

Lymphogranuloma venereum[b]

Pyogenic (pus-producing infections)

Scabies[a]

Syphilis[d]

Trichomoniasis[a]

NONINFECTIOUS CAUSES

Behget's syndrome (a recurring ulceration of the genitalia)

Drug reactions

Leukoplakia (formation of white spots on tongue or cheek surfaces)

Tumors

Injury to genitalia

[a]Chapter 9; [b]Chapter 6; [c]Chapter 7; [d]Chapter 5

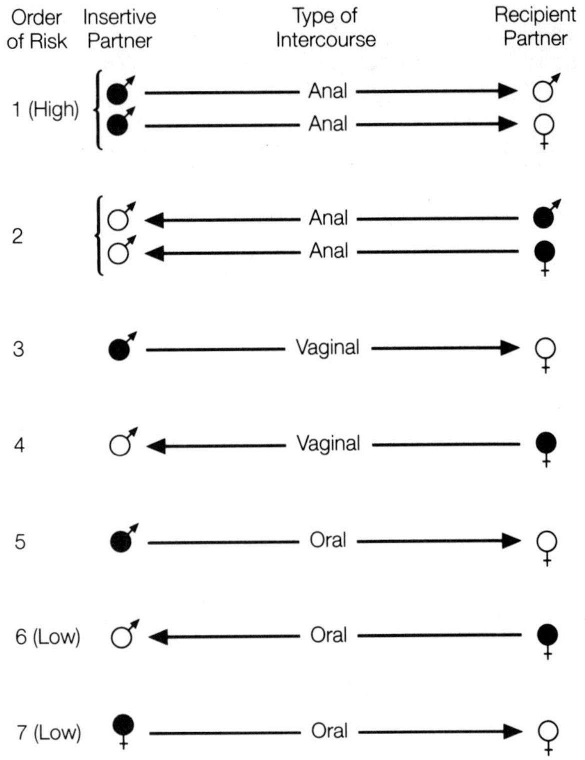

FIGURE 12.6

The order of risk of HIV infection for an uninfected partner (open circle) or from intercourse with an infected partner (closed circle). The presence of uncovered genital sores (chapter 4) increases the possibility of infection of either partner. ♂, male; ♀, female.

HOW EFFECTIVE IS THE CONDOM?

AIDS is still considered a relatively new disease and in many parts of the world it remains largely confined but not limited to individuals practicing high-risk sexually-related activities. One response to this disease, as well as to STDs in general, has been an increase in condom usage. In the United States alone, following the surgeon general's recommendation of condom usage, sales increased 20.3 percent from 1986 through 1987. On a global level, the highest rate of condom usage is in Japan. Japan, like many European countries, seems to have a tradition of condom acceptance dating back to the second world war, when all members of the armed forces serving overseas were issued condoms. Other factors contributing to the high usage of condoms in Japan include an attractively packaged product by Japanese manufacturers and a high proportion of condom sales to *housewives* made by door-to-door *saleswomen*.

Much can probably be learned about the effectiveness and future potential of condoms in controlling the spread of HIV infection by looking back to how condoms have performed since their introduction.

Condoms actually were first developed against syphilis. As described in chapter 5, this STD was apparently imported into Europe from the New World by the sailors of Christopher Columbus's returning fleet at the end of the 15th century. The great Italian anatomist, Gabriel Fallopio, described the alarm and effects syphilis caused throughout Europe. His publication also contained the first account of a *condom*. It was made from a linen sheath that fitted around the glans penis as protection against the much feared "Great Pox," or syphilis. It was only some time later that the birth control potential of condoms was recognized and people began to make them from natural animal membranes which would not be penetrated by male sex cells, or spermatozoa.

The earliest rubber condoms were made from sheets of rubber, and the finished product had a seam along its entire length. Today, condoms are made by dipping glass shaped in the form of a penis, into latex. Finished products are tested in a variety of ways to check for leakage. Laboratory studies clearly show that HIV and other viruses of comparable size will not penetrate intact latex condoms. Moreover, while information on condoms interrupting the spread of STDs is limited, nearly all studies indicate a protective effect. Beneficial effects have been reported by heterosexual married couples, prostitutes, and HIV-negative wives of HIV-positive hemophiliacs who used condoms on a regular basis. It should be noted that such protection is poor with condoms stored under hot, humid conditions.

One of the challenges facing the world at the end of the 20th century is the development of an integrated approach to three great problems, namely, effective family planning, prevention of HIV infection, and sexually transmitted disease control. More educational programs and greater correct use of condoms may hold the key to all three.

FIGURE 12.7

Human immunodeficiency virus I. (a) An electron micrograph of a number of HIV particles showing their general organization. Envelopes (e), capsids (c), and nucleic acid care can be seen in different particles. (Courtesy of Dr. T. Katsumoto). (b) A detailed view of the structure and organization of human immunodeficiency virus (HIV). Various protein (*p*), and glycoprotein (*gp*) parts as well as the nucleic acid core (RNA) and the characteristic enzyme *reverse transcriptase* are shown.

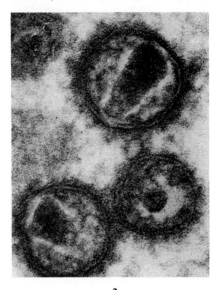

a

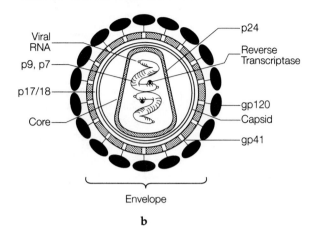

b

VIRUS STRUCTURE AND ORGANIZATION

On examination in an electron microscope HIV exhibits a compact, cylindrical, somewhat centrally-related **core** containing **ribonucleic acid (RNA),** and the **reverse transcriptase enzyme.** These features serve to qualify HIV as a retrovirus. Figure 12.7 shows both the electron microscopic and diagrammatic views of the virus.

GENETIC ORGANIZATION (GENOME) OF HIV-1

A distinguishing property of the lentiviruses is their unusually complex genetic makeup. HIV has a genetic organization or *genome* (JĒ-nōm) consisting of at least nine genes (fig. 12.8). These include the genes "gag," which codes for the formation of capsid proteins; "pol," which codes for reverse transcriptase; and "env," which codes for envelope proteins. Other parts of the genome are involved with the regulation of viral activities and processes. Figure 12.8 and

table 12.6 provide additional information about the HIV genome and its functions.

HUMAN IMMUNODEFICIENCY VIRUS–2 (HIV–2)

HISTORICAL ASPECTS AND GEOGRAPHICAL DISTRIBUTION

Human immunodeficiency virus–2 (HIV-2) is one of the two distinct, but related human viruses known to cause acquired immunodeficiency syndrome, or AIDS. This virus was first isolated in 1986 from AIDS patients and healthy individuals in western Africa, and more recently from Europe and the western hemisphere.

The great majority of HIV–2 infections recognized in Europe have been in individuals from West Africa, in Europeans who had travelled in West Africa and the former Portugese colonies, or in those who had contact (mostly heterosexual) with such people. In the United States and Canada most HIV–2 infected persons were originally from West Africa.

TABLE 12.6 | THE PARTS OF THE HIV GENOME

GENE	ACTIVITY ASSOCIATED WITH PROTEIN PRODUCTION
env	Production of virus envelope structure protein
qaq	Production of virus core (structural) proteins
pol	Production of specific enzymes, including reverse transcriptase and integrase

GENE	ACTIVITY ASSOCIATED WITH GENE REGULATION
nef	Participates in regulating the genes in the genome
rev	Increases production of *gag* and *env* genes
tat	Increases production of viral structural proteins in infected cells
vif	Participates in regulating the genes in the genome
vpu[a]	Role not specifically known, but is related to making a virus infectious
vpx[b]	Role not specifically known, but is related to making a virus infectious
Long terminal repeats (LTR)	Regulates the activity of the genes in the HIV genome

[a]For HIV–1 only
[b]For HIV–2 only

HIV–2 infections found in Brazil occurred in homosexual men and in hospitalized patients.

From the beginning, HIV–2 infection was closely associated with West Africa and in particular with previous Portugese colonies. Recent testing of stored blood specimens collected in 1980 of persons from these areas showed evidence of infection. In addition, on the basis of medical records and the results of blood tests HIV–2-associated-AIDS has been diagnosed retrospectively in several Portugese patients, some of whom exhibited symptoms in 1978. These individual's probably were exposed to the virus in the 1960s. A number of other reports describe the presence of HIV–2 antibodies in stored blood specimens collected in the mid-1960s. From such lines of evidence it is quite likely that HIV–2 has been circulating in West Africa at least since the 1960s.

TRANSMISSION

HIV–2 appears to be spread in the same way as HIV–1. Evidence for its sexual transmission is pro-

vided by the high rates of HIV–2 infection in people with STDs and in female prostitutes, and the occurrence of infection in the heterosexual partners of HIV–2-infected persons. Occasional cases of HIV–2 infection have been found in homosexual men. To date, no evidence of nonsexual transmission has been found in households with HIV–2-infected members.

Several reports suggest that blood and blood products, by transfusion or through exposure to contaminated needles, can spread HIV–2. Such findings include increased rates of HIV–2 infection in children and adults who had received single or multiple blood transfusions, and isolated cases of HIV–2 infection in European hemophiliac patients and intravenous drug users.

Mother-to-child transmission also has been shown to occur. Evidence for this route comes from reports of the isolation of HIV–2 from infants born to HIV–2-infected mothers.

FIGURE 12.8

The genes of HIV–1 together with the specific virus parts associated with them. See table 12.6 for an explanation of the gene symbols and activities.

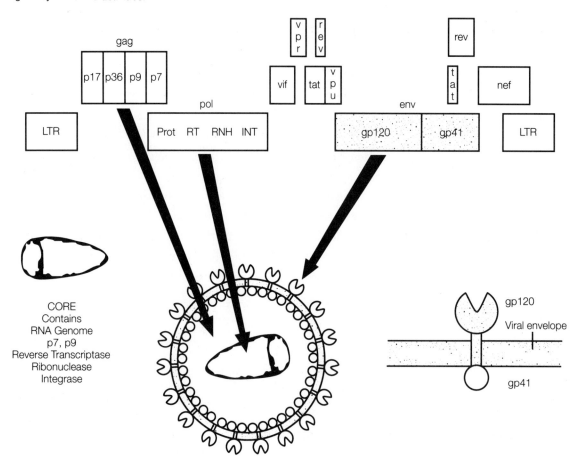

THE LIFE CYCLE OF HIV-1

HIV type–1 is a remarkable disease agent. First, this virus produces a crippling immune deficiency primarily by its unique ability to seek out and to destroy T helper or CD_4 cells. These cells, as chapter 10 emphasized, form the Achilles heel of the body's entire immune response since they serve essential roles contributing to both humoral and cell-medicated immunities. Secondly, HIV–1 is capable of increasing the rate of new virus particle formation by involving host mechanisms for nucleic acid and protein synthesis. Finally, this virus is capable of establishing a hidden or persistent state of infection within a susceptible host which may last for long periods of time. With its activation, HIV enters into a destructive phase leading to the death of the host cell. The cycle of HIV replication and activities will now be presented not only to show how this virus is able to achieve its various relationships, but to indicate where the virus might be attacked by drugs or chemicals during treatment.

STARTING FROM RNA TO DNA AND BACK AGAIN

The first step in the replication cycle of HIV–1 is the *attachment* of the infectious virus to the CD_4 antigen on the surface of human T helper lymphocytes. HIV

FIGURE 12.9

The locations of the body containing cells susceptible to HIV infection. With the possible exception of the supportive tissues of the brain made up of glial cells and special staining cells in portions of the gastrointestinal tract, every cell that can be infected has CD_4 surface receptors.

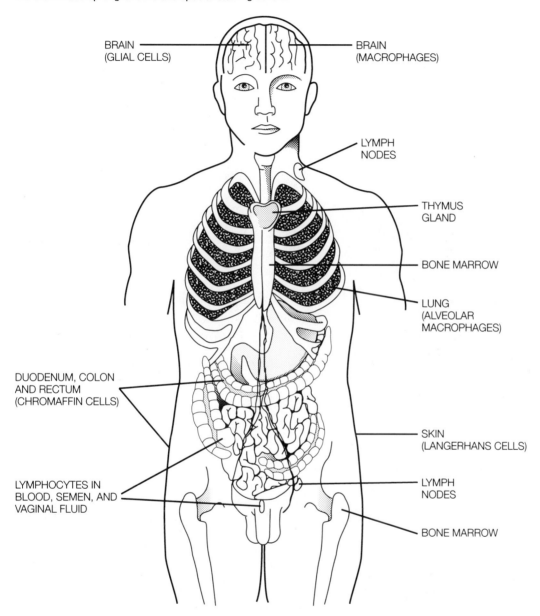

BRAIN
(GLIAL CELLS)

BRAIN
(MACROPHAGES)

LYMPH
NODES

THYMUS
GLAND

BONE MARROW

LUNG
(ALVEOLAR
MACROPHAGES)

DUODENUM, COLON
AND RECTUM
(CHROMAFFIN CELLS)

SKIN
(LANGERHANS CELLS)

LYMPHOCYTES IN
BLOOD, SEMEN, AND
VAGINAL FLUID

LYMPH
NODES

BONE MARROW

has a specific attraction for cells bearing this antigen which include macrophages, glial cells of the brain cells, intestinal surface cells, and certain non-lymphoid cells (fig. 12.9).

The susceptibility of non-lymphoid cells is believed to possibly contribute to the nervous system abnormalities and the diarrhea-associated dramatic weight loss or wasting conditions that develop in

FIGURE 12.10

The replication cycle of HIV. Refer to the text for a general
description of the events involved.

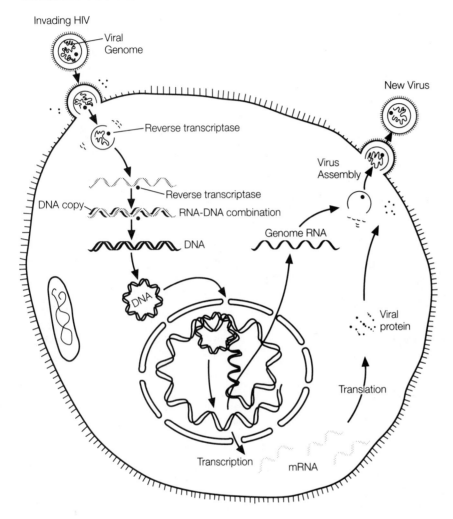

some HIV-infected persons. HIV attachment takes
place between the *gp* (glycoprotein) *120* envelope
part of the virus and specific sites of the CD$_4$ antigen. After this binding step the viral envelope
unites with the host cell membrane and the virus is
ushered into the cells. As the virus penetrates, it
sheds its outer envelope and releases its RNA
genome into the host cell (fig. 12.10).

Once safely inside the cell, HIV converts the viral
genome into the DNA complex described earlier.

HIV–1, like other retroviruses, begins the replicative cycle by forming a DNA copy. The process requires *genetic information* to *flow from RNA to DNA* in
a reverse, or *retro*, direction. This event is critically
dependent on the action of the retroviral enzyme
reverse transcriptase, which uses the HIV RNA as
a pattern to form a complementary single strand of
DNA resulting in an *RNA–DNA combination* referred
to as a **hybrid** (HĪ-brid). The reverse transcriptase
next causes the elimination of the RNA pattern and

FIGURE 12.11

The course of the disease from the time of HIV infection to the development of the symptoms of AIDS. The appearance of antibodies or *seroconversion* is also shown.

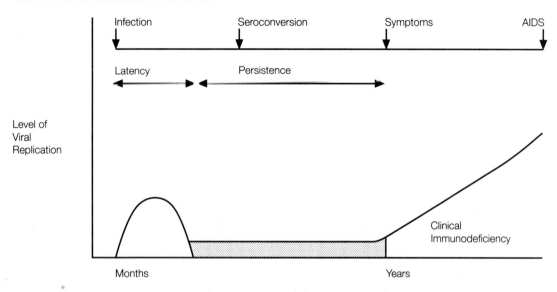

brings about the construction of another single DNA strand that is complementary to the first one formed. The resulting *double DNA strand* quickly forms a circular structure known as a **provirus** (pro-VĪ-rus), which enters the infected cell's nucleus. Here this proviral DNA may remain independent, or become a part of the chromosomal DNA of the host cell (integrated), by a viral enzyme known as an **integrase.** In the integrated situation, the provirus may remain latent (hidden) until it is activated. While in its hidden state, the virus is replicated during the division of the infected cell. This means that all of the descendants of the originally infected cell will contain the virus.

Once activated, the proviral DNA is transcribed into viral RNA by the action of specific host cell enzymes. This viral RNA, which includes both the viral RNA genome and messenger RNA, is transported to the host cell's cytoplasm. Here the messenger RNA is translated to form viral proteins that are in turn adjusted as needed by host and viral enzymes. The viral genome and proteins are then assembled into complete viruses that are released from the cell's membrane surface by a *budding process.* This release

of virus particles from the infected cell's membrane promotes the spreading of HIV to other cells bearing the **CD₄ antigen,** and also contributes to the death of the originally infected cell. Figure 12.11 shows the general steps in the HIV replication cycle.

AIDS is clearly viewed as a fatal disease. However, new insights have been gained from research studies dealing with the life cycle, and interactions between HIV and host cells offer some promise for treatment and control. Knowing the stages in HIV development and replication (table 12.7) provides the bases for the future design of effective antiviral agents with which to attack specific target sites.

Knowing the features of HIV–1 structure as well as its replicative cycle also has provided the foundation for tests to detect infections. The next section deals with general approaches to this topic.

DETECTING HIV INFECTIONS

Given the medical, psychological, and social significance of a positive antibody test for human immunodeficiency virus infection, not only must test

TABLE 12.7 | EXAMPLES OF TARGET SITES FOR ANTIRETROVIRAL THERAPY[a]

Virus surface receptor

Virus entry

Reverse transcriptase

Virus integration into host cell genetic material (genome)

Viral transcription and translation processes

Viral parts production and assembly into infectious viruses

Virus budding process

[a]See figure 12.12. It shows these various target sites as they relate to viral replication.

results be accurate, but the interpretation of such results must be correct as well. Serologic or blood tests for the detection of antibody to HIV were first licensed by the Food and Drug Administration in 1985. They were mainly used for the screening of donated whole blood and plasma. Today, HIV antibody tests are used not only for the screening of donated blood, in blood and plasma collection centers, but they are performed in counseling and testing centers, in medical facilities, in correctional institutions, and for such purposes as screening active duty military personnel and military service applicants.

The presence of an antibody against HIV indicates a current infection though a number of infected persons may have limited or no clinical evidence (visible signs and symptoms) of disease for several years. Antibodies can be detected in a variety of body fluids from infected individuals. These include blood, saliva, cerebrospinal (ser'-ē-brō-SPĪ-nal) fluid (the watery material surrounding and protecting the brain and spinal cord), and secretions from the cervix. Detection of antibodies in blood specimens, however, still remains the most sensitive method.

Most individuals develop detectable levels of antibodies against HIV within six weeks to six months after infection. However, such **seroconversion** (development of antibodies) may take up to three years to occur (fig. 12.11). This hidden or latent period can result in false negative antibody test reports in rare

instances, and present a public health danger by falsely reassuring an individual who is infected and a source of HIV, that he or she is free of infection. On the other hand, there are also rare instances of false positive test results that may lead to unnecessary anxiety in an individual who is, in fact, uninfected. Some of the sociological, psychological, and legal aspects of HIV testing are discussed later in chapter 16.

Serologic testing to confirm HIV infection has two important functions: to establish a basis for diagnosis, and to decrease the transmission of the virus. The counseling and testing of persons who are infected, or at risk for acquiring HIV infection, is an important part of the current prevention strategy. In addition, early diagnosis carries with it the possibility of earlier treatment and prolonging the life of the infected individual.

THE TESTS—GENERAL INFORMATION

The tests currently available and licensed in the United States for HIV antibody testing are enzyme immunoassays **(EIA)** and the **Western blot (WB) assay.** These tests and more specific ones use viral parts (antigens) that are obtained from disrupted whole virus particles cultured in human tissue culture cell lines, or newly developed genetically engineered viral proteins. The Public Health Service (PHS) emphasizes the point that an individual can be considered to have serologic evidence of HIV infection only after an enzyme immunoassay (EIA) screening procedure such as the enzyme-linked immunosorbent assay (**ELISA**) is repeatedly reactive, and a supplemental confirmatory test such as the Western blot assay, or indirect immunofluorescence test, support the EIA findings. In these tests, the terms "reactive" or "nonreactive" are used to describe the results before a final interpretation is made. The terms *"positive"* and *"negative"* are used to describe the interpretation of EIA results indicating that the blood specimen is either repeatedly reactive (*positive*) or repeatedly nonreactive (*negative*). The terms *positive, indeterminate,* and *negative* used in the interpretation of WB assays indicate that the specimen tested is: reactive (positive) for a definite pattern of viral proteins referred to as specific bands (fig. 12.12); reactive for a nonspecific pattern of viral proteins (indeterminate); or nonreactive (negative). Figure 12.13 shows the testing paths followed in the diagnosis of HIV infection.

METHODS TO MEASURE THE RELEASE OF VIRUS FROM INFECTED CELLS

These approaches are used primarily in research studies and include procedures to detect infectious virus, viral proteins, and viral RNA (fig. 12.14) in body fluids. A relatively new test, the polymerase (pol-IM-er-ās) chain reaction, is extremely sensitive and permits reliable detection of very small quantities of virus in body fluids.

EPIDEMIOLOGY OF HIV INFECTION

While the origins of human immunodeficiency virus type I (HIV–1) remain uncertain, the available evidence indicates that the current HIV–1 pandemic probably started, silent and unnoticed, during the mid-to-late 1970s. The recognition of AIDS in 1981, the discovery of HIV–1 in 1983, and the wide availability of diagnostic tests for antibodies to HIV–1 since 1985, have led gradually to a clearer picture of the worldwide extent and distribution of HIV–1 infection.

FIGURE 12.12

The appearance of a Western blot analysis. Lane (column) 1 is a negative control. Lane 2 is a positive control and shows the appearance of specific proteins (*p*) when they are present in specimens. Lanes 3 through 8 show the presence of these proteins in various specimens. (Courtesy of Dr. O. Lyon-Caen, Hospital de la Sal Petriere, Paris, France)

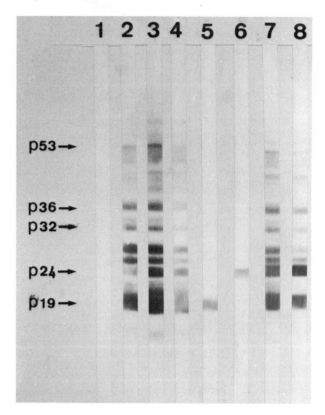

The majority of HIV infections continue to be transmitted by voluntary human behaviors; predominantly sexual intercourse and intravenous drug use. Thus, HIV infections are not uniformly distributed in any population, but disproportionately affect certain identifiable groups of individuals whose behavior places them at greater risk of HIV infection. Such groups of individuals are likely to remain the major source which will continue the pandemic (fig. 12.15).

As of July 1988 there were 108,176 AIDS cases reported from over 140 countries to the *World Health Organization* (**WHO**). An international surveillance

FIGURE 12.13

The testing paths for the diagnosis of HIV infection. Explanation
of abbreviations: ELISA=enzyme=linked immunosorbent assay.
This is an example of an enzyme immunoassay.

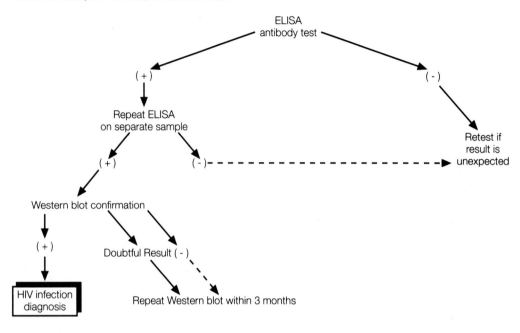

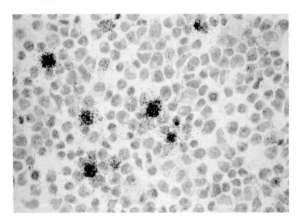

FIGURE 12.14

The result of a deoxyribonucleic acid probe showing the
presence of HIV nucleic acid (RNA) within infected cells (arrows).
(Courtesy of T. Folks, National Institutes of Health)

of HIV infection and the acquired immune deficiency syndrome (AIDS) is maintained by the *Global
Programme on AIDS of the World Health Organization.*
This agency maintains that between five and ten
million persons may be infected with HIV–1, and
projects that between 500 thousand and 3 million
AIDS cases will occur over the next five years. The
virus will probably be spread to every country in the
world.

The finding of HIV–1 in a particular geographical
area appears to depend on an unusual combination
of individual behaviors, social practices, and the date
of entry of the virus into a population. From the information available as of 1989, four broad but distinct epidemiologic patterns of HIV–1 infection and
AIDS in the world can be distinguished. Three major
patterns are compared in table 12.8. Figure 12.16
shows four patterns, one of which indicates a shift
from pattern I to pattern II.

FIGURE 12.15
The epidemiological chain of events with HIV infection.

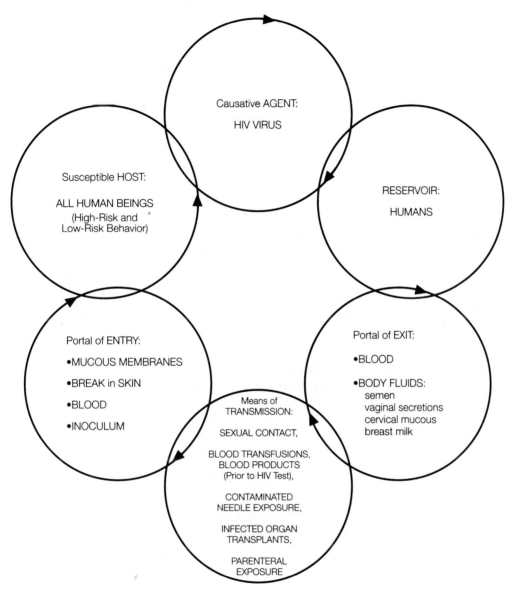

Causative AGENT:

HIV VIRUS

Susceptible HOST:

ALL HUMAN BEINGS
(High-Risk and
Low-Risk Behavior)

RESERVOIR:

HUMANS

Portal of ENTRY:
• MUCOUS MEMBRANES
• BREAK in SKIN
• BLOOD
• INOCULUM

Means of
TRANSMISSION:

SEXUAL CONTACT,

BLOOD TRANSFUSIONS,
BLOOD PRODUCTS
(Prior to HIV Test),

CONTAMINATED
NEEDLE EXPOSURE,

INFECTED ORGAN
TRANSPLANTS,

PARENTERAL
EXPOSURE

Portal of EXIT:
• BLOOD
• BODY FLUIDS:
  semen
  vaginal secretions
  cervical mucous
  breast milk

TABLE 12.8

TABLE 12.8 | HUMAN IMMUNODEFICIENCY VIRUS–1 (HIV–1) INFECTION PATTERNS IN THE WORLD

PATTERN I	PATTERN II	PATTERN III
Major Affected Groups		
Homosexual/bisexual men; intravenous drug abusers	Heterosexuals	Individuals with multiple sexual partners
Geographic Distribution		
Western Europe, North America, some areas in South America, Australia, New Zealand	Africa, Caribbean, some areas in South America	Asia, the Pacific Region (minus Australia and New Zealand), the Middle East, Eastern Europe, some rural areas of South America
Time of Introduction or Extensive Spreading		
Mid-1970s or early 1980s	Early-to-late 1970s	Early to mid-1980s
Means of Transmission: Sexual Activities		
Mainly homosexual; limited heterosexual involvement (expected to increase)	Mainly heterosexual	Both homosexual and heterosexual
Means of Transmission: Mother-to-Newborn (Perinatal)		
Primarily among female intravenous drug abusers; sex partners of intravenous drug abusers; women from HIV–1 endemic areas	In areas where 5–15% women are positive for HIV–1 antibody	Currently not a problem
Means of Transmission: Parenteral[a]		
Intravenous drug abusers[b]	Contaminated needles and syringes account for an undetermined portion of HIV infections.	A small number of infections are caused by imported blood or blood products.

[a]Refers to routes other than those associated with the digestive system. Examples include intravenous and intramuscular.
[b]HIV-contaminated blood and blood products were sources of infection before 1985.

SELECTED FEATURES OF THE EPIDEMIOLOGIC PATTERNS

Pattern I is principally in North America, western Europe, Australia, New Zealand, and many cities and small towns of Latin America. In these areas, the sexual transmission of HIV-1 occurs mainly among homosexual and bisexual men. In certain locations more than 50 percent of homosexual men have been found to be infected. Heterosexual transmission also occurs and appears to be increasing slowly. In pattern I transmission through blood occurs primarily as a result of intravenous drug abuse. Pediatric infection is less common because relatively few women in these areas of the world have been infected thus far.

FIGURE 12.16

Four global epidemiologic patterns of HIV infection and AIDS as of 1989. Pattern I is found in North America, western Europe, Australia, and New Zealand. About 80–90 percent of the cases in these areas are in homosexual and bisexual men or intravenous drug users. Pattern II is found in sub-Saharan Africa and parts of the Caribbean. The primary form of transmission in these areas is heterosexual, and the ratio of infected males to infected females is approximately equal. Latin America is shifting from Pattern I to Pattern II and is now considered as a separate Pattern I/II. Pattern III consists of areas where few cases or infections have occurred to date.

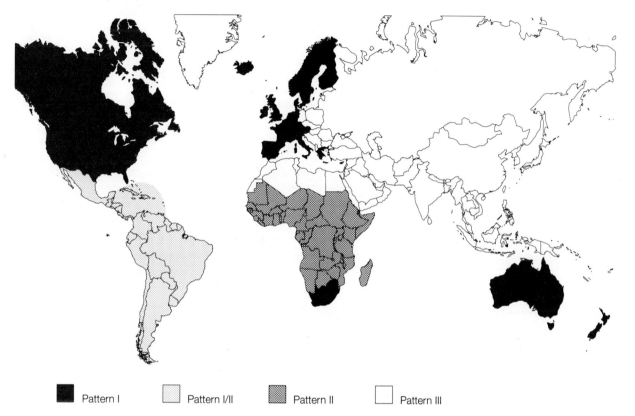

Pattern I   Pattern I/II   Pattern II   Pattern III

Pattern II is found in sub-Saharan Africa and increasingly in Latin America, especially in the Caribbean. The sexual transmission of HIV–1 here is predominantly heterosexual. While up to 25 percent of sexually active adults and the majority of female prostitutes in some large cities are infected, the overall ratio of infected males to infected females is about equal. Transmission through blood transfusions continues in areas where the blood is not yet routinely tested. Where intravenous drug abuse is uncommon, the use of unsterile needles or other skin-piercing instruments may contribute to the spread of HIV–1. Infected mother-to-infant (perinatal) transmission is a major problem in pattern II regions.

It is quite apparent that epidemiologic patterns can change over time. Various lines of evidence suggest that this may be true for Latin America. This area appears to be changing or shifting from pattern 1 to pattern II. Thus, the designation of I/II is used for the region. As in patterns I and II, extensive spread of HIV occurred around the late 1970s or early 1980s. At first, the burden of HIV infection was more or less confined to: 1) homosexual or bisexual men with multiple male sexual partners, 2) intravenous drug abusers sharing injection equipment, and 3) recipients of HIV-contaminated blood or blood products. In the middle or late 1980s, increasing transmission among heterosexuals with multiple

DISEASE

HIV INFECTION; ACQUIRED IMMUNE DEFICIENCY SYNDROME (AIDS); AIDS-RELATED COMPLEX (ARC); AIDS-RELATED DEMENTIA (ARD); PERSISTENT GENERALIZED LYMPHADENOPATHY (PGL).

CAUSE

HUMAN IMMUNODEFICIENCY VIRUS TYPE 1 (HIV–1)

Source/Transmission

Humans. Viral transmission occurs through specific sexual activities (both anal and vaginal intercourse); use of contaminated blood and blood products; use of contaminated needles; perinatally from an infected mother to her newborn.

The mean interval between HIV infection and the beginning of AIDS is about 7–8 years.

Epidemiology

HIV infection is found worldwide. Populations at high risk of infection include: homosexually/bisexually active males; intravenous drug abusers; recipients of contaminated blood or blood products; sexual partners of persons from each of these groups; newborns of mothers infected with HIV.

Diagnosis

Laboratory diagnosis includes blood tests for antibodies to HIV or its parts, such as enzyme-linked immunosorbent assay (ELISA) and the Western blot assay; virus culture; detection of viral nucleic acid in infected cells (probes) and finding decreased levels of T helper cells in blood specimens.

Prevention and Control

HIV transmission can be slowed or stopped by reducing or eliminating behaviors that place persons at risk for infection.

---

sexual partners was noted to the extent that heterosexual transmission has increasingly become the main form of HIV transmission in pattern I/II area. The male-to-female ratio for HIV infections in recent years has been found in some pattern I/II areas to be close to equal. As heterosexual transmission increases in these areas an increased number of pediatric AIDS cases can be expected.

The pattern III areas include North Africa, the Middle East, Eastern Europe, Asia, and the Pacific, where HIV–1 does not seem to have been present until the early to mid-1980s. These regions account for only 1 percent of the AIDS cases reported to date. The first cases here resulted from contact with people in patterns I and II areas or from exposure to imported, contaminated blood. HIV–1 has not yet spread to the general population in the pattern II countries, where the positive blood tests among blood donors ranges from 0–2 per 100,000. The transmission of HIV–1 infection is increasing, especially among prostitutes and intravenous drug users native to these regions. These geographic epidemiologic patterns show that HIV–1 has entered and spread within various populations and subpopulations at different times and rates. Unless changes in behavior occur, local, national, and global patterns will continue to shift and create a situation that may threaten all communities with explosive outbreaks of HIV infection.

Other features of HIV are given in the accompanying **STD FACT FILE.**

CHAPTER 13 | THE SPECTRUM OF HIV INFECTION

I think I probably will die of AIDS. I lived a good life, and I've no regrets. I've made my will, and made a tape for my memorial service: good poems and country music . . .

—*Person with AIDS*

In June 1981, M.J. Gottlieb and his co-workers reported an unusual form of pneumonia in five homosexual men in Los Angeles, California, not knowing that this event marked the beginning of a worldwide epidemic that in less than ten years would cause the death of more than 100,000 persons and be spread among millions. Similar findings on the cases of an aggressive form of cancer known as Kaposi's (KAP-ō-shēs) sarcoma were soon reported from New York City and San Francisco.

The Centers for Disease Control in Atlanta, Georgia, established a case-definition for the new disease, which later became known as **acquired immune deficiency syndrome,** or **AIDS.** Physicians were asked to report new cases so that information about the spread of the disease could be obtained. It soon became evident that AIDS was an infectious disease which could be transmitted by sexual and/or blood contact and from an infected mother to her unborn child. Since in these respects the disease was similar to hepatitis B virus infection, the measures used for protection against hepatitis B were applied for the prevention of AIDS.

By the beginning of 1989, the World Health Organization estimated that there were over 400,000 persons with AIDS and that more than 50 percent of these individuals were already dead of the disease (fig. 13.1). Currently, worldwide estimates of HIV-infected persons range between 5 and 10 million.

FIGURE 13.1

Two panels of the *Names Quilt* on display at WHO on World AIDS Day, December 1, 1988. The *Names Project* includes the making of a quilt representing the person with AIDS who died. Individual quilts tell a little bit of the individual's personal history. (Courtesy of World Health Organization)

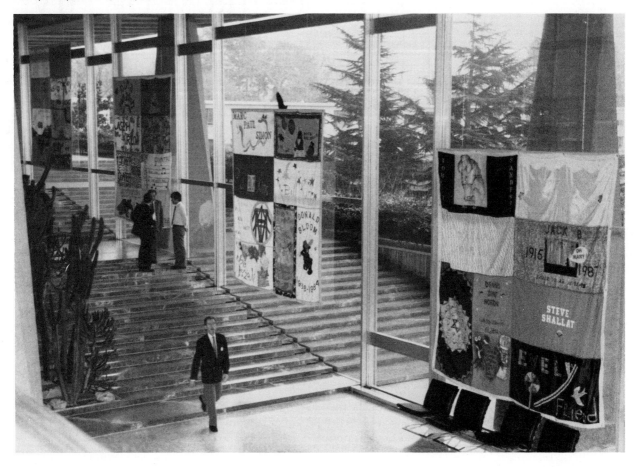

This chapter will describe the scope of HIV infection and the general features of AIDS, AIDS-Related Dementia (ARD), AIDS-related complex (ARC), and pediatric AIDS (PAIDS). Attention is also given to the laboratory tests used to detect and to follow disease development.

FIGURE 13.2

A general indication of how HIV infection progresses. It should be noted that an individual may be able to transmit the virus from the time they are first infected by any of the routes described in this chapter.

THE HIV SPECTRUM OF INFECTION				
HIV INFECTION	ANTIBODY POSITIVE	MILD SYMPTOMS	ARC	AIDS
Infection with HIV. Antigens detectable. No symptoms; person feels well.	Production of specific antibodies that can be detected by blood screening tests (seropositive). Asymptomatic	Unexplained mild fatigue. Intermittent symptoms; night sweats, fever.	Unexplained prolonged and severe diarrhea, weight loss, and night sweats.	Full blown disease; and includes opportunistic infections and malignancies

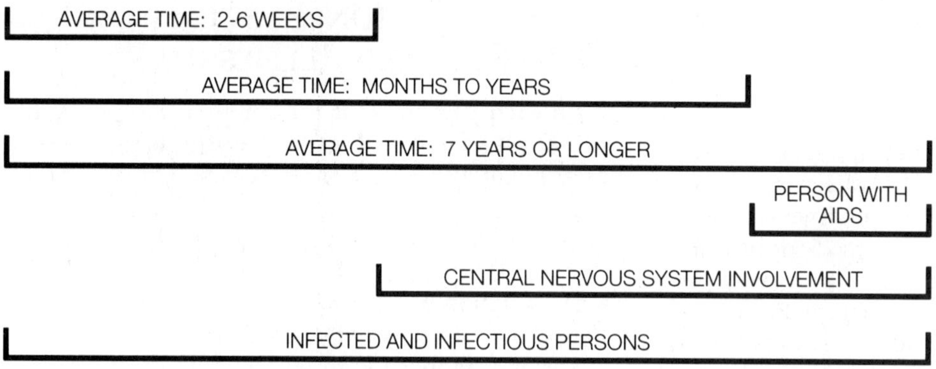

AVERAGE TIME: 2-6 WEEKS

AVERAGE TIME: MONTHS TO YEARS

AVERAGE TIME: 7 YEARS OR LONGER

PERSON WITH AIDS

CENTRAL NERVOUS SYSTEM INVOLVEMENT

INFECTED AND INFECTIOUS PERSONS

THE SCOPE OF HIV INFECTION

The scope of HIV-associated diseases has increased significantly since the time of the first reports of AIDS. Unfortunately, the designation of AIDS has been inappropriately applied to the entire spectrum of HIV-related disease conditions. It is important to note that AIDS is the terminal or final stage of HIV infection and is generally distinguished by the presence of a complicating opportunistic infection or cancerous process (fig. 13.2). Although AIDS is the most visible stage, concentrating on these late complications seriously draws attention away from the range of conditions and symptoms associated with HIV infection. Included among the various conditions that should be noted are: the asymptomatic carrier stage, AIDS-related complex or, ARC (an HIV infection with some of the symptoms of AIDS), neurological abnormalities such as mental deterioration and physical destruction of the nervous system, abnormal kidney function, developmental defects in an unborn child, and irritation and inflammation of the lungs.

Opportunistic Infections

A striking feature of *persons with AIDS* (**PWA**) is the frequency of opportunistic infections, which are mostly caused by microorganisms that have the potential to produce infections if they accidentally gain access to the tissues of HIV-infected individuals. Such opportunists take advantage of the weakened immune system to become established so that they can cause their life-threatening conditions in *immunocompromised hosts.* Frequently, opportunists are normal residents in or on the bodies of such hosts.

HIV Infection and Cancers

HIV-infected persons are also known to have an increased risk to develop several types of cancers or malignancies (ma-LIG-nan-sēs). These include at least three types of human tumors: **carcinomas** (kar'-si-NŌ-mas) such as skin cancers often seen in the mouth or rectum of infected individuals, **tumors or abnormal masses** originating in B lymphocytes known as **B cell lymphomas** (lim-FŌ-mas), and **Kaposi's sarcoma** (KAP-ō-shēs, sar-KŌ-ma). Carcinomas are tumors associated with **epithelial** (ep'-i-THĒ-lē-al) tissue cells that form the outer surface of the body, and line body cavities and passageways leading outside of the body. Kaposi's sarcoma is a pigmented tumor composed of blood-vessel tissue in the skin (color photographs 22 and 23) or internal body organs. Before AIDS, the condition was primarily seen in elderly men of Eastern Europe or Mediterranean descent. Additional features of the more aggressive forms of Kaposi's sarcoma and other related conditions are described later in this chapter.

The Incubation Period

The interval between contracting HIV infection and the appearance of disease generally varies according to the means of virus transmission. For example, the incubation period in recipients of infected blood (transfusion-related AIDS) appears to be greater than six to seven years, while the incubation periods for sexually acquired AIDS may range from eight to twelve years. In the case of pediatric AIDS, young infants born to mothers with HIV infection may exhibit an incubation period as short as six months or less.

Associated Clinical or Medical Conditions

The full range of clinical or medical conditions associated with HIV infection is now recognized to be far greater than when the first cases of AIDS were identified in 1981. In September 1987, the Centers for Disease Control officially adopted a comprehensive classification system for grouping patients infected with HIV virus according to certain clinical states. The system includes the range of identified virus-associated conditions and is intended to provide a more unifying and effective approach to the medical care of HIV-infected persons.

Once HIV infection occurs there is a great threat of the disease progressing to serious illness. Such conditions include opportunistic infections, Kaposi's sarcoma and other cancerous conditions, kidney abnormalities, and psychological and central nervous system disorders (table 13.1).

Classification System for HIV-Related Illnesses

With each passing year the range and types of illnesses associated with HIV infection increases. For example, new types of infections and/or variations in disease conditions are reported regularly. Whether this situation reflects changes in viral actions, host susceptibility, environmental factors, or a combination of such factors is unknown. To cope with the broad range of diseases, and because of the need for a standard with which to detect, diagnose, and to follow epidemiologic patterns of HIV infections, several classification systems have been proposed. One of the most widely used has been the classification adopted by the Centers For Disease Control (CDC) in 1987. This classification system covers the entire range of HIV-1 infection and is designed to aid in the surveillance of HIV-1-associated diseases. It is also applicable to epidemiologic studies, prevention and control activities, and public policy and planning. According to the CDC's definition of HIV infection, individuals can be placed into four broad groups. This classification system is based largely on clinical findings with subgroups based upon laboratory findings (during early stages),

TABLE 13.1 | THE HIV INFECTION PATHWAY TO AIDS

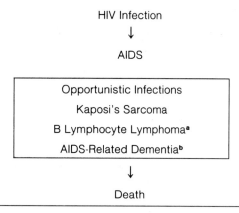

HIV Infection

↓

AIDS

| Opportunistic Infections |
| Kaposi's Sarcoma |
| B Lymphocyte Lymphoma[a] |
| AIDS-Related Dementia[b] |

↓

Death

[a]A cancerous state
[b]One of several psychological disorders

or specific disease symptoms (during later stages of illness). HIV infection is considered to exist in any individual with a repeatedly reactive (positive) blood screening test, such as with ELISA, supported by another specific method of laboratory analysis, i.e. Western blot assay, DNA probes, immunofluorescence, etc. The CDC system emphasizes that persons with such results should be considered both infected and infectious. (Finding low numbers of T helper lymphocytes in laboratory blood specimens also is considered by the Centers for Disease Control as an indicator of AIDS.)

The *Centers for Disease Control Classification System* consists of four mutually exclusive groups which are arranged so that HIV-infected patients can move to a higher group number (categories), never to a lower one. It should be noted that this system applies only to individuals diagnosed by means of clinical and laboratory findings as having HIV infection.

THE GROUPS

The features of Group I occur within the first few weeks after exposure and include those instances in which there is known exposure such as a contaminated needle accident, or a known sexual or contaminated needle-sharing experience. Individuals show

the symptoms of a mononucleosis condition, such as enlarged and tender lymph nodes, an enlarged spleen, and an abnormal number of nontypical lymphocytes.

Group II is the stage at which most HIV-infected persons are in the course of the current pandemic. These individuals show no significant clinical signs or symptoms as a consequence of HIV infection. The immune system at this time has not yet been seriously damaged. It usually takes at least one or two years from the time of the initial infection until the immune system actually starts showing the effects of HIV infection. There may also be a great variation in the time a person stays in Group II before progressing to Groups III or IV.

Group III is the stage of HIV infection in which there is a generalized involvement and enlargement of the lymph nodes. Individuals can remain in this category for several months to many years before moving to Group IV.

Group IV includes all the symptoms and diseases associated with AIDS or AIDS-related complex (ARC). When the individual enters Group IV, the immune system is sufficiently suppressed for the clinical signs of the secondary diseases to develop in the immunodeficient person. When a person is in

INCREASING AIDS CASES AMONG WOMEN

In November 1990 federal health officials reported that AIDS cases among women in the United States have been steadily increasing. Moreover, the disease is expected to be among the five leading causes of death among women in 1991. The others are cancer, accidents, heart disease, and homicide.

According to the Centers for Disease Control (CDC) in Atlanta, Georgia, AIDS cases among women increased by 29%, compared to 18% in men, from 1988 to 1989. In addition, women accounted for 11% of the 152,271 reported cases in adults.

According to the CDC, "Many women in the United States are unaware they are at risk for HIV infection, and HIV-infected women often remain undiagnosed until the onset of AIDS, or until a perinatally infected child becomes ill." Adding to the problem is a recent finding by the World Health Organization (WHO) that the number of women infected with the human immunodeficiency virus "may well double as heterosexual transmission becomes the predominant mode of spread . . . in most parts of the world."

WHO projected that a cumulative total of 600,000 women will have developed AIDS by 1992 and that the disease will kill at least 2 million women during the 1990s, most of them in sub-Saharan Africa. An estimated one in 40 women in sub-Saharan Africa carries the HIV virus. Moreover, about one in three children receives the virus from their mothers, and those spared the disease face life alone if their parents die. The WHO forecasts that the deaths from AIDS will cause nearly 10 million African children to be orphaned in the 1990s.

The increasing number of AIDS cases in U.S. women has largely resulted from the widespread transmission of HIV among drug abusers and their sexual partners. HIV infection has disproportionately affected minority women, reflecting to a large extent the intravenous drug connection. Although Blacks and Hispanics make up 19% of all U.S. women, they represent 72% of all U.S. women diagnosed with AIDS. Eighty-five percent of these cases occurred among those of childbearing age, and about 25% of these women were in their 20s at the time of diagnosis—meaning that many were probably infected as teenagers.

Group IV and certain of its subgroups, any one or more of the serious opportunistic infections or cancerous conditions that pose the life-threatening aspects of the HIV disease spectrum are present.

THE QUESTION OF SURVIVAL AFTER HIV INFECTION

The development of HIV infection varies significantly. It ranges from the development of AIDS and death within a year after infection to an absence of any disease effects many years after infection. While the proportion of HIV-infected persons progressing to AIDS is still not known, several studies support the finding that a very high proportion of HIV-positive persons will eventually develop the fatal disease. After the diagnosis of AIDS is made, approximately 72 percent survive the first year, and about 47 percent survive the second year. With each succeeding year the percent surviving become significantly fewer. Research findings reported in 1990 suggest bacteria known as *Mycoplasma* may possibly cooperate with HIV in producing the symptoms of AIDS.

The following section presents the various complications and disorders associated with HIV infection.

TABLE 13.2 | FORMS OF KAPOSI'S SARCOMA

	CLASSIC FORM	AFRICAN FORM	EPIDEMIC FORM
Sex	Male (common)	Male & female	Male (usual)
Age	Elderly	Young	Adult
Organ	Skin	Lymphatic	Diffuse
Behavior	Inactive	Aggressive	Aggressive
Outlook	Good, 8–13-years survival	Poor	Poor, 2-years survival
Immunosuppression	No	Yes (possibly viral)	Yes, HIV

KAPOSI'S SARCOMA — THE FIRST TUMOR TO BE CONNECTED TO AIDS

A broad range of cancers or malignancies (ma-LIG-nan-sēs) has been seen in the background setting provided by AIDS and the large number of HIV infections. Malignancies such as cancers of the testes, the liver, and of pigment-producing skin cells known as malignant melanoma (mel'-a-NO-ma) have been frequently found among the HIV-infected. While little evidence currently exists to show that these cancerous conditions result from an HIV-caused immunodeficiency, a direct relationship has been proposed for a cancer known as Kaposi's sarcoma.

Kaposi's sarcoma (KS) in the presence of HIV infection has been considered to be diagnostic of AIDS. However, in 1990, reports appeared indicating a microbial disease agent, separate and distinct from HIV, as the possible sexually transmitted cause of KS. These and other features of the malignancy are discussed in the following section.

HISTORICAL BACKGROUND

Kaposi's sarcoma was first reported by the Hungarian skin specialist Moritz Kaposi in 1872. The condition, which generally appeared in the form of numerous pigmented tumors or growths on the skin, was primarily seen in elderly men of Eastern European or Mediterranean descent. Today, this type of "classic" Kaposi's sarcoma is considered one of the least life-threatening forms of cancer.

In the early 20th century, certain parts of Africa, such as Kenya and Uganda, had unusually high numbers of KS cases. Certain features of the condition, such as the age group affected and its appearance and course, however, differed from classic KS. This version of Kaposi's sarcoma is currently one of the most common tumors found in Kenya and Uganda and is referred to as the "African form" (table 13.2).

Before AIDS made its appearance in the United States, KS was a very rare disease. Annual cancer statistics indicated that three persons out of one million might develop the condition. Today, besides persons with AIDS, Kaposi's sarcoma is most commonly seen in Italian and Jewish men over the age of 50. In addition, the sarcoma can develop in persons with some form of immune deficiency and in kidney disease patients given drugs to suppress the normal functioning of their immune systems (immunosuppression) in order to guarantee the success of a kidney transplant.

The development of KS and other forms of cancer in persons with AIDS is one of the most frightening aspects of the immunodeficiency. The sarcoma found in such individuals appears to be much more destructive, and is referred to as the "epidemic form."

FIGURE 13.3

Kaposi's sarcoma at a site of a local infection. (From M. Janier, P. Morel, and J. Civatte, *Journal of American Academy of Dermatology* (1990) 22:124–125.)

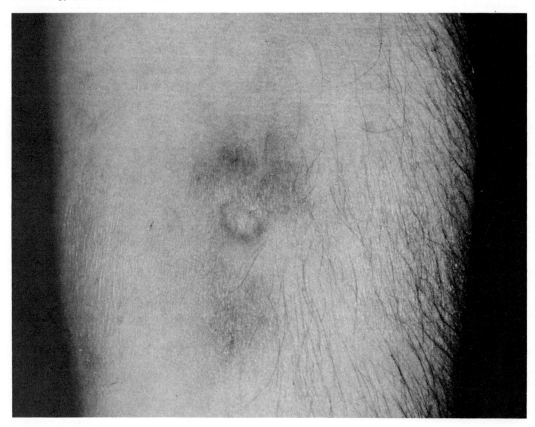

The Modern Forms of KS. The tumors generally seen in KS are red-to-purple, and consist of distinctive cancer cells called "spindle cells," large numbers of newly formed, small blood vessels, and spaces filled with blood (color photograph 22).

While KS is commonly thought of as a skin disease, autopsy findings have revealed the involvement of other body parts. Thus, KS should be considered to be a *systemic* (body system) disease. With this point in mind the forms of this cancerous condition can be described and summarized as follows.

First, the disease may be a relatively harmless, slowly progressing skin condition, with highly red-to-violet pigmented surfaces, patches, or lumps (nodules) located beneath the surfaces of the skin on the arms or legs (fig. 13.3). Individuals generally survive as long as twenty-five years, and death in such persons is caused by unrelated problems.

Second, the disease can appear as progressively increasing numbers of tumors that tend to penetrate into the body and grow rapidly. Such tumors spread to the lymph nodes, bones, and internal organs, especially those of the gastrointestinal tract. Since these tumors contain blood vessels, internal bleeding can occur and may end in death. This form of KS is seen with immunosuppressed kidney transplant patients, persons with AIDS, and in individuals with treated or untreated cancers of the lymph system known as *lymphomas*. One of the most alarming findings associated with Kaposi's sarcoma in persons with AIDS is that more than one-third of such cases develop another kind of cancer.

A COMBINATION OF KAPOSI'S SARCOMA AND OPPORTUNISTIC INFECTIONS

It is estimated that the occurrence of Kaposi's sarcoma (KS) in persons with AIDS ranges from 26–77 percent. Here is an actual report of a case with lung involvement.

A 31-year-old Hispanic male homosexual without any history of intravenous drug use complained of chest pains and difficulty in breathing. He underwent an examination of the respiratory system and was found to have a *Pneumocystis* infection. Further examination revealed the presence of Kaposi's sarcoma involving the skin and gastrointestinal tract, and a cryptococcal meningitis (an infection of the coverings of the brain and spinal cord). Treatments for the respective infections were given accordingly. Six months later the patient was admitted to the local medical center. He was experiencing fever, harsh cough, and difficulty in breathing. Numerous purple growths were scattered over his entire body and on the roof of the mouth. A chest X-ray showed many small masses scattered throughout various parts of the lungs (fig. 13.4). Later examination of lung specimens were positive for KS.

Unfortunately, within a short time the patient's condition worsened and ended in death three weeks later.

Third, Kaposi's sarcoma is found in the lymph nodes of children in equatorial Africa, or as a rapidly spreading and often fatal cancerous form in young adults. The latter condition originates in the skin and/or lymph nodes of the individual.

A fourth form of the disease appears in epidemic numbers and resembles the spreading form seen in African young adults. Male homosexuals are the primary victims here.

KS CAUSE AND TRANSMISSION — THE BIG MYSTERY

The cause of Kaposi's sarcoma has long been a puzzle. In the early 1980s a number of reports indicated that homosexual men with AIDS had a high risk of developing the condition. Some investigators proposed that KS was triggered by the use of chemicals such as nitrite (NĪ-trīt) inhalants known as "poppers." Recent reports appear to disprove this suggestion and provide strong evidence for an infectious agent, probably a virus, as the cause.

KS appears to be far more common among persons who developed AIDS after having sex with homosexuals or bisexuals than among people who became infected with HIV through exposure to contaminated blood. For example, in one study 21 percent of homosexual men with AIDS had KS, while this cancer was found in only 1 percent of persons with AIDS with hemophilia. Many hemophiliacs were infected with HIV in the early 1980s, before the virus was shown to be transmitted by contaminated blood or blood products. Another line of support for the sexual transmission theory of the KS agent is provided by reports of six homosexual men who had the cancer but showed no evidence of HIV infection.

Diagnosis. The tumors of KS are easily recognized (color photograph 23). However at times the condition must be distinguished from other states producing similar lesions. In such cases laboratory diagnosis is necessary and includes the microscopic examination of a tumor's contents.

Treatment. A number of approaches are used for treatment. These include radiation, cell destroying (cytotoxic) chemicals such as vinblastine (vin-BLAS-tēn) and vincristine (vin-KRIS-tēn), and biologic

FIGURE 13.4

A chest X ray showing many small masses of Kaposi's sarcoma in the lower lungs (arrows). (From P. G., Hamm, M. A. Judson, and C. P. Aranda, *Cancer* (1987) 59:807–810.)

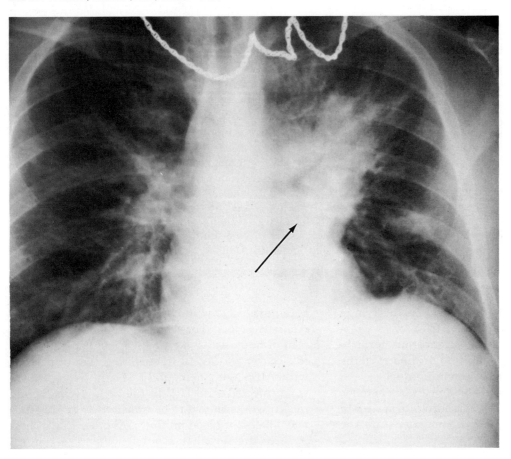

agents such as alpha interferon and azidothymidine, known also as AZT. Surgery also may be used to control bleeding. The decision to start any form of treatment is a hard one to make. This is especially the case since some individuals with KS may have only a few tumors and will do well for months or even years without treatment. Others with KS will rapidly deteriorate and die either of the cancer itself, or of some type of opportunistic infection (fig. 13.5 and color photograph 25).

Newer treatments or combinations of the approaches mentioned continue to be explored in the hopes of at least stopping further progression of the cancerous tumors.

ORAL INVOLVEMENT

As HIV begins to attack the body's immune system common opportunistic oral infectious agents are quick to take advantage of the situation. Over 250 oral opportunistic infections, cancers, and other types of conditions associated with HIV infection now have been recognized. The three most common of these illnesses are oral candidiasis (kan'-di-DĪ-a-sis), hairy leukoplakia (loo'-kō-PLĀ-kē-a), and periodontitis (per'-ē-ō-don-TĪ-tis).

FIGURE 13.5 ·

An AIDS patient showing both the skin sores of the fungus infection sporotrichosis, and the tumors of Kaposi's sarcoma. (From I. C. Shaw, W. Levinson, and A. Montanaro, *Journal of American Academy of Dermatology* (1989) 21: 1145–1147.)

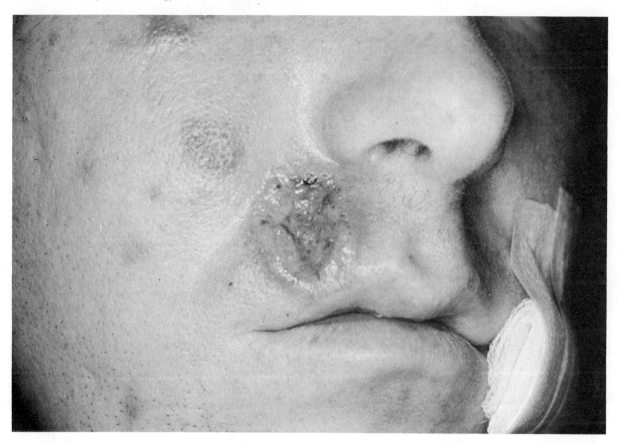

ORAL CANDIDIASIS

This condition is caused by the yeast *Candida albicans* (KAN-di-da, AL-bi-kans) already described in chapter 9. In most infected individuals white and/or red spots appear anywhere on the inner surfaces of the mouth. This condition, which sometimes is not obvious, can vary in appearance and thus may go unnoticed. Many persons with oral candidiasis experience changes in their ability to taste, a sore throat, and at times pain and difficulty swallowing.

The presence of a creamy film, sometimes referred to as a *pseudomembrane* (soo'-dō-MEM-brān) on the tongue is often the first symptom of HIV infection, and a predictor for the development of AIDS. Treatment of this yeast infection requires the use of an appropriate antifungal drug.

PERIODONTAL DISEASE

This condition is a highly progressive, and potentially dangerous form of gum disease that rapidly destroys the gum tissue and bone needed to support the teeth. The HIV- or AIDS-related type of this gum disease not only takes unusual forms, but is also resistant to the usual approaches to treatment. Frequently a combination of treatments, is needed.

FIGURE 13.6

A well-developed case of hairy leukoplakia. The whitish patches with a rather hairy surface can be seen on the side of the tongue.

(From E. Alessi and colleagues, *Journal of American Academy of Dermatology* (1990) 22: 79–86.)

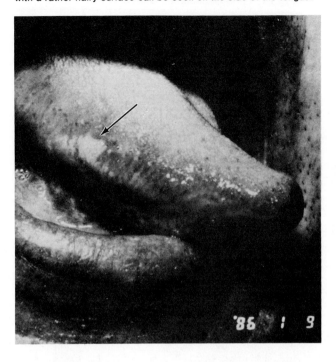

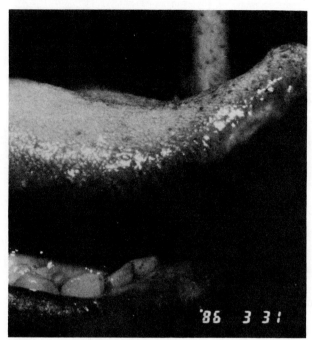

Oral Hairy Leukoplakia — A Reliable Indicator of AIDS. Infections involving the mouth or oral cavity are among the most common features of the immunodeficiency in HIV disease. They include the yeast infection, oral thrush, or candidiasis, gum inflammation caused by herpes simplex virus type 1, and the formation of painless, fuzzy white patches on the sides of the tongue, known as hairy leukoplakia. Frequently, oral lesions associated with these conditions are the first signs of a problem recognized by the individual, and which serve as the reason used to seek medical or dental advice.

Oral hairy leukoplakia (fig. 13.6) occurs almost exclusively in HIV-infected persons and is highly predictive for the development of AIDS. This condition, which was first described in 1984, is the result of an infection caused either separately or jointly by Epstein-Barr and human papilloma viruses.

HIV AND KIDNEY DISEASE

HIV infection can be associated with abnormalities of kidney function beginning from the asymptomatic positive blood test stage to the advanced form of AIDS. Many of these complications are the result of infectious or cancerous diseases due to the immunocompromised condition of the individual. Recent findings however, now show that HIV can produce kidney, or renal, disease that is distinct from other forms of kidney involvement. The disease has been named *HIV-associated nephropathy* (ne̅-FROP-a-the̅) or **HIVAN.** In addition, HIV infection can occur in patients with an existing renal disease and those with *end stage renal disease* (**ESRD**) who are treated with long term dialysis and transplantation. The length of survival in HIV-infected patients with renal disease appears to be much shorter than in other HIV-infected individuals. Unfortunately, HIV

TABLE 13.3	EXAMPLES OF PSYCHOLOGICALLY RELATED CONCERNS AND EFFECTS OF PERSONS WITH AIDS

Anger	Guilt
Anxiety	Loss of self-esteem and control
Anticipation of grief and loss	Personality changes
	Shock
Altered views of body, sexual function, and body function	Fear of pain, abandonment, and death
	Feelings of unfinished business
Denial	Suicidal thoughts
Depression	
Dependency	

disease may progress more rapidly in those individuals. Information on treatment of both renal disease and HIV infection is limited, and no effective treatment for HIVAN is currently known.

THE PSYCHOLOGICAL IMPACT

The life-threatening illness caused by HIV usually is accompanied by a devastating impact on the infected individual. This effect is made worse by the special attraction of the virus for brain and nervous system tissue. Persons with AIDS are no different from other individuals with life-threatening conditions and experience a number of psychological effects including feelings of anger, guilt, self-pity and anxiety. Table 13.3 lists additional concerns of persons with AIDS. In reviewing the events in their lives such individuals may go through a period of distress and confusion.

During this time, lowered self-esteem and changes in their sense of identity, belonging, and values, as well as alienation from families and loved ones can lead to ideas of suicide. Personal anger can be directed inward and accompanied by withdrawal and depression. Anger also may be projected onto family members, loved ones, and others directly involved with caring for the strickened individual.

Accepting the change from being in a state of good health to one of a life-threatening illness is difficult and may be catastrophic.

AIDS-Related Dementia. The most common of the nervous system problems caused by HIV infection is **AIDS-related dementia,** or **ARD.** This neurological condition is currently included in the Centers for Disease Control definition for AIDS. While AIDS-related dementia occurs most often in individuals who have already been diagnosed with AIDS, it can also appear at the same time or before the development of any opportunistic infection.

Diagnosis of ARD involves noting an individual's cognitive (ability to perceive), and/or motor (muscular movement), and/or behavioral patterns. The early complaints of persons with ARD include cognitive changes such as: difficulty remembering names, appointments, and telephone numbers, and impaired concentration, making it hard to follow a conversation or the plot of a book or movie. Some individuals notice a mental slowing which shows up as a "less quick to catch on" or a marked slow response to questions or situations.

Behavioral changes typical of ARD include a general lack of feelings, withdrawal, and a loss of interest in socializing. As the condition progresses

TABLE 13.4 | SOME SIGNS AND SYMPTOMS OF AIDS RELATED DEMENTIA

SIGNS AND SYMPTOMS	BRIEF EXPLANATION OR DESCRIPTION
Difficulty in concentrating	Cannot focus on conversation; individual is easily distracted
Forgetfulness	Misplacing objects; forgetting recent events and familiar names; losing track of time
Impaired coordination	Clumsiness; worsening handwriting
Impaired judgement	Poor decision-making, impulsive behavior
Leg weakness or hand trembling	Difficulty in standing; uncontrolled shaking of hands
Mental slowing	Response time much slower than usual
Mood changes	Emotional outbursts, anger, rage; extreme highs and lows (happy one time, then rapid change to depression)
Personality changes	Disinterest; irritability; withdrawal
Psychotic behavior	Hallucinations (ho-loo-sin-NĀ-shuns)[a], paranoia (par-a-NOY-a)[b], or grandiose (GRAN-dē-os) thoughts[c]

[a]Perception of sights and sounds not actually occurring
[b]Refers to persistent abnormal feelings of persecution
[c]Refers to one's unrealistic and exaggerated view of self-worth importance, ability, and even wealth

individuals tend to become easily disturbed and confused. Psychoses (sī-KŌ-ses), severe forms of mental disturbance in which gradual personality breakdown and loss of contact with reality occur, also become apparent, especially when the individual exhibits some inappropriate behavior or begins to hallucinate.

Motor abnormalities, which usually develop later than the cognitive changes, include unsteady walking, uncontrolled shaking of the legs and hands, and a loss of fine motor coordination in picking up objects or during writing. Table 13.4 summarizes the features of ARD.

Determining if HIV-infected persons have ARD requires ruling out all other possible causes of mental or behavioral changes. This is an important process since there are many treatable conditions known to cause similar symptoms (table 13.5). Examples include treatable opportunistic infections, drug side-effects, and psychiatric disorders such as depression.

Management. Persons in the early phases of ARD along with their care-givers must be made aware of the coming changes and how to cope with them. For example, memory problems can be lessened by writing things down and making and keeping lists as reminders. Small doses of antidepressant drugs or psychologically stimulating medications are also frequently useful.

In later stages, the surrounding environment of the person with ARD becomes the major point of focus. Measures generally are needed to eliminate any and all factors that could cause confusion. These include a greater organization and structure in daily routines. Drugs used in later stages of ARD are generally directed to controlling depression and irritability. AZT has shown some promise in reversing the effects of ARD.

TABLE 13.5	TREATABLE CAUSES OF CENTRAL NERVOUS SYSTEM (CNS) CHANGES IN HIV INFECTIONS

INFECTIONS[a]

Cryptococcosis

Herpes virus-caused inflammation of the nervous system

Nontuberculosis infection

Papilloma virus infection known as progressive multifocal leukoencephalopathy (prō-GRES-iv, mul-ti-FŌ-kal, loo-kō-en-sef'-a-LŌP-a-thē)

Toxoplasmosis

Widespread (disseminated) tuberculosis

CANCERS

Burkitt's lymphoma[b]

Primary sarcoma of the brain

Widespread Kaposi's sarcoma

OTHER CAUSES

Depression

Drug-related injuries

Nutritional deficiencies

Psychosis[c]

[a]Most of these conditions are described in chapter 11.
[b]A form of cancer that involves body sites other than lymph nodes.
[c]Conditions in which personality breakdown and loss of contact with reality occur.

DIAGNOSIS OF HIV INFECTION
LABORATORY ASPECTS

Certain aspects of the approach used to diagnose both asymptomatic HIV infection and AIDS are quite similar. Diagnosis of HIV infection usually depends on the finding of repeated positive HIV antibody screening tests such as *ELISA*, confirmed by more specific procedures such as the Western blot assay. (chapter 12 describes these tests.) Additional laboratory findings important to diagnosis include low levels of T helper or T_4 lymphocytes, and a reduction in the number of platelets (blood clotting units). The ratio of T_4 (T helper) to T_8 (T suppressor) cells may become inverted. Normally T_4 cells outnumber T_8 cells. Unfortunately, such laboratory results lead to an unfavorable outcome.

Effective in January, 1992, according to the Centers for Disease Control a person will be considered to have AIDS if he or she has fewer than 200 T_4 (CD4) cells per cubic milliliter of blood. Healthy persons have about 800 to 1,000 of these cells in the same volume of blood.

CLINICAL SIGNS

The clinical course in HIV-infected persons varies. Many HIV seroconverters (positive for HIV antibodies) are asymptomatic for several years, whereas others progress to AIDS shortly following infection.

Table 13.6 | Clinical Findings of Diseases which May Indicate HIV Indications

Condition	Formal Term for Condition (if Applicable)
Blood Disorders	
Abnormal decrease of white blood cells	Leukopenia (loo'-kō-PĒ-nē-a)
Unexplained decrease in blood platelets (blood clotting units)	Idiopathic thrombocytopenia (id'-ē-ō-PATH-ik, throm'-bō-si-tō-PĒ-nē-a)
General Body Signs and Symptoms	
Inflammation of the face	Dermatitis (der'-ma-TĪ-tis)
Unexplained fever	
Unexplained sudden and large weight loss	
Yellowing of toenails	
Increased Involvement (Disease) of Lymph Nodes	
Long-lasting unexplained swollen lymph glands	Lymphadenopathy (lim-fad'-e-NOP-a-thē)
Increased size of tonsils in adults	
Malignancies	
Includes Kaposi's sarcoma (color photographs 22 and 23), carcinomas of the liver, throat, and lungs, and Hodgkin's disease■	

Table 13.6 lists a number of clinical findings or diseases which may indicate HIV infection. Four of the conditions listed, when they occur together, seem to be reliable predictors of AIDS (fig. 13.7). They are dermatitis of the face, yellowing of toenails, hairy leukoplakia, and oral candidiasis.

In the early stages, HIV infection produces different signs and symptoms in female patients than doctors are used to seeing. Physicians trying to determine who has HIV infection or AIDS generally rely on a list of opportunistic infections which does not include any of the diseases or conditions commonly seen among infected women. As a result women tend to be diagnosed later than their male counterparts. HIV-infected women often suffer a range of recurring diseases or disorders including cervical cancer, chronic yeast infections, pelvic inflammatory disease, irregular or stopped menstrual periods, and early menopause. Although these signs and conditions also are found with many uninfected individual's, HIV-infected women experience them again and again. Other features of HIV infection and AIDS are given in the accompanying **SIGNS & SYMPTOMS ¡OX.**

Treatment

Strategies for the treatment of patients with AIDS, AIDS-related complex (ARC), or pediatric AIDS have focused on the development of drugs with activity

TABLE 13.6 | (CONTINUED)

CONDITION	FORMAL TERM FOR CONDITION (IF APPLICABLE)
Infectious Diseases Suggestive of Cellular Immunity Defects	
Inflammation of central nervous system	Encephalitis (en'-sef-a-Lī-tis)
Inflammation of the covering of the brain and spinal cord	Meningitis (men-in-Jī-tis)
Inflammation of the intestines, especially the large intestine or colon	Enterocolitis (en'-ter-ō-kō-Lī-tis)
Sore-forming conditions caused by microorganisms generally of little consequence to persons with normal immune systems	
Mucous Membrane Disease	
Oral candidiasis (yeast infection)[b] with esophagus involvement (color photograph *24*)	
Oral hairy leukoplakia	
Worsening vaginal candidiasis	
Recurring or Non-Healing Skin Infections	
Progressive herpes simplex virus, fever blisters or sores,[c] shingles,[c] and molluscum contagiosum[d] virus infections	

[a]A cancerous condition in which enlarged lymph nodes, spleen, and liver typically occur.
[b]See chapter 9 for further details.
[c]See chapter 7 for a description of this condition.
[d]See chapter 8 for a description of this virus.

against HIV and on agents that may restore immunity, the **immunomodulators** (im'-ū-nō-MOD-ū-lā-tors). The development of such AIDS-related drugs continues to be a priority for the research-based pharmaceutical industry. Over fifty companies are involved in this activity. Table 13.7 lists examples of potential AIDS-related drugs. These products are in various stages of development, ranging from their use during early research studies in laboratory animals to clinical testing in humans.

Antiviral chemotherapy for HIV infections has been quite limited. In 1987 zidovudine (azidothymidine, or AZT) became the first AIDS treatment approved by the Federal Drug Administration (FDA). This drug interferes with HIV replication *in vitro* by inhibiting reverse transcriptase and interfering with the activities of other enzymes important to virus replication.

Other promising drugs under study or in limited use include: dideoxycytidine (dī-dē-oks-ē-Sī-ti-dīn), or ddc, a more potent relative of AZT; and alpha and gamma interferons (antiviral proteins currently being manufactured by genetic engineering techniques).

FIGURE 13.7

Four notable clinical signs of progression towards AIDS or opportunistic infections with a variety of microorganisms. (See chapter 13.) (a) A dermatitis, or inflammation, of the face. Note the involvement around the nose and lips. (b) Yellow toenail changes on the first toes. (c) The condition of white spots on the sides of the tongue, known as hairy leukoplakia. (d) Widespread oral candidiasis or yeast infection. (From L. Morfeldt-Manson, I. Julander, and B. Nilsson, *Scandinavian Journal of Infectious Diseases* (1989) 21:497–505.)

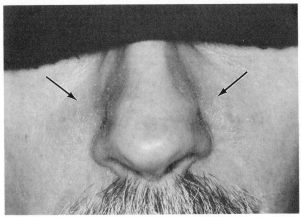

a

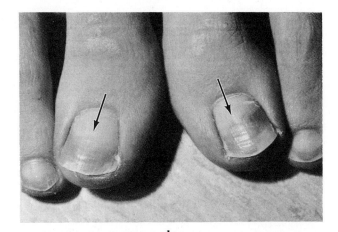

b

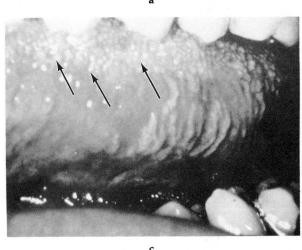

c

d

SIGNS & SYMPTOMS BOX

DISEASE
HIV INFECTION
INCUBATION PERIOD
VARIABLE, BUT GENERALLY WITHIN 7 YEARS AFTER INITIAL INFECTION

First Signs & Symptoms Usually Appear:
Primary (the first) symptoms may appear within one to eight weeks after HIV infection.
Secondary symptoms, including opportunistic infection, cancerous states, and abnormal functioning of the immune system may develop within 7 or more years.

Primary Signs
1. Flu-like illness; running nose
2. Fever
3. Enlarged lymph nodes
4. Sore throat
5. Involvement of the central nervous system
6. Rash

Secondary Signs[a]
1. Weight loss greater than 10 percent of normal body weight
2. Diarrhea for over 1 month's time
3. Persistent fever
4. Night sweats
5. Yeast infection of the mouth and esophagus (passageway connecting the throat to the stomach)
6. Various skin infections
7. Kaposi's sarcoma
8. Dementia
9. Various psychological and neurological disorders
10. Oral hairy leukoplakia
11. Various cancers

Complications
Opportunistic infections

[a] Refer to Table 13.6 for other indications of HIV infection.

TABLE 13.7 | EXAMPLES OF AIDS-RELATED DRUG PRODUCTS IN DEVELOPMENT

DRUG TRADE NAME	GENERIC (GENERAL NAME)	GENERALLY USED TO TREAT
Betaseron	beta interferon	AIDS, ARC, and Kaposi's sarcoma
ddA	Dideoxyadenosine	AIDS, ARC
ddC	Dideoxycytidine	AIDS, ARC
Foscarnet	trisodium phosphonoformate	HIV infection, CMV eye infection
Peptide T	octapeptide sequence	AIDS
Virazole	ribavirin	AIDS, ARC, Kaposi's sarcoma
Wellferon	alpha interferon	HIV infection, Kaposi's sarcoma

NEW TREATMENT OPTIONS

Physicians can now obtain investigational new drugs (IND) not yet approved by the United States Food and Drug Administration to treat qualified persons with AIDS. This new option was made possible by the Treatment IND regulation, entitled "Investigational New Drug, Antibiotic, and Biological Drug Product Regulations; Treatment, Use, and Sale; Final Rule." This regulation, which was enacted June 22, 1987, is intended to help treat and diagnose individuals with life-threatening or serious diseases. Drugs that have either been tested for effectiveness in humans, or undergone extensive clinical trials in humans can be used for treat-

ment, provided the FDA grants approval for use and the following requirements are met:

1. The drug will be used to treat life-threatening or serious diseases;
2. No satisfactory alternate drug or other treatment exists to treat the disease;
3. The drug is or has been under study in a controlled clinical trial; and
4. The developer of the drug is actively seeking marketing approval.

The IND regulation clearly has treatment, and not simply approval of a drug, as its goal.

The treatment of HIV-infected individuals and persons with AIDS also includes dealing with opportunistic infections. Chapter 13 presents these diseases together with some of the medications used for treatment. Unfortunately, several of the drugs used for either HIV and/or opportunistic infections have undesirable side-effects such as loss of appetite, confusion, headache, and depression. Many of them disappear or can be lessened by reducing dosages or treating the particular side-effect symptom. Some side-effects are of a mild nature and do not pose any major discomfort (fig. 13.8).

As indicated earlier, another approach being explored is the use of drugs that help to strengthen a failing immune system. Since persons with AIDS suffer a defect in the normal functioning of T helper cells, efforts to restore the immune function of these cells seem reasonable. Proteins such as interleukin-2 and various other drugs capable of restoring immune activity are being tested.

FIGURE 13.8

One of the possible side effects of AZT treatment. Pigment deposits, in the form of bluish or brownish discoloration, can involve an entire nail or only appear as a longitudinal line. (From C. A. Fisher and P. R. McPoland, *Cutis* (1989) 43:552.)

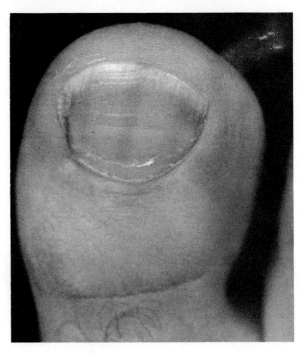

ZIDOVUDINE (AZT) RESISTANCE

The use of zidovudine (zi-DŌ-vū-den), also known as AZT, has become widespread since the drug has been shown to be of benefit in the treatment of individuals infected with HIV and persons with either AIDS or advanced AIDS-related complex (ARC). In these individuals with immune deficiencies, long-term and continuous treatment with zidovudine is necessary if the effects of HIV are to be controlled. In 1989, HIV isolated from several patients being treated with zidovudine for six months and longer showed a lowered sensitivity to the effects of the drug. On the other hand, virus isolated from untreated persons or from individuals treated with the same drug for six or less than six months showed a consistent sensitivity.

The basis for the observed zidovudine resistance appears to be the accumulations of several permanent genetic changes or mutations in the gene that encodes the information for the enzyme **reverse transcriptase** (RT). As indicated in chapter 12 this enzyme is essential for the replication of HIV and its spread in infected hosts. When RT is made nonfunctional by zidovudine, the virus can be controlled. From studies of viral drug resistance, the associated mutations develop within six months. Rapid testing procedures to identify drug-resistant HIV are being designed. Such tests are of major importance since they can be used to evaluate the effectiveness of zidovudine on the progress and control of HIV infection.

A WORD ABOUT AIDS-RELATED COMPLEX (ARC)

While no formal definition of ARC exists, it is frequently described as a stage of HIV infection when an infected person exhibits a combination of two physical signs or symptoms and two laboratory abnormalities typical of AIDS (table 13.7). Persons with ARC frequently show some form of T lymphocyte defect, a mucous membrane disease such as oral candidiasis, and/or any number of opportunistic virus- or fungus-caused skin infections typically found with persons with AIDS. In addition, these individuals also may have prolonged constitutional symptoms such as fever, night sweats, difficulty in breathing, long-lasting fatigue, persistent enlarged lymph nodes, weight loss, and unexplained diarrhea. Figure 13.9 shows the general features of ARC and its position in relation to AIDS and HIV carriers.

In many cases, persons with ARC may experience even more severe emotional problems than those faced by persons with AIDS. Suspended in limbo somewhere between being infected with HIV and developing AIDS, ARC persons are uncertain if they will live or die. Moreover, such individuals are confronted with many of the same problems as persons with AIDS, which include social isolation, depression, and anxiety.

PEDIATRIC ACQUIRED IMMUNE DEFICIENCY SYNDROME (PAIDS)

Human immunodeficiency virus type 1 (HIV-1) infection and disease in infants and small children have been recognized since 1983. The first reports of pediatric AIDS (PAIDS) described children with nonspecific conditions such as yeast infections of the mouth, swollen lymph glands, enlarged livers and

FIGURE 13.9

The course of AIDS relating to the loss of T helper cell
effectiveness, ARC (AIDS–related complex), and the HIV carrier.

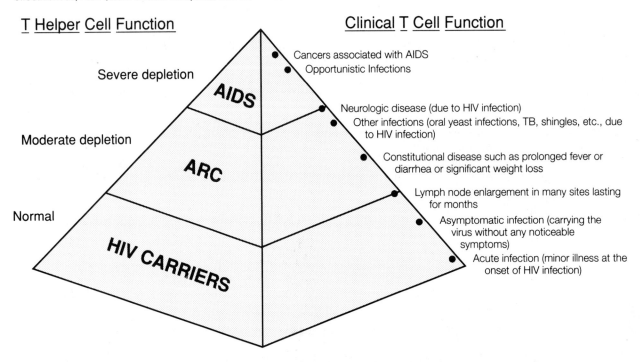

T Helper Cell Function

Clinical T Cell Function

Severe depletion

Moderate depletion

Normal

AIDS

ARC

HIV CARRIERS

Cancers associated with AIDS
Opportunistic Infections

Neurologic disease (due to HIV infection)
Other infections (oral yeast infections, TB, shingles, etc., due
to HIV infection)

Constitutional disease such as prolonged fever or
diarrhea or significant weight loss

Lymph node enlargement in many sites lasting
for months

Asymptomatic infection (carrying the
virus without any noticeable
symptoms)

Acute infection (minor illness at the
onset of HIV infection)

spleens, a failure to develop normally, and recurring infections of various kinds (fig. 13.10). In the United States and third world countries, the majority of documented cases have occurred as a result of mother-to-offspring transmission of infection during pregnancy or the perinatal period, which extends from the 28th week of pregnancy through 28 days following birth. In the United States at least 80 percent of children with PAIDS are known to have a parent who either has AIDS or is at risk for the disease and presumably infected with HIV.

TRANSMISSION

Human immunodeficiency viruses may be transmitted from infected women to their offspring by three main routes: 1) to the fetus during pregnancy by the maternal circulation; 2) to the infant during labor and delivery by inoculation or ingestion of blood or other body fluids containing HIV; and 3) to the infant shortly after birth through breast milk containing HIV. The probability of an HIV-infected

mother giving birth to an infected child is about 20 to 50 percent for the first child, and 50 percent to 65 percent if the mother has already given birth to an infected child.

SIGNS AND SYMPTOMS

In general, newborns of HIV-infected mothers are generally born at full term of pregnancy and with normal features and measurements. Particular signs of HIV infection are only rarely observed at birth. Symptoms generally occur from 2 to 18 months after birth. However, longer time periods have been reported. Most infants show signs of disease within the first year of infection.

The range of symptoms found in cases of PAIDS include the major and specific features such as severe opportunistic infections (fig. 13.11), neurological abnormalities, abnormally small head size, malignancies, salivary gland enlargement, and lung inflammation. Among the common and/or nonspecific

FIGURE 13.10

A double tragedy of AIDS. Both the mother and child shown here are infected with HIV. (Courtesy of World Health Organization, Photo by E. Hooper)

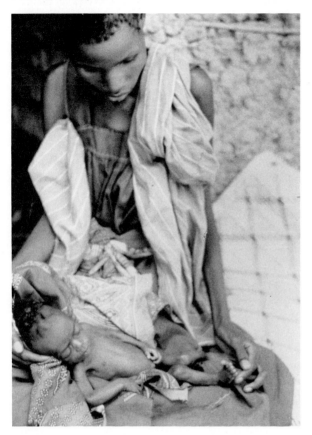

FIGURE 13.11

The presence of blood-filled pimples, or papules, on the legs of an HIV-infected nine-year-old. Some of these lesions have developed into open sores. (From M. M. Chren, R. A. Silverman, R. U. Sorensen, and C. A. Elmets, *Journal of American Academy of Dermatology* (1989) 21:1161–1164.)

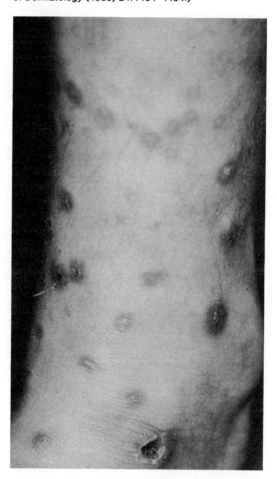

features, the following have been reported: enlarged livers, spleens, and lymph glands; recurrent middle ear infections; oral thrush and/or diaper rash associated with the yeast *Candida;* failure to develop normally; diarrhea and an abnormal curvature of the nails and enlargement of fingertips, known as *clubbing.* Additional aspects of PAIDS are given in the accompanying **SIGNS & SYMPTOMS BOX.**

PREVENTING THE SPREAD OF AIDS

Providing individuals with information with which to reduce the risk of HIV infection by using safer sex practices is of major importance. This is currently the

case since no effective cure for AIDS, antiviral agent for HIV, or vaccine is available. Prevention through practicing safer sexual practices appears to be the best means available for reducing the risk of HIV infection and controlling the spread of AIDS. Table 13.8 lists a number of safer sexual activity guidelines, which include the recommendations of the American Association of Physicians for Human Rights and the National Coalition of Gay STD Services.

SIGNS & SYMPTOMS BOX	**DISEASE** PEDIATRIC ACQUIRED IMMUNE DEFICIENCY SYNDROME (PAIDS) **INCUBATION PERIOD** VARIABLE

First Signs & Symptoms Usually Appear:
Between 2 and 18 Months After Birth.
However, Longer Time Periods Have Been
Noted

Signs
1. Abnormal development or weight loss
2. Diarrhea lasting longer than one month
3. Prolonged fever
4. Kaposi's sarcoma may be present
5. Persistent cough
6. Detectable enlarged lymph nodes
7. Generalized skin rash
8. Yeast infection involving the mouth and throat
9. Abnormal curling of nails and enlarged fingertips

Complications
Repeated ear infections and sore throats

There is a risk of infection in all forms of penetrative sexual activity involving infected persons. The degree of risk varies, however. For example, vaginal and anal intercourse are high-risk activities. However, using a barrier device such as a condom that does not break, tear, or come off during sexual activity will provide protection. With other activities such as unprotected oral sex the risk of HIV infection is lowered if ejaculation does not occur.

It becomes quite obvious from various studies and reports that the current epidemic of, not only HIV infection but of other STDs as well, is the result of many interacting factors and circumstances involving individuals, infectious agents, and society at large.

TABLE 13.8	GENERAL MEASURES TO CONTROL THE SPREAD OF AIDS (SAFER SEXUAL ACTIVITY GUIDELINES)

Know the health status of your sex partner, and exchange information so that future contact can be made in the event a health problem develops.

Avoid unprotected vaginal or anal intercourse.

Avoid oral sex.

Avoid *rimming and fisting.*[a]

Reduce the number of sexual partners.

Avoid the sharing of sex apparatus pieces or "toys," which include vibrators and dildos.

Avoid any form of sexual activity if either partner has a viral infection or unexplained disease symptoms such as swollen lymph nodes, fever, respiratory symptoms, or diarrhea.

Change sex practices to avoid the exchange of any body materials such as semen, vaginal secretions, blood, urine, and/or feces.

Seek medical services for any symptoms which indicate the presence of an infection or a problem with the immune system.

[a]*Rimming* refers to the sexual practice of using the tongue to stimulate the anus.
Fisting refers to the sexual practice of inserting a fist or fingers into a sex partner's rectum.

CHAPTER 14 | VACCINES—PROBLEMS AND PROSPECTS

An ounce of prevention is worth a pound of cure

—Anonymous

As the number of reported cases of AIDS continues to mount, the magnitude and severity of the problem becomes increasingly evident, and the need to develop effective strategies to prevent and control HIV infection becomes ever more urgent. One of the simplest, safest, and most effective forms of prevention and control is vaccination.

THE BEGINNINGS OF IMMUNIZATION

It has been recognized for centuries that individuals who recovered from certain infectious diseases were protected from reinfection. The first attempt to imitate such a natural phenomenon began with **variolation** (var-ē-ō-LĀ-shun), or **inoculation,** a procedure that was practiced in China, India, and probably Africa for centuries before being introduced into Europe and North America in 1721. This procedure involved injecting healthy individuals with pus from the skin blisters of smallpox victims. Even though inoculated individuals acquired resistance to the disease, the material used was potentially dangerous to their well-being. Edward Jenner, an English physician during the 1790s, substituted fluid from the blisters of individuals infected with a virus related to smallpox called cowpox (vaccinia). Jenner's approach to protecting against smallpox contributed to the realization that the causative agent of an infectious disease need not be present to stimulate the immune system. Only specific parts of microorganisms and other cells considered to be foreign by the body trigger an immune response. Such parts and substances are called **antigens.** (Immune responses, antigens, and related factors are described in chapter 10). Jenner's contribution also ushered in the modern era of immunization (fig. 14.1). It also was an important step in the eventual eradication of smallpox in 1978 by the World Health Organization.

The well-documented effectiveness of vaccines against smallpox and yellow fever, as well as against infections by polio, measles, and mumps viruses, caused many in the medical community to believe that vaccines could prevent *all* virus diseases. Unfortunately, this does not always appear to be the case. The unsuccessful results in attempting to develop vaccines against human papilloma viruses, herpes viruses, and HIV, clearly emphasize some of the obstacles that must be overcome before effective vaccines can be developed. If the immune system is to defeat a pathogen, it must be capable of attacking the invader freely in the blood and other body locations as well as the cells infected by the invader. Viruses such as the herpes viruses and HIV have the ability to insert their genetic information into that of the invaded host cell, thus protecting themselves from the immune responses of the host. Such responses, as chapter 10 described, may be either *nonspecific* or *specific.* Nonspecific immunologic responses are quite general and represent the first defenses used by the body to protect itself against foreign cells and substances. Specific immunological responses such as the production of immunoglobulins provide resistance to particular disease agents and/or their products. Other contributors to this category of responses include B and T lymphocytes and macrophages which are responsible not only for detecting but for eliminating the cells and related factors that have penetrated the defenses of the body.

Clearly, immunization is a proven approach to provide protection against many infectious diseases, and prevents significant numbers of deaths. However, the development of an effective and safe vaccine is not always a simple matter.

How does a vaccine provide protection? What goes into the making of a vaccine? What are the prospects for not only an AIDS vaccine but for STDs in general? These questions as well as related topics will be the main focus of this chapter.

ACQUIRED IMMUNITY
NATURALLY ACQUIRED ACTIVE IMMUNITY

An individual successfully recovering from a natural infection usually acquires a specific natural resistance to the causative agent. Such immunity includes the availability of specific immunoglobulins (**Igs**) and the services of specialized T lymphocytes to attack the pathogen. Because immunity is not always lifelong, *a naturally acquired form of active immunity* may last from a few months to several years. Persons having it are protected against reinfection or ordinary future attacks by the disease agents responsible for its production. Some of the familiar diseases to which an individual can develop sufficient protection include chicken pox, measles, mumps, and influenza (the flu). Unfortunately, immunity to reinfection by certain other disease agents is either insufficient or nonexistent. This group of

FIGURE 14.1

The original vaccination procedure performed by Edward Jenner (1749–1823). It was done by removing some fluid from a blister of cowpox on the hand of a dairymaid and injecting it into the arm of a small boy. The successful outcome of Jenner's vaccination against smallpox established a firm basis for the value of artificial immunization.

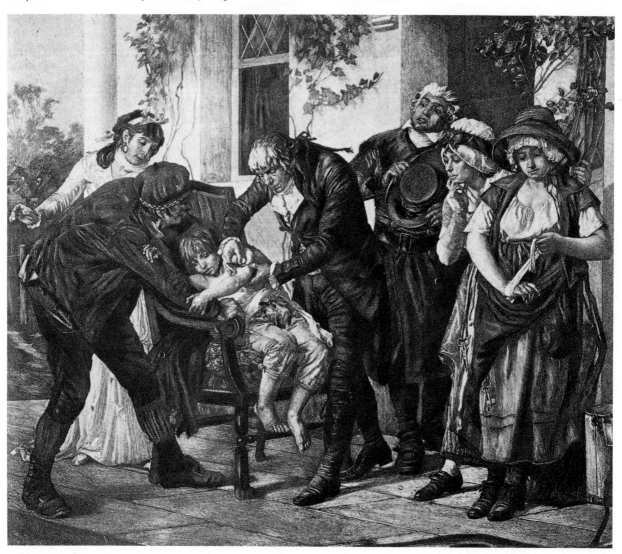

diseases includes several STDs such as gonorrhea, syphilis, and chlamydial infections. Vaccines are, however, under development.

NATURALLY ACQUIRED PASSIVE IMMUNITY

This form of immunity involves the natural transfer of antibodies from an immunized person to a non-immune recipient. For example, an expectant mother can pass some of the Igs from her circulation to that of her fetus across the placenta, a single layer of cells separating the two systems. Thus, if the mother has antibodies against diseases such as diphtheria, lockjaw (tetanus), or polio, a share of these protective proteins will be transferred *passively* to her offspring to protect it during the first months after birth.

Naturally acquired passive immunity also can occur by means of colostrum (kō-LOS-trum), a protein-rich fluid produced by the mother before the appearance of true breast milk. During nursing, certain Igs and white blood cells are passed from the mother to her newborn infant in this breast fluid.

ARTIFICIALLY ACQUIRED ACTIVE IMMUNITY

Active immunity here results from the process known as active immunization (vaccination), in which carefully prepared, special antigens in the form of vaccines are introduced into the body. Such antigenic exposure imitates a natural infection by provoking a primary immune response, without causing the severe effects of the actual disease. Subsequent exposures to the antigen, such as booster shots, stimulate a secondary immune response of the type that would occur following exposure to a disease agent to which some immunity has already developed in the individual.

Vaccines or preparations used to produce an *artificial active immunity* include: (1) **killed microorganisms;** 2) inactivated bacterial exotoxins, known as **toxoids;** (3) living but **attenuated** (weakened) **microbes;** (4) **parts of microorganisms;** and (5) **genetically engineered** (modified) **products.** (The nature of specific types of vaccines and descriptions of the processes involved with their production are presented later.)

In general, active immunity requires about one to two weeks to develop, and in most cases it is relatively long-lasting. However, it should be noted that active immunization cannot be used to prevent a disease after a person has been exposed. This is because the time period needed for active immunity to develop is longer than the incubation period of the disease.

ARTIFICIALLY ACQUIRED PASSIVE IMMUNITY

Protection against some diseases can be obtained by the injection of specific Igs against the disease agent or its products. Such passive immunization gives a nonimmune person exposed to a disease agent almost immediate protection, or reduces the severity of the disease. Individuals exposed to infected persons with diseases such as measles, hepatitis A or B infections, or mumps are treated in this way. The immunoglobulins used in such situations come from a human or animal already immune to a specific disease. The protection provided is only temporary, since no active production of Igs towards the specific disease agent or its products occurs.

A general summary of the different forms of active and passive immunity is given in figure 14.2.

CURRENTLY AVAILABLE IMMUNIZATION PREPARATIONS

The various preparations used for immunizations can be grouped into two general categories: (1) agents for active immunization, which include suspensions of bacteria, protozoa, viruses, and/or their parts and toxoids; and (2) preparations for passive immunization, consisting mainly of the Ig-rich part of blood serum known as **gamma globulin** and **immune serum globulins.**

PREPARATION OF REPRESENTATIVE VACCINES

Vaccines for active immunizations include preparations of either pathogens or certain of their parts or products, such as toxins, which are inactivated before use. Microorganisms used in vaccines may be either killed, or only weakened to the point where they no longer are capable of causing disease, but can still provoke an immune response such as the production of Igs.

The effects of living or attenuated vaccines tend to imitate the results of an actual infection, and usually produce a better and longer-lasting immunity than that provided by killed preparations. The long-lasting effectiveness of attenuated vaccines is related to the fact that the living microorganisms in such preparations continue to reproduce in the body for a short time, and thereby prolong the stimulation of the immune response. Specifically, growing organisms provoke the immediate production of Igs

FIGURE 14.2

A summary of the acquired forms of immunity.

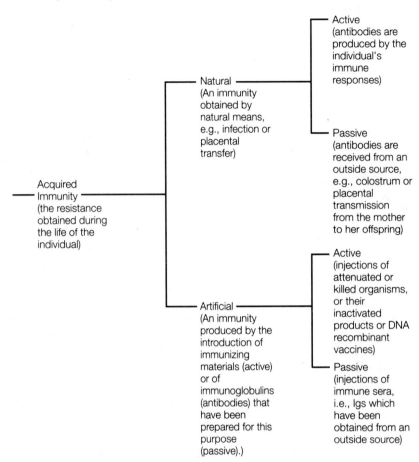

Acquired Immunity (the resistance obtained during the life of the individual)

Natural (An immunity obtained by natural means, e.g., infection or placental transfer)

Active (antibodies are produced by the individual's immune responses)

Passive (antibodies are received from an outside source, e.g., colostrum or placental transmission from the mother to her offspring)

Artificial (An immunity produced by the introduction of immunizing materials (active) or of immunoglobulins (antibodies) that have been prepared for this purpose (passive).)

Active (injections of attenuated or killed organisms, or their inactivated products or DNA recombinant vaccines)

Passive (injections of immune sera, i.e., Igs which have been obtained from an outside source)

to neutralize the infection, stimulate the cells needed to kill infected cells, and also generate the immune memory (**recall**) that guarantees a swift and lasting response in cases of future infections. Examples of attenuated vaccines, which are mostly viral, include the measles, mumps, rubella, and the Sabin polio vaccine.

Microorganisms used for killed vaccines are inactivated by exposure to chemicals such as formalin. Organisms are first grown, harvested after a suitable incubation period, and then killed. Heat is not used to kill these microorganisms since it is likely to change or damage their surface parts and thus reduce the immunizing effectiveness of vaccines. Commonly used killed vaccines include those used to

protect against influenza, whooping cough, and polio (Salk vaccine).

The toxins of several bacteria can be converted into nontoxic, but still Ig-stimulating toxoids. Heat or chemicals such as formalin are used in the preparation of toxoids. Examples of such preparations include diphtheria and tetanus (lockjaw) toxoids.

The preparations used for passive immunization are either **antitoxins** or **immune globulins.** Antitoxins are Igs capable of neutralizing the toxins that stimulated their production but do not affect the microorganisms that produced the toxin. Antitoxins are available for several diseases, including tetanus and diphtheria.

Immune globulins come in two forms, gamma globulin and specific immune globulins. Both types of preparations are obtained from human blood. Specific immune globulins are higher concentrations of Igs specifically for a particular disease agent. They are used in cases of measles, mumps, chicken pox, and hepatitis A and B infections.

THE SAFETY OF LIVE VERSUS INACTIVATED VACCINES

The acceptability of a vaccine depends upon the general need for the preparation and the degree of protection it can provide. Live vaccines produce a high level of immunity, usually in a single dose. However, while such immunizing preparations have obvious advantages when compared to inactivated ones, the use of live vaccines is subject to certain potential problems. These include the following possibilities: (1) the presence of infectious agents because of insufficient weakening; 2) the spreading of such disease agents from the immunized individual to susceptible contacts; (3) the presence of unknown or contaminating disease agents in the vaccine; (4) a mutation (a permanent genetic change) causing the microorganism in the vaccine to become highly destructive and capable of infecting various body areas; and (5) inactivation of the vaccine when not stored under refrigeration. Inactivated vaccines, on the other hand, are free from most of these potential problems. However, larger doses of such vaccines and several injections are needed to acquire the protection that is comparable to that obtained with live vaccines.

VACCINE SAFETY

An elaborate series of tests are used to ensure the safety and effectiveness of vaccines. For example, vaccines containing live viruses and/or their parts are checked for their immunological and disease-producing properties at all stages of preparation. The fate of viruses in the immunized individuals is also studied. In addition, if viruses from a vaccine are shed by the immunized individual, the possibility that they might cause disease in susceptible contacts is investigated. These and other safeguards are checked and, if necessary, corrected before a vaccine is released for immunization of the public.

THE STAGES OF VACCINE DEVELOPMENT—SOME BARRIERS FOR STD VACCINES

In asking the question of why vaccines are not or will not be available for a particular STD, one needs to look at the steps in vaccine development that may pose problems or barriers. The first step in developing any vaccine is identifying the targeted disease in all of its stages, and the causative agent. After the pathogen is known, it is necessary to learn as much about the agent as possible. If the pathogen can be grown in the laboratory and infect readily available animals, prospects are bright for the development of tests with which to detect the disease, and to uncover the secrets of the disease process. On the other hand, if cultivation of the pathogen is difficult or impossible, and infection of animals is limited to rare forms or to none at all, then prospects for vaccine development are not too bright. Some of the newer technologies, however, may reduce or even eliminate this problem.

The next step in vaccine development is to understand the disease process. How and where does the pathogen cause its damage? Are there several types of the causative agent? What host defenses contribute to recovery? Does immunity follow recovery? If it does, how long does it last? These are samples of the challenging and important questions which have had a significant impact on the attempts to produce vaccines for STDs such as syphilis, genital warts, and, of course, HIV infection.

The next step in vaccine development is the selection of the **candidate vaccine** preparation. This choice requires taking into consideration such things as the nature of the pathogen and the available technology. In other words, should the candidate vaccine contain live, attenuated organisms, killed organisms, or subunits of the pathogen in some form? For any type of vaccine, the road from development and preparation of the first batches of a vaccine for field testing trials to approval for licensure and widespread usage is often a very long one. It is

THE IMPACT OF HIV INFECTION ON STANDARD IMMUNIZATIONS

The appearance of HIV in epidemic form in the United States, Africa, and other parts of the world has raised concerns regarding the potential impact of HIV infection on the use of standard vaccines to prevent diseases such as tetanus, mumps, measles, and poliomyelitis. HIV-positive individuals who receive standard vaccines may not respond with an immune response that is protective. Moreover, the vaccinated persons in such cases may experience more frequent or severe reactions to vaccines. In short, then, should an HIV-infected person, adult or child, be immunized against the diseases mentioned earlier?

On balance, it appears, on the basis of available information, that vaccination of HIV-positive individuals is a generally safe procedure, even with live, attenuated vaccines. Such individuals tend to respond to these vaccines with the production of antibody levels believed to be protective. It appears also that the ability to respond immunologically depends upon the degree of immunosuppression.

HIV-positive children generally respond, but not as well as comparably-aged noninfected children, to the common childhood live vaccines such as those used to protect against polio, measles, mumps, and rubella. These childhood vaccines provide essential protection from infectious diseases that kill many hundreds of thousands of children annually on a worldwide basis. Such preparations are considered to be remarkably safe for all children and are generally recommended for routine immunization of HIV-infected children. One exception to the vaccines for HIV-infected individuals is the preparation containing live, but weakened, polio virus.

interesting to note that it took over 450 years from the first recorded reports of plague (the Black Death) to the development of a vaccine against the disease. Consider the state of affairs in the case of the modern plague AIDS. Because of the rapid accumulation of information and the progress made related to the features of the disease and HIV, a vaccine may become available before the end of the 1990s. The total time that could elapse in this case would be, at worst, nineteen years after the first recorded accounts of the disease.

Once a candidate vaccine has been shown to meet the requirements of an appropriate agency (in the United States this is the Food and Drug Administration), and the plan for its testing has been approved, it is tested for safety and immunizing properties in a small number of volunteers. If successful, the testing trials are expanded to larger groups of volunteers in various age groups. Finally,

if the vaccine is approved for the population for which it was developed, the preparation is put into large-scale production.

A number of obstacles to vaccine development, production, distribution, and general use are always possible. These include excessive production costs to prevent any commercial firm from undertaking the vaccine project, the possibility of substantial liability costs to threaten profits, and a fear of and/or indifference to the vaccine once it becomes available for general use on the part of a target population.

WHAT'S HAPPENING WITH THE AIDS VACCINE?

Among the first questions asked about each infectious disease brought to the attention of the public is, *When will a vaccine be available?* This question recognizes the effectiveness of existing vaccines and

VACCINE LIABILITY — AN OBSTACLE OF A HUMAN KIND

About twelve years ago, four drug companies developing a vaccine for swine flu gave the U.S. government an ultimatum: Unless they were granted protection (immunity) from all lawsuits associated with the use of their product, the firms said they would not sell the vaccine to the public. The threat worked. The U.S. Justice Department assumed full responsibility for more than 4,000 lawsuits. Approximately $100 million was paid to Americans who experienced unexpected side effects from the vaccine. Not one penny was paid by the drug companies.

Now in light of the great public concern over the AIDS pandemic and the cries for an HIV vaccine, the drug companies find themselves in a similar situation. Drug company officials and legal experts are warning the government that if an HIV (AIDS) vaccine is developed, companies may be unwilling to make it available to the public without some protection against lawsuits arising from its possible side effects. Over the past ten years a number of unique legal problems have made it impossible for drug companies to get insurance against lawsuits. Many officials argue that the unknown risks associated with an HIV vaccine could make it foolhardy for them to market the product commercially. Moreover,

because a vaccine of this kind would be given to large numbers of individuals, the possibility of unexpected, unfavorable reactions would be much greater than if the vaccine would be given to a smaller segment of the population. In an effort to cover anticipated legal expenses some of the companies remaining in the vaccine business have increased their prices. Others are in the process of evaluating their vaccine projects to see if they are financially feasible.

Another consideration to be evaluated is the financial reward to be gained from an HIV vaccine. Beginning with individuals practicing high-risk behaviors, and then extending gradually into the lower-risk segments of the population, the market for a vaccine that protects against HIV infection will probably be very large. The financial payoff appears to be so great for a company to develop a vaccine that the incentive to go forward is overwhelming.

It is quite clear that there is no drug or vaccine that does not pose some risk to the individuals taking it. However, the important issue in the HIV vaccine saga is not the liability problem, but whether the benefit outweighs the risk for the population as a whole.

expresses the expectation that today's biotechnologies will make possible the development of new and better vaccines. Theoretically, vaccines could be developed and used to control and eventually eliminate any infectious disease. In practice, however, development of vaccines for several diseases including most of the STDs, has proved to be quite difficult. For many infectious diseases such difficulties result from not fully understanding what happens during natural infections, and not having an appropriate laboratory animal or other means with which

to grow the disease agent and to test and evaluate a vaccine's safety and effectiveness. In the case of HIV infection other obstacles, including moral, ethical, and medicolegal considerations, and the shortage of uninfected human volunteers to test the vaccine, are among the major problems confronting researchers as they grapple with the main task, the development of a safe and effective vaccine. Table 14.1 lists several problems associated with the development of an HIV vaccine.

TABLE 14.1 | PROBLEMS ASSOCIATED WITH THE DEVELOPMENT OF HIV VACCINES

Biological properties of the virus are not completely understood.

The development of the disease is not completely understood.

No specific indicators (markers) are available to show a favorable immune response.

Virus exists both outside of cells and in a hidden form within infected cells.

HIV infections are mainly silent but advance to severe and life-threatening stages.

HIV infection cripples or destroys the immune system.

Surface antigens are numerous and are subject to periodic change.

Animal models for vaccine testing are inadequate.

Identification of volunteers to evaluate vaccine effectiveness is difficult.

Vaccine must prevent infection.

Vaccine must be safe.

Evaluation of the long-term safety of the vaccine must be performed.

Perhaps the most frustrating obstacle interfering with development of a successful vaccine is HIV itself. This virus hides in cells, undergoes permanent genetic changes (mutations) regularly, and survives despite many immune responses that would normally rid the body of an invading virus. Mutations of the envelope gene, which controls the protein architecture of HIV's outer parts, are common and result in enough antigenic differences among viruses isolated from infected persons to make vaccine development even more frustrating. Thus, the Igs formed against the surface parts of one strain of HIV may fail to recognize or neutralize newly mutated strains.

The persistent dilemma found with HIV-infected persons is that they develop Igs that inactivate the virus in laboratory tests, yet they become sick and die anyway. This leaves researchers in the position of trying to design a vaccine without knowing what kinds of immune responses will protect a person from HIV infection.

Nevertheless, one unifying approach to the development of an HIV vaccine has emerged: to make a preparation that stimulates the production of Igs against the envelope protein that encloses the virus. This strategy worked with the polio, measles, and hepatitis B vaccines, but unfortunately, it is not working for HIV, at least so far. HIV is an elusive enemy since it can be transmitted in infected cells as well as by free virus particles. Thus, an ideal vaccine must be able to trigger the immune system not only to produce Igs which would interfere with viral attachment and penetration into susceptible cells, but also to destroy HIV-infected cells. This may be a tall order to fill since the HIV infects some of the same cells (T helper lymphocytes) that need to be activated to stop the infection.

SOME HIV VACCINE CANDIDATES

To be effective an HIV vaccine would need to imitate or improve on the immunological response that occurs during a natural infection, cause few if any side effects, be highly stable, and relatively easy to produce and use. Toward this end a number of preparations are being considered as vaccine candidates. Table 14.2 lists several examples.

Killed or Attenuated HIV. Traditionally, viral vaccines have been made from whole viruses that have been killed or from an attenuated strain that stimulates antibody production but does not cause

TABLE 14.2 | HIV VACCINE CANDIDATES

Live, attenuated HIV

Killed, inactivated HIV

Purified envelope glycoproteins

A blend of viral proteins produced by recombinant DNA techniques

Vectors (viruses, bacteria) containing envelope glycoproteins (gps)

Anti-idiotypic vaccines

disease. Killed vaccines have been effectively used to combat a number of viral diseases, including polio and influenza. In addition, some promising results have been obtained in experiments with inactivated simian immunodeficiency virus (SIV) vaccines. SIV is a virus normally found among certain types of monkeys and is capable of causing an illness similar to AIDS in these animals. Despite the various successes of killed preparations investigators are hesitant to use whole HIV because they do not want to risk the possibility of live, disease-producing virus particles accidentally finding their way into vaccine preparations. Another objection to the use of whole killed virus for a vaccine has been raised by some researchers based on the concern for injecting viral nucleic acids that might integrate into the genetic material of the recipient's cells and cause problems such as the activation of cancer-causing genes.

Live, attenuated HIV, also a logical vaccine candidate, probably will not be acceptable, largely because a weakened viral strain might regain its disease-producing capability through mutation or some other genetic mechanism. In addition, attenuated HIV may still contain inactive genes having the potential to disrupt a cell's normal growth in such a way as to cause cancer. Vaccine developers are clearly not certain that truly harmless forms of HIV exist or whether it is possible to make the virus irreversibly harmless.

Subunits. Several vaccine-developing teams are dissecting the molecular architecture of different viral parts such as the outside envelope and the inner core in an effort to determine which part or sub-unit

of the part would be more likely to protect against HIV infection.

Sub-unit vaccines consist of antigenic parts or fragments rather than the entire pathogen itself. Their use thus eliminates the possible danger of an *inadvertent* infection. The first HIV vaccine candidate tested in humans in the United States contained a sub-unit from the viral envelope. The results thus far have been inconclusive.

Sub-units are generally less effective than the whole pathogen in stimulating an immune response. Thus, the choice of an antigenic sub-unit for a vaccine is critical. Several viral sub-unit vaccines consist of a viral antigen combined with a substance known as an **adjuvant** which increases the vaccines' antibody-stimulating capability. In other candidate vaccines, sub-units are produced by specially, genetically engineered microorganisms or animal cells. This approach is described in the following section.

Recombinant DNA Vaccines. Recombinant DNA technology is one of the newer methods of modern science used to manipulate the genetic composition and properties of different forms of life. In the case of vaccines, only the genes from the disease agent that contain the information for the production of immunologically important protein sub-units or related proteinlike antigens of viruses and bacteria are introduced into the genetic system of another bacterium, yeast, or animal cell. These genetically changed microorganisms now can produce the desired sub-unit in quantity under the direction of the newly acquired genes. The sub-units are collected and purified for use as a **sub-unit vaccine.** The hepatitis B vaccine is a product of this new technology.

A Bright Spot among Vaccines

Dr. Jonas Salk, the developer of the first polio vaccine, working with Dr. Alexandra Levine at the University of Southern California in Los Angeles, injected an experimental vaccine into nineteen volunteer patients suffering from AIDS-related complex. The vaccine contained killed HIVs stripped of their outer coats. More than a year later, in 1989, ten of the nineteen patients showed a major improvement in the production of T lymphocytes. Although none of the injected individuals demonstrated a significant production of Igs, fifteen volunteers did exhibit other forms of an immune response. This study and related ones indicate that this vaccine might one day be used to prevent HIV-infected individuals from developing full-blown AIDS.

Despite the arguments against a living vaccine in the case of HIV, researchers are trying to get around the problem by inserting selected antigen-producing genes from HIV into another living microorganism such as vaccinia virus, the agent used to immunize people against smallpox (fig. 14.1). The modified virus, generally referred to as a **vector,** would be expected not only to produce the desired HIV antigens but also to present the antibody stimulating antigens to the immune system in a more natural manner, thereby possibly provoking a wider range of immune responses such as those described earlier in chapter 10. Since vaccinia virus is a large virus, several genes can be inserted into it.

Injecting a vaccinia-HIV sub-unit vaccine into chimpanzees produced specific immune responses. While such results are promising, the use of vaccinia virus is not totally free of problems. The live virus has the potential to cause a range of severe complications in immunocompromised hosts, such as HIV-infected persons.

Several other viruses and microorganisms are being used as **recombinant DNA vaccine** candidates. For example, in 1989 British scientists using recombinant DNA techniques produced a vaccine consisting of a live attenuated poliovirus (similar to that used in the Sabin polio vaccine) with sprouts of HIV envelope sub-units hanging on its outer surface. The sub-unit vaccine was in reality a living poliovirus with an outer surface resembling HIV. Since preliminary tests in laboratory animals resulted in an anti-HIV immune response, this genetically engineered or recombinant DNA product may have potential as an HIV vaccine.

Anti-idiotype Vaccines. Among the most novel vaccine candidates are those consisting of **anti-idiotypes.** An *idiotype* is the specific part of an antibody to which an antigen attaches or binds. By means of a rather complicated procedure an antibody is formed that not only resembles the antigen but can provoke an immune response to that antigen. An anti-idiotype vaccine would be specific, harmless, and capable of blocking the sites on cells to which viruses attach. In short, this type of vaccine has the potential to induce a high level of immunity in newborns and in others exposed to HIV.

Immunoglobulin Vaccines. Passive immunization with high levels of neutralizing immunoglobulins (antibodies) may have a role in the prevention of HIV infection in selected populations such as newborn infants and HIV-positive mothers. This approach has not yet been shown to be effective in any animal model for AIDS. However, since passive immunization has been found to be an effective preventive measure with other infectious diseases such as hepatitis B, measles, and mumps, studies are continuing.

SPECIFIC OBSTACLES

Developing a vaccine candidate takes a great amount of time, effort, and money. Even though a potentially effective preparation is in-hand, the problems are not over. In the case of an HIV vaccine, certain barriers stand in the way of showing that it genuinely protects against HIV infection. Two examples of such barriers are the lack of an ideal animal model and the availability of volunteers for human vaccine testing trials.

Animal Models. A major barrier to the development of a safe and effective vaccine against HIV infection is the lack of a readily available animal model to evaluate whether primary HIV infection and the development of AIDs can be prevented by immunization with candidate AIDS vaccines. Chimpanzees appear to be the only animal system in which experimental infection is successful. After inoculation with HIV, chimpanzees show a specific immune response and the virus can be isolated from various specimens. However, HIV infection does not produce an AIDS-like disease in these animals. Moreover, the number of chimpanzees for HIV testing in the United States is currently low, making extensive testing of vaccine candidates difficult.

The Problem of Volunteers for HIV Vaccine Testing. Would anybody volunteer to test such a vaccine? Many researchers believe that a lack of appropriate volunteers might be a significant problem. (Such volunteers must be HIV-negative and must be counseled to avoid all high-risk behaviors which may affect vaccine testing results throughout the trial period.) In all probability there would be no volunteer opposition to tests with live vaccines using the proven, safe vaccinia virus or other carriers. However, a live unknown HIV vaccine, no matter how weakened, would be very threatening since there is a possibility that the virus might regain its disease-producing capability through mutation or other genetic mechanism.

Other major issues affecting the recruitment of volunteers for the testing of HIV vaccines will be maintaining the confidentiality of all information of vaccine-caused positive blood tests (**seroconversion**). Confidentiality will have to be continued for the duration of the trial because volunteers may be identified as belonging to groups practicing the high-risk behaviors associated with HIV infection — a factor that potentially could lead to various types of discrimination or other socially damaging situations. In addition, vaccine-caused seroconversion may lead to difficulties in donating blood, obtaining insurance, travelling internationally, or entering the military or foreign services. Vaccine-stimulated HIV antibodies may last a significant length of time. Even though volunteers would be given some form of paperwork that certified their participation in vaccine test trials, and that their antibodies were the result of immunization and not an HIV infection, the positive blood test issue may have a major impact on the current and future recruitment of vaccine trial participants.

VACCINES FOR OTHER STDS

Despite the fact that many of the obstacles interfering with HIV vaccine development also apply to other STDs, the future does hold some promise for certain STD vaccines. For example, in the case of syphilis immunization of rabbits with a live, attenuated preparation of the causative agent produced some protection. Moreover, the injection of antibodies into infected laboratory animals lessened the effects of the disease, but did not provide complete protection. Whether humans will respond as the laboratory animals did is still an open question.

Immunization against gonorrhea is being pursued quite aggressively since even a partially effective vaccine could be helpful in reducing the incidence of this STD. Although field testing may be a specific barrier, attention is being focused on parts of the disease agent and a DNA recombinant preparation as vaccine candidates.

Another STD for which a vaccine is being actively sought is genital herpes. Even though the antibodies formed during natural herpes infections do not protect against subsequent episodes of the disease they may change the course of the infection. A DNA recombinant vaccine using the vaccinia virus into which genes from both HSV-1 and HSV-2 have been inserted is likely to be the most promising vaccine candidate.

Vaccine development with other STDs have been limited largely because of a lack of knowledge regarding the immune responses involved with the disease. For example, with genital warts it is not known if an infection with one type of human papilloma virus (HPV) provides protection against a later reinfection with the same virus type. Recurrence of genital warts is common, but it is not clear whether this condition results from an incomplete recovery from a previous infection, reactivation of a latent infection, a new infection with a different type of HPV, or reinfection with the same HPV type. If a natural infection does not protect against reinfection with the same type of HPV the development of an effective vaccine is questionable. Adding to this perplexing situation is the absence of suitable laboratory systems with which to grow HPV and to test vaccine candidates. Despite such problems research is still continuing, especially in the area of DNA recombinant vaccine development.

PROSPECTS FOR THE FUTURE

Ever since the eighteenth-century physician Edward Jenner found an effective means of combating the dreaded disease of smallpox, vaccines have been indispensable, when available, in the battles against various infectious diseases. It is no small wonder, then, that researchers and people the world over are turning toward a vaccine in hopes of conquering HIV infections as well as other STDs. What we are now experiencing is both the technical possibility and economic feasibility for vaccines that would have been impossible on both counts just a few years ago. In fact, it is now possible to develop vaccines against agents that cannot even be grown in the laboratory. It appears that if identification of the specific antigens of the disease agent needed to produce protective antibodies is possible, then it seems that the question is no longer whether a vaccine can be made, but when. Vaccines for HIV, CMV, syphilis, and genital herpes are likely to be developed within the 1990s, but will they be accepted by the public? Vaccines are only of value when they are used.

CHAPTER 15

HIV INFECTION IN AND OUT OF THE WORKPLACE

One day on a road in the English countryside, a clergyman happened to meet Plague. "Where are you bound?" asked the clergyman. "To London," responded Plague, "to kill a thousand." . . .
When they chanced to meet again some weeks later, the clergyman inquired, "I thought you were going to kill a thousand. How is it that two thousand died?" "Ah, yes," replied Plague. "I killed only a thousand. Fear killed the rest."

—Anonymous

People should not worry about contracting HIV at their place of work. Such fears are fanned by gossip and rumors, even though the vast majority of the 2.3 billion or so working people in the world face little or no risk of acquiring or transmitting HIV at the workplace. These were among the conclusions of the conference sponsored by the World Health Organization, with the International Labor Organization, in June 1988. The meeting, attended by medical, public health, labor, government, union, and business representatives from 18 countries, however, raised a number of issues related to the concerns of workers. Several of these focused on the responsibility of employers to inform, educate, and develop policies important to the well-being of both HIV-infected and non-HIV-infected working personnel. This chapter considers these topics and focuses on occupations and HIV infection/AIDS exposure, and the precautions and practices used to prevent and control the spread of HIV infection. Some of these are also applicable to day-care centers, the home, and other locations or situations.

Workplace Policy—What Should It Be?

In a society where the workplace is not just a source of income, but also a source of community, where fellow workers frequently are friends, there is no way to build a wall around HIV-infected persons. Executives or managers of various businesses or agencies who think that HIV/AIDS is not a concern of their employees, either are not aware of the extent of the problem or are frightened to acknowledge the facts. HIV/AIDS affects both afflicted workers and their colleagues. Employees afraid of infected co-workers have walked off the job. In some areas workers have even refused to share tools or use the company truck driven by a fellow employee rumored to have died of AIDS until it was sterilized. Still others would not sit in the company cafeteria next to a stricken co-worker.

What is the business community or a service agency to do? HIV/AIDS is not the so-called garden variety type of disease that calls for standard responses and ordinary policies. The disease is not only new and frightening, but the publics' perception is loaded with bias and misinformation. HIV/AIDS requires a rethinking of the boundaries between the business enterprise or service agency and the public domain. Moreover, the relationship between the employer and employees also needs a careful re-examination.

Employees have a particular challenge and responsibility to develop workplace policies that are humane, fair, scientifically accurate, and legally sound. These policies should address legal issues such as antibody testing, discrimination and confidentiality; treatment issues such as health insurance benefits and affordability of care; and prevention measures such as AIDS education for all employees, clientele, and suppliers. Table 15.1 lists several items proposed by the World Health Organization that should be included in an HIV/AIDS policy for the workplace. To be effective, such a policy should involve employers, employees, and their organizations, and where appropriate, governmental agencies.

The developers of a workplace policy should use an approach which treats AIDS like any other disease and shows compassion for the person with HIV infection or AIDS. This is not only the right policy but it is also legally required, at least in the U.S.

Policies Do Not Reach Everyone—The Differences between Large Corporations and Small Businesses

Approximately 10 percent of all American businesses have a policy (either written or unwritten) with respect to HIV infection/AIDS and employment. Most of such businesses are large corporations with a large force numbering over 1,000 employees, who are predominantly white, well educated, and relatively well paid. A 1989 survey revealed that about 20 percent of 151 Fortune 500 firms have AIDS-related policies. A majority of these organizations, which include the Bank of America, the Levi Strauss Company, and Pacific Bell, have offices in or around the San Francisco Bay area, where the HIV/AIDS epidemic has been largely confined to gay men. Because these companies were the first employers in the private sector to respond in an organized way to the disease, the issues and concerns surrounding AIDS have usually been defined in terms of corporate hiring, firing, and employment of gay men with AIDS.

Nationally, at the present time gay men and intravenous drug users (IVDUs) make up the greater percentage of all reported AIDS cases. Gay men and IVDUs, and their sexual partners represent separate at-risk populations.

Small businesses are more likely than their larger counterparts to have people who are infected with HIV, and individuals who practice high-risk behaviors. Quite obviously, then, small businesses have a greater need for HIV/AIDS-related policies and employee education programs. However, because of limited resources these employers are probably less likely to have such policies and programs, and less able to respond in a socially responsible way to HIV/AIDS-related employment problems and concerns.

TABLE 15.1	SPECIFIC AREAS THAT SHOULD BE COVERED BY COMPANY OR AGENCY WORKPLACE HIV/AIDS POLICIES

CONDITIONS FOR EMPLOYMENT

HIV/AIDS screening or inquiries about tests already taken should not be a requirement for employment.

CONDITIONS DURING EMPLOYMENT

1. A policy should be developed and in place before HIV-related questions or issues arise in the workplace.
2. As established HIV/AIDS policy should be distributed to all employees.
3. An information and education program should be provided for all employees.
4. Confidentiality of all medical information, including HIV/AIDS status, must be guaranteed and maintained for all employees.
5. An employee should not be required to inform the employer of his or her HIV/AIDS status.
6. Employees affected by or perceived to be affected by HIV/AIDS must be protected from stigma and discrimination not only from co-workers and employers, but also from clients.
7. Employees and their families should have access to information and education programs on HIV/AIDS, as well as to relevant counseling and appropriate referrals to needed services.
8. HIV-infected employees should not be denied standard social security and and/or occupationally related benefits.
9. Provisions should be in place to provide reasonable working arrangements for HIV-infected employees unable to perform in their usual working capacity.
10. Procedures must be in place to provide appropriate first aid to reduce the risk of transmitting any blood-related infections.
11. HIV infection should not be a basis for termination of employment.

EMPLOYEE EDUCATION PROGRAMS

Large and small businesses, public service agencies, school systems, and other employers have a major responsibility to educate their employees about HIV infection and AIDS. Efforts should be directed to prevent the groundless hysteria that sometimes develops when a co-worker contracts the deadly disease. Many educational programs have been launched by employers to persuade their employees to stop smoking, to eat properly, to avoid drugs, and to stop drinking. Adding to these persuasion efforts, attempts to educate and to develop policies dealing with HIV/AIDS is not a quantum leap. Depending on the particular business or agency, most education programs are quite similar in purpose and concentrate on what employees need to know.

Most concerns and fears of employees are expressed in terms of specific questions about personal risk and HIV infection. Other blood-related diseases such as hepatitis B also raise similar concerns. Here are some common examples:

- How is HIV spread?
- How is HIV not spread?
- How can I protect myself against infection on the job?
- Who is at risk?
- What do I do if I become exposed to an HIV-infected person?
- If I am or become infected, can I bring HIV home and infect loved ones and friends?
- How can I protect myself and those close to me?
- What is the company policy as far as health care and insurance if I become exposed or infected on the job?

AIDS AND THE FASHION INDUSTRY

Fashion businesses, which include Yves Saint Laurent, Calvin Klein, and Anne Klein, make a sizable contribution to the U.S. economy. The total apparel and accessories sales for 1989 amounted to $91.2 billion, thus making fashion businesses one of the nation's major industries. Also in this year American companies exported $2.6 billion worth of apparel. Such large volumes of exports and good financial returns have attracted the attention of many corporations and banks in both the United States and Japan. Their investments in major houses of fashion provide the necessary cash for operating expenses and funding ambitious new projects. The glamour associated with the fashion industry gives such corporations good profiles and visibility in the financial world.

With the unfortunate deaths of several top designers caused by AIDS a dark cloud has formed over the fashion industry. This industry is known to employ the creative talents of many men, which include top designers, hairdressers, make-up people, and window-dressers. While it is difficult, if not impossible, to determine exactly how many AIDS-related illnesses and deaths have occurred in the fashion world, a number of well-known leaders in the industry have died since 1986 of the immunodeficiency. These include Perry Ellis, Angel Estrada, and Willi Smith. A more recent addition to the list is Halston, who introduced U.S. women to the pillbox hat, slinky jerseys, and Ultrasuede.

The fashion industry is becoming extremely nervous about its image, not only with investors, but with consumers as well. The industry is struggling to find a new direction despite the fact that its creative energy is being dampened by AIDS. Many designers are finding it more difficult to finance their fashion lines, while others complain they cannot get life or medical insurance.

The sales of certain houses of fashion have not been affected since the deaths of their namesakes. Others have struggled. In addition, individuals in the workplace have had to cope with AIDS on a different level. Many are worried that their co-workers will disappear into the hospital from one day to the next. Such concerns easily can demoralize a firm's staff and ruin an entire fashion collection. It is quite clear that AIDS is blurring the images that expensive clothes so carefully emphasize: beauty, health, vitality, and, of course, sex appeal. One cannot help but wonder what direction the fashion industry will take over the next ten to fifteen years.

Because of the concern about the vulnerability to AIDS associated with men in the fashion industry, greater interest in women designers is beginning to emerge among members of the financial community. Investors are looking at women from a different point of view.

Employers frequently need to stress how HIV infection is not spread (table 15.2), and why the stigma that accompanies HIV infection leads to irrational and unfair behavior at the workplace. Employees must understand that an individual who is at high risk or known to be infected is not necessarily immoral, bad, unclean, or unpleasant. Employee education programs should also stress avoiding or modifying specific risk-related activities and not avoiding or isolating persons at risk for HIV infection or those already infected with the virus.

TABLE 15.2 | How You Won't Get AIDS

You Won't Get AIDS . . .

1. . . . from everyday contact.	8. . . . from food.
2. . . . from a mosquito bite.	9. . . . from a towel.
3. . . . from a public pool.	10. . . . from a telephone.
4. . . . from a toilet seat.	11. . . . from a pimple.
5. . . . from a haircut.	12. . . . from a kiss.
6. . . . by donating blood.	13. . . . from a classroom.
7. . . . from tears.	14. . . . because someone is different from you.

Source: America Responds to AIDS poster: "Stop Worrying About How You Won't Get AIDS, and Worry About How You Can"

Employer approaches and strategies to increase the employees' knowledge of HIV/AIDS may take various forms and include in-service training sessions and brochures (fig. 15.1). The language used should be easily understood and tailored to the audience. In addition, situations may require the use of sexually explicit examples in order to avoid any misunderstandings. This can be done tastefully and effectively. Providing accurate, current, and adequate information to employees is probably the best weapon currently available to control the spread of HIV infection and to reduce irrational fears in the workplace. In all presentations, the names of any infected co-worker must be kept confidential to prevent unfair treatment or discrimination from occurring.

OCCUPATIONS AND HIV/AIDS EXPOSURE

A number of occupations carry with them the possibility of exposure to HIV. These include health care, law enforcement, rescue and/or fire-fighting, and various forms of social services such as drug abuse treatment and counseling. During the course of normal routines, many workers in these occupations find themselves in situations involving direct contact with blood and other body fluids and secretions. Naturally, faced with job-related risks of HIV exposure, workers have particular concerns about their personal safety and well-being. Knowing and using certain *universal precautions*, whenever and wherever applicable can greatly reduce or even prevent the possibility of, not only HIV infection, but other blood-related diseases such as hepatitis B. Nowhere is this more evident than with health care workers.

HEALTH CARE WORKERS

Health care personnel at all levels need to know about and take precautions against HIV-associated diseases, because they are likely to see infected persons in the course of their work. Thus, such health care practitioners, which include doctors, nurses, dentists, respiratory therapists, and medical laboratory personnel, are at a slightly higher risk than other workers of occupationally acquired HIV exposure and possible infection. This situation is largely the result of coming into contact with a large number and variety of patients, and being in situations in which there is a likelihood for exposure to blood and other body fluids.

FIGURE 15.1

An example of a brochure used to inform health care personnel about exposure situations and safety precautions to follow. Most health care facilities have developed similar types of publications. (Courtesy of World Health Organization)

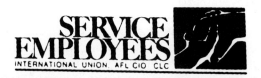

AIDS
AND THE HEALTHCARE WORKER

Fourth Edition
March, 1987

SERVICE EMPLOYEES
INTERNATIONAL UNION, AFL CIO CLC

(This brochure also available in Spanish)

A wide range of HIV-infected persons are likely to seek health care services. Many of such individuals may or may not be aware of their HIV condition and/or stage of infection, and actually be without symptoms. Some clearly may need care because of a worsening state of health or complications of HIV infection. Still others may not be able to communicate information about their condition, or for various reasons, including the fear of discrimination, may choose not to share information with the person providing health care services.

While HIV infection is currently the most feared, there are several other blood-related diseases that can be spread by contact with body fluids and secretions. These include hepatitis B, syphilis, and cytomegalovirus infection. The development and application of an employee disease prevention program can effectively reduce the spread of all blood-related infectious agents to health care workers. Effective programs generally depend on at least three factors: 1) the use of appropriate precautions; 2) availability of appropriate supplies in sufficient quantity; and 3) employees fully informed about and using appropriate universal precautions (fig. 15.2).

Universal Precautions. Fortunately, HIV is difficult to transmit in a health care setting, partly because the virus is killed by common disinfectants. *Most* studies have shown no proven seroconversions to a HIV positive state after simple or even repeated needle-sticks or mucous membrane or skin exposures in health care workers.

Unfortunately, accidents do occur and can cause acute illness and/or HIV antibody response. Reports in 1986 documented that two nurses who received intramuscular injections of HIV-contaminated blood and one mother, who when caring for her infant with AIDS and handling bloody stools seldom wore gloves or washed her hands, developed HIV antibodies. Other reports documented that three nurses who had non-needle-stick exposures to HIV-antibody-positive patients developed HIV antibodies themselves. Since the risk of the unknown is always present in health care the possibility always exists for the development of HIV antibodies (seroconversion) and illness in health care workers with only work-related exposure to HIV.

FIGURE 15.2

An example of safety guidelines for health care personnel. (Courtesy of Burroughs Wellcome Co.)

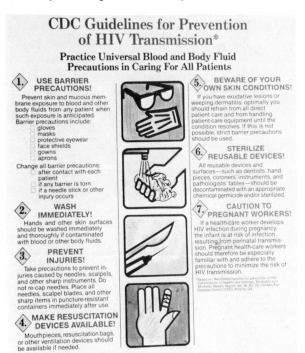

To protect health care workers as much as possible it is generally assumed that every patient is a potential source of disease agents, and appropriate infection control measures must be taken. This is particularly true with HIV/AIDS since seroconversions may take at least one year, and patients who do not have HIV antibodies can still transmit the virus.

The body substance isolation or universal precautions approach makes the health care workplace safer for both health care workers and for their clients. Table 15.3 lists a number of the precautions followed by health care workers. Employers are responsible for monitoring the work setting to make certain that protective measures are being observed. If they are not, either more education or disciplinary actions usually are implemented.

Since most precautions are aimed at preventing punctures by sharp objects and exposure to the splash and splatter of blood and other body fluids,

TABLE 15.3 | UNIVERSAL PRECAUTIONS

PRECAUTION FACTOR	APPLICATION
Protective apparel and related barriers	*Gloves* should be worn to protect hands from coming into direct contact with blood or other possible infectious body fluids or secretions. They should be changed and disposed of after each contact or use. *Gowns, face masks, and protective eyewear,* should be worn, whenever practical, during procedures that generate droplets or other splatter of blood and other body fluids.
Hand-washing	Hands and skin surfaces should be washed immediately and thoroughly if contaminated with blood or other body fluids or secretions. Hands also should be washed immediately after gloves are removed.
Needle and other sharp object disposal	Care should be taken to prevent injuries by needles or other sharp objects. Needles should not be recapped, bent, or broken by hand. After use needles should be disposed of in puncture-resistant containers.
Open and/or weeping cuts	Workers with open, weeping skin cuts or sores should not give direct care to patients or handle equipment used in such care situations until the cuts heal. Cuts should be covered with appropriate bandages that repel liquids.
Ventilation devices (e.g., mouthpieces)	Ventilation devices should be available for use during resuscitation and testing procedures. Disposable devices should be used whenever possible.
Pregnancy	Pregnant employees should be especially familiar with and strictly follow the universal precautions.

various types of barriers are used. Such barriers generally serve to prevent, restrict, or stop entry and include safe hypodermic needle disposal containers (fig. 15.3), latex or vinyl gloves, drapes, gowns, face masks, and eye shields.

Historical records indicate the use of protective clothing or apparel dates back to about 1721. At that time, the fear of contagion during the plague epidemics in Europe was a legitimate concern, and physicians wore special garments to avoid infection from coming into contact with fleas and the body fluids of their patients (fig. 2.5). Today an extensive selection of protective apparel is available, usually in the form of drapes and gowns. Such apparel is designed to truly keep blood and other potentially infectious material away from health care workers. Special repellent fabrics (fig. 15.4) or plastic or polyethylene to reinforce fabrics are used for this

FIGURE 15.3

An example of a needle disposal container. (Courtesy of Becton Dickinson Vacutainer Systems, Rutherford, New Jersey)

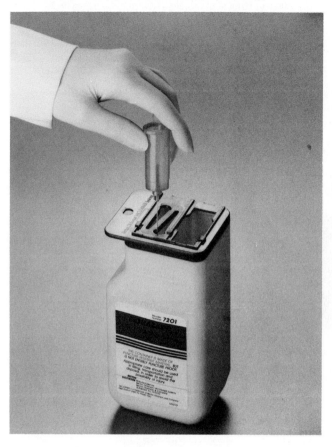

FIGURE 15.4

What a difference a fabric makes. Two examples of fabrics used in cover gowns for health care workers. A laboratory test designed to simulate actual conditions of use when beef blood is applied to the material. On the left, 68.6 percent (arrow) of the blood gets through. With the material shown on the right only 1.4 percent (arrow) gets through. Cover gowns made of the fabric on the right clearly are more protective against blood penetration.[1] (Courtesy of Kimberly-Clark)

[1]These breathable fabrics are not totally impervious. The **absence of visible blood penetration is not a guarantee of zero penetration.**

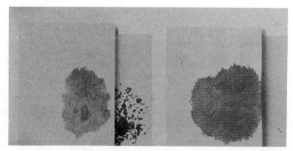

Gloves are worn in a number of patient situations, especially those associated with anticipated contact with blood and other body fluids or secretions, broken skin, and moist body surfaces. The appropriate use of gloves protects not only the health care worker, but the patient as well. A wide selection of different latex and vinyl gloves is available to meet a broad range of needs. Because of the concern about HIV and HBV infections, health care personnel are using more gloves than ever before.

PUBLIC SAFETY WORKERS

Individuals in law enforcement, and rescue and firefighting services are referred to as **public safety workers.** While most of these professionals are not considered to be health care workers, many of them are the first to arrive at the scene of an emergency accident, crime, or other situation which frequently involves direct contact with blood. Knowing and applying the appropriate universal precautions should enable public safety workers to perform effectively on the job and lessen the risk of infection with HIV, HVB, or other blood-related disease agents. (See table 15.3.)

purpose. Sheets consisting of repellent fabric also are used to cover patients, personnel, and equipment during operations.

Accidental needle-sticks represent a common problem and one that is associated with needle disposal. Several types of containers are in use and are intended to provide a system of safe needle and syringe disposal. Another solution for safe needle disposal is the high-risk needle device. This device consists of a standard hypodermic needle with a unique plastic cover that locks in place when the procedure involving the needle is completed (fig. 15.5). Once locked, the cover protecting the needle tip helps to reduce the chance of an accidental stick.

FIGURE 15.5

The Shamrock Safety Blood Collection Set, a disposable system designed to prevent accidental needle-stick injuries. (a) The Shamrock (arrow) is used in a standard way. (b) Once the procedure is completed the needle is simply pulled back into the protective Shamrock shield, and the unit is ready for disposal. (Courtesy of Ryan Medican, Inc., Brentwood, Tennessee)

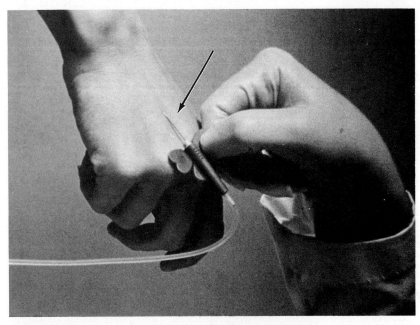

a

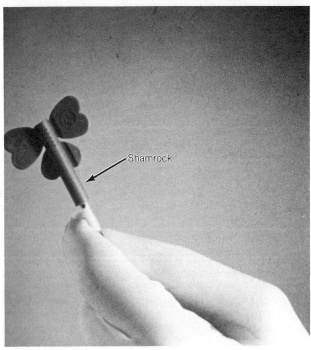

Shamrock

b

TABLE 15.4 | RECOMMENDATIONS FOR CHILD OR DAY-CARE CENTER FACILITIES

1. Disinfect bathrooms, kitchens, and sleeping quarters with household bleach.
2. Clean and disinfect toilets on a daily basis.
3. Disinfect toilets after each use if person has diarrhea.
4. Rinse dishes and eating utensils in a bleach solution before the final rinse.
5. Dispose of food and other waste (paper plates, plastic eating ware, etc.) carefully and frequently. Place all items in covered containers away from the food preparation area.
6. Use liquid soap dispensers.
7. Wash towels and linens in hot water with detergent and bleach.

Source: Based on the 1983 recommendation of the County of Los Angeles Department of Health Sciences, Drug Abuse Program Office

CHILD-CARE AND RELATED FACILITIES

An HIV-infected child in any child-care facility, preschool program, or grade school has raised and continues to raise several questions and concerns. Such questions and concerns are of importance not only to parents, but to the personnel staffing these facilities. Deciding whether an HIV-infected child should be encouraged or allowed to attend preschool or grade school is generally based on two considerations: 1) Will an HIV-infected child be a source of infection to other children and personnel of the facility?; and 2) Is the HIV-infected child at risk of contracting a serious infection from other children? Infectious diseases are not a surprising fact of life in child-care centers or preschools. Microorganisms are readily spread among groups of young children.

In general, there is no evidence that HIV can be spread by casual contact or by the ordinary activities in child-care facilities or in preschools. This includes any kind of activity that takes place in a classroom, gym, or playground. Thus, an HIV-infected child does not pose a hazard to other children or to a facility's personnel. Nevertheless, if an HIV-infected child does attend, an education program should be established for the staff as well as the parents of other children attending the facility. Particular attention should be given to correcting

misconceptions and providing accurate information. In addition, staff members should be trained in the applications of the universal precautions listed in table 15.3 that are appropriate for the child-care or preschool facility. Additional guidelines are given in table 15.4.

HIV/AIDS OUTSIDE THE WORKPLACE
HOME CARE PROVIDERS

HIV-infected persons or persons with AIDS in the home can raise questions and concerns on the part of relatives, friends, and other individuals who provide care. Such care-givers need to keep in mind several aims, the most important of which is to avoid exposing themselves or others to potentially infectious materials from the patient, and to protect the patient from possible infections from others. Suggested guidelines are listed in table 15.5.

SELF-CARE

While HIV-infected individuals or persons with AIDS may safely share household and public facilities with others there still is a need to exercise certain precautions in the home to avoid exposure to opportunistic disease agents. For example, HIV-infected persons should avoid contact with pets such

THE HAZARD OF INFECTION FROM THE SHARED COMMUNION CUP

While the possibility of acquiring an infection whenever wine is received via a common communion cup has been repeatedly discussed, the current AIDS pandemic has renewed the fears about the religious practice.

The act of Holy Communion consists of persons gathered together receiving bread and wine from a minister or other member of the clergy officiating at the ceremony. Participants receive a wafer or a piece of bread, the wafer often being placed directly on their tongues by the minister or the bread being placed in their open hands before they themselves transfer it to their mouths. The former method of distribution occasionally involves the exchange of very small amounts of saliva between communicants since the minister's fingers touch either the lips or the tongue when placing the wafer in the recipient's mouth.

The wine is received either through drinking from a common cup, by dipping the bread or wafer into the wine before eating it, or by pouring the wine into individual cups for drinking. With the shared communion cup it is often believed that the risk of transferring saliva and any associated microorganisms is minimized by the disinfecting power of the silver from which cups are usually made, a similar effect of the alcohol in the wine, rotating the cup between each communicant, and wiping the rim of the cup both inside and out with a cloth between use by each communicant. Various studies have shown that only the use of a cloth to wipe the rim of the cup reduces the likelihood of transmitting microorganisms.

Even though an infectious disease attributable to the shared communion cup has never been reported, some churches have discontinued its use. While HIV continues to be studied, future reports may strengthen but could also change the conclusion that the shared communion cup does not act as a means for the transmission of an infectious disease.

TABLE 15.5 | GUIDELINES FOR HOME CARE PROVIDERS

1. Wear gloves when handling blood, other body fluids, excretions, or any items soiled or contaminated by potential infectious materials.

2. Disinfect any visibly contaminated surface, object, or container with a disinfectant such as a household bleach solution consisting of one part bleach and ten parts water.

3. Wear some form of protective clothing or covering to guard against spillage or splatters of blood or body fluids. Such protective clothing should cover the arms and street clothing.

4. Remove protective clothing and gloves before leaving the patient's room, and place them in a strong plastic bag that can be tied securely.

5. All disposable items soiled with blood or other possibly infectious material should be placed into a suitable container, such as a plastic bag, or burned.

6. Wash hands thoroughly with adequate soap and hot water, whether they have become contaminated or not.

as tropical and domestic birds or their cages, since they may be a source of certain bacterial and fungal disease agents. Cat litter boxes and even tropical fish may pose additional hazards.

With respect to food, unpasteurized milk and other dairy products, including yogurt and various cheeses, should not be eaten. Although the possibility is generally low, such foods because of their unpasteurized nature may be contaminated with various potential bacterial disease agents. Organically grown vegetables fertilized with human or animal waste should not be eaten unless they are thoroughly cooked. Organically grown fruits may be eaten if they are washed well and can be peeled.

Other possible sources of opportunistic disease agents in the home include showers and hot tubs since they may support the growth of various fungi and bacteria. These home areas can be easily cleaned, disinfected, and maintained safely with the use of a household bleach solution usually made in the proportion of one part bleach to ten parts water.

The inside surfaces of refrigerators also should be cleaned periodically with soap and hot water to reduce the possibility of contact with fungi and bacteria. Any spoiled food should be disposed of promptly since such material can be a source of unwanted microorganisms.

Infection control guidelines for HIV-infected individuals and persons with AIDS have been established. These guidelines are based on commonsense hygienic practices designed to reduce exposure to most infectious disease agents transmissible in the home. Examples of such practices followed by HIV-infected individuals and persons with AIDS are given in table 15.6.

THE IMPORTANCE OF COMMON SENSE

Even though HIV-infected persons can pose a small risk of infection for health care workers and others coming into contact with them in the workplace, they can be safely and properly cared for by such personnel. The risk of contracting, as well as transmitting HIV infection can be significantly reduced by following appropriate procedures when working with needles and other sharp objects, and using barriers such as gowns, gloves, and face masks when handling blood and other potentially infectious body fluids. Family members, friends, and volunteers caring for persons with AIDS are not in any danger of acquiring HIV infection through casual contact. Common sense practices work to protect everyone.

TABLE 15.6	EXAMPLES OF COMMONSENSE HOME HYGIENIC PRACTICES FOR HIV-INFECTED PERSONS
PERSONAL HYGIENE	1. Bathe or shower regularly. 2. Wash hands after using the bathroom. 3. Cough or sneeze into disposable tissues or handkerchiefs. 4. Keep fingernails and toenails clean and cut appropriately to prevent fungus infections.
TRASH AND WASTE DISPOSAL	1. Sturdy bags should be used for all trash. 2. Lined trash containers should be used for the disposal of any and all potentially contaminated materials such as dressings, diapers, tissues, and sanitary napkins. 3. Flush liquid wastes down the toilet.
FOOD PREPARATION	1. Hands should be washed before and after food preparation. 2. HIV-infected persons may safely prepare foods for others provided hands are washed before beginning. 3. Spoons, forks, etc. used to sample food during its preparation should be thoroughly washed with soap and hot water. 4. All meats should be cooked well and thoroughly. 5. Raw milk and partially cooked eggs should be avoided in the daily diet.
SHARING OF FACILITIES AND UTENSILS	1. Kitchen and bathrooms may be shared. 2. Dishes, forks, knives, etc. should not be exchanged or shared while eating. 3. Toothbrushes, razors, enema materials, etc. potentially contaminated with body fluids, secretions, or excretions should not be shared. 4. Towels and washcloths should not be exchanged or shared without first being laundered.
CLEANING AND DISINFECTING	1. Sponges, clothes, brushes, etc. used to clean bathroom floors, sinks, etc. should not be used for the cleaning of kitchen areas. 2. Bathroom floors should be cleaned at least once per week. 3. A 1:10 solution of household bleach should be used to disinfect sinks, showers, toilets, etc.
CLOTHING, BED LINENS, AND TOWELS	1. Hot water and household bleach should be used for laundering clothing, bed linens, etc. 2. Items soiled with fecal matter, urine, blood, semen, etc. should be washed separately.

PART 4 | PUBLIC HEALTH CHALLENGES AND SOCIETY'S RESPONSIBILITIES

The current HIV epidemic presents a tremendous challenge to public health and society. Planning for the management of AIDS at a national as well as local levels has assumed a greater importance in view of the increases of newly diagnosed cases. The economic effect of the disease is substantial and is predicted to increase in many communities as the future number of cases grow. The economic aspect is only one of the complex factors that must be considered in molding society's response to this pandemic.

Surveys indicate that public awareness of AIDS is high. Most people know how HIV is transmitted. However, there are still many people who believe that the virus can be acquired by donating blood or through casual contact. Among teenagers, the misunderstanding about HIV transmission has been complicated by ignorance related to sexuality in general. The problem is reflected by the high rates of pregnancy and STDs that occur within this age group.

The first three parts of this book focused on aspects of the epidemiology and general features of disease, the characteristics of STDs, and history and findings associated with HIV and the AIDS pandemic. This final section will attempt to expand the focus somewhat by considering relevant economic, ethical, political, and educational issues, as well as future prospects for the treatment and prevention of all STDs.

A World Health Organization poster picturing the world as a fragile egg sitting on the edge of a wall and about to have a "great fall." (Courtesy of World Health Organization)

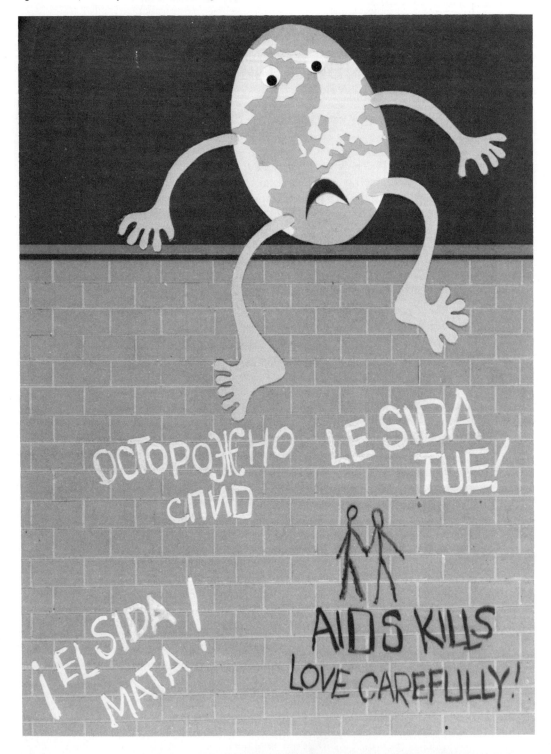

CHAPTER 16 ECONOMIC, ETHICAL, AND POLITICAL ISSUES

HIV infection cannot be spread by casual contact. There is no justified medical reason for discrimination. Fear and ignorance must be overcome, not accommodated.

—100th Shattuck Lecture
May, 1989

Most people in the world have heard about AIDS and have opinions about who develops the disease and what should be done to prevent more persons from being infected with HIV. These perceptions are important because they determine how people with HIV infection and AIDS will be treated in their communities and what kinds of measures will be developed and used to prevent the further spread of HIV.

Unfortunately, persons with AIDS or those who fear that they may be infected with HIV may hesitate to seek health care when they are concerned about discrimination. The situation gets worse when people most in need of prevention information, counseling, or health care avoid seeking them out of fear of being labeled as either someone with AIDS or someone who has engaged in high-risk behavior.

This chapter examines public attitudes towards AIDS and the economic, ethical, and political issues raised by this and related sexually transmitted diseases.

Economic Impact of AIDS on Health Care

In 1940, pneumonia was a life-threatening disease, most babies were born at home, and Americans could expect to live sixty-three years. Today, most pneumonia cases can be controlled by antibiotics, nearly all babies are born in hospitals, and the average American lives seventy-five years. Quite obviously, medicine has made astonishing progress in this century. But now it is being hard hit in all of its aspects—health care, research, and education—by economic limits.

Spending on health care in the United States has risen from 9 percent of the gross national product (GNP) in 1980 to 12 percent in 1990, which amounts to $600 billion and does not provide care to everyone. This figure could reach 15 percent by the year 2000, according to the Health Care Financing Administration. In contrast, Canada provides care to everyone at 8.6 percent of its GNP. Other Western countries spend even less, since, like Canada, they have national health insurance.

The Cost of Illness

Illness imposes a variety of financial costs and burdens upon individuals and society. These include both direct costs of prevention, diagnosis, and treatment, and the indirect costs associated with lost productivity and income caused by increased morbidity and mortality resulting from illness.

The total costs of health care for persons with AIDS is still small on a national scale relative to total national health expenditures and to the costs of all illnesses. This is true despite the fact that the per patient cost of AIDS is similar to the cost of other serious illnesses that are expensive to treat. However, the projected high lifetime medical cost per AIDS case raises important issues concerning the United States' system for financing health care. The need to address these issues is intensified by the high concentrations of HIV infections and AIDS cases in specific geographical locations such as New York City, and San Francisco, and by the high prevalence of HIV infection among individuals who are already most likely to fall through the cracks in the existing health care system—the young, ethnic minorities, the poor, the jobless, and the homeless. According to public health officials, persons with HIV infection and/or AIDS, and especially intravenous drug users, will place an enormous drain on the nation's resources during the next five or more years.

Compared to totals spent on medical care, or deaths from all illnesses, the national economic impact of AIDS in the early 1990s will be small. Its impact on San Francisco, New York City, and some other large cities, however, will be quite serious. Residents of those cities may be required to pay higher taxes and health insurance premiums to finance a portion of the medical costs of local persons with AIDS and HIV infections, and may have increasing difficulty buying health insurance for themselves.

Direct and Indirect Costs— What Are They?

The direct costs of HIV infection and AIDS include personal medical care expenditures, as well as nonpersonal costs for educational and preventative programs and campaigns, vaccine and drug development, and other forms of research. Other costs associated with HIV infection and AIDS are more subtle and not as obvious. For example, most hospitals and other types of health care facilities and offices have or are in the process of adopting universal precautions. (See chapter 15 for a discussion of this topic.) Depending on the circumstances, adopting universal precautions can require the use of disposable items such as gloves, masks, and gowns, following special blood-screening and laboratory procedures, and establishing educational and counseling programs for staff members. In health care facilities the associated costs are built into the bills of all recipients of health care services and are not found in the charges of only those individuals diagnosed as being HIV-infected or having AIDS.

What Are the Projected Lifetime Costs?

Total personal medical expenditures for AIDS will depend both on the cost per person with AIDS and the number of such individuals. The U.S. Public Health Service estimates that approximately 450,000 cases of AIDS will be diagnosed by the end of 1993, thus extending its earlier prediction of 270,000 cases of the disease by the end of 1991. Personal medical costs for all persons with AIDS during 1991 have been projected to reach levels between $4.5 billion and $8.5 billion.

According to a 1987 study by the Rand Corporation, the projected lifetime medical cost of a person with AIDS in his thirties is between $70,000 and $141,000. This is more money than the projected lifetime cost of treating someone in his thirties who has a heart attack ($67,000), digestive system cancer ($47,000), or leukemia ($29,000). Treating persons with AIDS is expected to cost tens of billions of dollars each year of the 1990s.

Certainly numbers such as those mentioned have caused some to accuse the government of misplaced priorities and attention, especially in light of findings that show breast cancer, high blood pressure, and diabetes killing more people than AIDS. However, there are certain points to consider here which are frequently not too well known or appreciated. First, while heart disease and various cancers usually strike people who have lived full lives, AIDS is by now the third largest killer of men in their prime. In 1987, 8,867 men aged 25 to 44 died of AIDS—just 364 fewer than the number in this age group who died of cancer. Heart disease is recognized as the second largest killer of men aged 25 to 44, claiming 11,769 of them in 1987. Two-thirds of the people who die of cancer are aged 65 or older, while over half of those who die of heart disease are aged 75 or older. Most of the people who die of AIDS have not yet reached their 40th birthdays. Thus, because of AIDS society loses many years of potential contributions persons with AIDS could make.

WHO BEARS THE DIRECT COSTS?

On the surface, the direct costs of AIDS appear to be borne by a wide range of payers: persons with AIDS and their families, employers of individuals with AIDS and their insurance companies, public and private hospitals, and the federal, state, and local governments. However, since the AIDS crisis began

in the early 1980s some of these payers have been engaged in debates with governmental agencies over who should foot the bill for medical costs. Shifting the financial burden of AIDS onto others becomes increasingly important as the number of cases increase. There is a possibility that the burden of the direct costs associated with AIDS may be largely distributed among persons with AIDS or individuals who are perceived as practicing high-risk behavior, other users of the health care system, and federal, state, and local taxpayers.

In 1989, the direct costs of AIDS amounted to $3.75 billion. Federal and state governmental programs paid 40 percent of the bill, while private insurance companies took care of another 40 percent. The remaining 20 percent fell into the self-pay (often meaning no pay) category. AIDS patients without private insurance coverage must pay for the cost of treatment themselves. After they have spent nearly all their assets down to less than $2,000, and are medically indigent, they become eligible for Medicaid coverage in most but not all states. Income and asset limits for Medicaid vary both across and within states. The federal government pays 50 to 70 percent of Medicaid costs, depending on per capita state income, with the state governments and in some instances local governments paying the remainder. A small fraction of the medical costs of treating persons with AIDS who are veterans, who have chronic disabilities or are elderly, or prisoners is borne by the U.S. Veterans Administration, the Medicare program (financially supported entirely by the federal government), and federal and state prison systems. Hospitals also absorb a major share of the costs. This occurs because Medicaid reimbursement rates are generally lower than hospital costs for treating persons with AIDS, and because individuals without private health insurance or Medicaid coverage may be unable or unwilling to pay their hospital bills.

Despite the substantial projected costs for the lifetime care for a person with AIDS, which amounts to $83,000 on the average, a fifth of those infected with HIV have no insurance at all. Increasingly, these people are flooding into over-burdened public hospitals and raising fears of bankruptcies.

Why No Insurance?

As the AIDS epidemic grows, it may become quite difficult for individuals to buy health insurance. Some businesses may even be refused group coverage for their employees. Several insurance companies currently refuse to sell insurance to persons with AIDS. This is not an unusual practice since firms are known not to sell insurance to new clients with a fatal disease. However, a significant number of insurance companies refuse to sell policies to individuals with positive blood tests for HIV. In the near future, insurance companies may insist on testing prospective customers for HIV infection (seropositive), just as they often require testing for high blood pressure today. Individuals who test positive for HIV could conceivably be offered coverage with premiums that equaled the expected value of the cost of treatment. In practice, however, such persons would be considered uninsurable. Testing would effectively prevent seropositive individuals from obtaining personal insurance, but insurance firms could continue to offer coverage to others in cities with large numbers of AIDS cases, or HIV-infected individuals.

If HIV testing is prohibited for insurance purposes, private insurance companies may begin to refuse to sell health insurance to *all* individuals in cities with many AIDS cases, or to write policies that limit the medical coverage and other benefits for HIV infection or AIDS. Insurance companies may choose this alternative approach instead of raising premiums to cover their increased costs, because low-risk individuals could conceivably begin to stop buying insurance if premiums were too high. However, individuals with a high probability of developing AIDS would continue to want full coverage, and the pecentage of persons with AIDS among those insured would rise. Under such circumstances insurance companies would raise their premiums further, and most low-risk individuals would probably discontinue their coverage. Ultimately only those individuals with the highest risk or probability of developing AIDS would want to buy insurance at the very high rates that insurance companies offering such policies would require.

Pointing the Way. AIDS has exposed and continues to expose a number of weak points of the U.S. health care system. These include shortages of facilities to treat chronic conditions and a lack of access to health insurance. The lack of insurance coverage among persons with AIDS and the requirement that they impoverish themselves before gaining eligibility for Medicaid, has led to proposals for more realistic federal coverage for persons with AIDS, and to calls for a broader system of government health insurance. Lack of private insurance coverage is not unique to people having a high probability of being infected with HIV or developing AIDS. Nearly one-fourth of the adult U.S. population under sixty-five is not covered by private health insurance, and federal health insurance is available only to the poor, the elderly, or the chronically ill or disabled.

Treatment Costs Versus Prevention and Non-AIDS Research

There is no question that the most effective means of controlling a contagious epidemic is through prevention. However, the AIDS movement in the United States has emphasized the need for the rapid development of treatment for persons with AIDS to be given top priority for federal funding. Consequently, spending on drug development has outpaced funding of prevention programs two to one. Some public health officials believe that the concentration on cures has been at the expense of educating individuals who remain at risk—primarily intravenous drug users (IVDUs), ethnic minorities, women, and adolescents. Thus, the epidemic in eastern inner cities and other areas is likely to grow. Focusing largely on treatment after infection may not be an adequate long-range strategy.

The emphasis on AIDS research is also beginning to draw fire from scientists whose non-AIDS research projects have been squeezed for funds. Traditionally, major public health issues and efforts have fueled broad basic research studies. Some scientists feel that funds for AIDS research are rather narrowly focused and could reduce the chances of spin-off discoveries for other diseases. Others, however,

SOCIAL ISSUES

AIDS phobia	Reactions of others
Fear of contracting disease by co-workers	Prejudice and/or stigma related to being diagnosed with HIV infection
Loss of job, and/or career	
Loss of public assistance	Prejudice related to life-style
Physical and social isolation	

ETHICAL AND LEGAL ISSUES

Confidentiality	Disclosure to third parties at risk
Antibody testing	Education
Informed consent	Health care
Relationship with sexual partner not recognized or protected by law	Quarantine

are emphasizing that AIDS research is providing a wealth of new knowledge about viruses, cancer, the brain, and the immune system.

SOCIAL, ETHICAL, AND LEGAL CONSIDERATIONS

In the 1990s HIV and AIDS-related disorders continue to pose significant social, ethical, and political issues. These include discrimination, confidentiality, the rights, responsibilities, and duties of both infected and non-infected persons, and the responsibilities of health care providers. Table 16.1 provides a more complete listing. Several of the issues mentioned will be explored here.

INFLUENCES ON HIV AND AIDS-RELATED ATTITUDES

Policies dominated by overreaction threaten to build walls around sick people and victimize them, and even the most robust democracy may not be strong enough to withstand such divisive forces. Since the early days of the AIDS pandemic it has been quite obvious that the clergy and political leaders, health care providers, and the mass media (newspapers, television, and radio) greatly influence the public's perceptions and attitudes toward HIV-infected individuals and persons with AIDS. For example, political leaders publically discussing AIDS have been few and far between. Twenty thousand people died of AIDS before a U.S. president delivered a speech which mentioned the disease. Far from the silence on the topic of AIDS-related attitudes by many, but not all, political leaders, some religious leaders have expressed hostility, rejection, and showered blame on persons with the disease. Such attitudes are not typical of all religons. The Catholic church and several other religious groups have taken a different approach. While they extend compassion and care to persons with AIDS, they continue to condemn some of the ways in which individuals become infected, and object to certain methods of prevention such as the use of condoms.

Anxiety about AIDS has not been limited to the general public. Health care workers have refused to provide care to persons with the disease. Why? The answer is partly related to the fears of such individuals. Some health care providers are clearly worried about their vulnerability, not only to HIV infection, but to an increased risk for hepatitis B infection as well. Certain others go out of their way to avoid treating infected persons because of personal attitudes and prejudices, especially against members of groups hardest hit by HIV infection. Such attitudes, which include discomfort with the homosexuality or intravenous drug use of patients, were also expressed in various surveys of United States medical and nursing students. The reluctance to treat persons with HIV infection or AIDS has been associated with limited knowledge and with misconceptions about HIV transmission, testing practices, and the ethical obligation of health care providers to treat AIDS patients.

The misconceptions about the transmission of HIV and AIDS-related factors present a major challenge to health care. Individuals involved with the delivery of health care, which include physicians, nurses, and others, must come to grips with the true facts and realities of the disease. This is especially important in light of the finding that people who either have AIDS, or fear that they may have been infected with HIV, may be reluctant to seek health care when they are concerned about discrimination. Moreover, those people most in need of prevention information and health care may avoid seeking them out of fear of being identified as either someone with AIDS, or someone who has engaged in high-risk behavior.

The mass media has had an especially important influence on the attitudes of the public and policy makers. Looking back over the course of the AIDS pandemic, it is clear that HIV infection spread far more rapidly than did the concern about AIDS. At least part of the blame for the slow response by the public should be placed on the shoulders of the mass media establishment. There were amazingly few newspaper articles about AIDS until 1983, when the question of household and casual contact as factors in transmission appeared.

When articles did appear, they clustered around spectacular events, such as the death of the actor Rock Hudson and the possible spread of HIV by household or heterosexual contact. For the most part, the mass media in the United States did not treat AIDS as very important, possibly because at the time it was not saleable to the general public until Rock

Hudson's death in 1985. Although coverage of AIDS has increased over the years, it is possible that there continues to be less reporting of it and related issues in many newspapers because of concerns over the sensitivities of the general public.

HUMAN RIGHTS AND WRONGFUL DISCRIMINATION

It can be seen that AIDS represents a human rights challenge in a number of important respects. First, in many instances it is a profound test of whether human rights are respected in practice and not just in theory. Persons with AIDS or HIV infection, those perceived to be infected, and members of groups in which high-risk behaviors are observed have, in practice and almost as a rule, suffered greatly from one or another form of discrimination, which can even be a result of the application of some laws. They have been, and are being, refused access to health care, employment, social services, and education; some have lost employment and housing. In addition, such individuals have been tested for HIV antibodies without consent, and in certain cases have been isolated, mistreated, forcibly quarantined, and even deported. In his press conference held in 1988, Retired Admiral James D. Watkins, chairman of the President's Commission on AIDS, stated that the threat of discrimination is "the most significant obstacle to progress" against the pandemic. "If the nation does not address this issue squarely," he said, "it will be very difficult to solve most other HIV-related problems."

Because they can be spread to others, a number of infectious diseases have been the subject of legal statutes and regulations, as well as court decisions imposing special limitations on an individual's freedom. The legality of measures to control the spread of such diseases is determined under principles of constitutional law that require the individual's rights to liberty and privacy to be balanced against the public's rights to health and safety. Balancing these interests in the context of AIDS is extremely difficult, because the rights on each side are so fundamental and so strongly affected by the nature of the disease. Concepts of human rights, including rights against wrongful discrimination, are

ISOLATION OF PERSONS WITH AIDS UPHELD (A VIEW FROM ANOTHER PART OF THE WORLD)

On December 24, 1989, the Bombay High Court upheld the government's exclusive right to isolate HIV-positive persons when it considers the situation to be appropriate. Three HIV carriers, who had been isolated for varying periods from February to October, challenged their segregation from society on the grounds that it was a violation of their human rights as provided under certain articles of India's Constitution. The Justices of the High Court dismissed the claims of the three petitioners, even though they conceded that isolation was "an invasion upon the liberty of a person." The judges also emphasized their position by stating that "in matters like this, individual right has to be balanced against public interest." They also felt that isolation would protect a person with AIDS from himself in the event he becomes "desperate and loses all hopes of survival."

All of the judges agreed with the World Health Organization guidelines that isolation was not "ideal" and, in fact, could be counter productive. But they pointed out that "ideal is not always practical in life." When a high risk to the public exists, "erring on the safer side may be permissible."

The judgement was praised by local authorities who had developed the health act which first made isolation mandatory and later optional. [On the other hand, one of the involved persons with HIV infection became more dejected and saw the court's decision as one more obstacle in his battle to get back into society and lead a normal life.

Since the decision was made, another of the HIV-infected individuals was dismissed from his job. This action depressed him greatly because he was the only breadwinner in his family.

Source: Portions of this report were printed in *The Times of India, New Delhi*, on Monday, 25 December 1989

---

major features of the current legal landscape or setting.

Legislation in relation to human rights and wrongful discrimination can be of two types: that which protects human rights and seeks to avoid or to prevent wrongful discrimination or its effects, and that which invades human rights and often extends wrongful discrimination and its effects. Examples of both types include: express actions that exclude persons with HIV infection or AIDS from access to health care, housing, schools, employment, or from purchasing insurance; and laws that require HIV antibody testing.

Emphasizing and incorporating human rights and antidiscrimination provisions into domestic law corresponds to similar developments in international legal documents, the most famous of which is the *Universal Declaration of Human Rights*. Articles 2 to 21 of this legal instrument reflect an individual's right to liberty and security; equality before and under the law; freedom of expression, conscience, religion, and mobility; and freedom from mistreatment and arbitrary detention.

A LOOK AT THE RIGHTS OF INFECTED PERSONS

From the public's point of view, AIDS continues to be a major menace and threat to well-being, especially since HIV infection still is spreading and often ends in death. Moreover, no vaccine or treatment has been found to prevent infection, reduce infectivity, or change the outcome of the disease. From the individual's standpoint, measures to control AIDS may invade privacy, infringe on personal liberty, and

AIDS-RELATED DISCRIMINATION

In June 1990 the American Civil Liberties Union (ACLU) reported the results of a detailed study concerned with AIDS discrimination in the United States. According to the findings of this comprehensive study, discrimination is on the rise against, not only those ill with the disease or infected with HIV, but also the relatives, close friends, and caregivers. Complaints of such AIDS-related bias nearly doubled in 1988, after an 88 percent increase from 1986 to 1987.

Most instances of discrimination were found to be related to employment, housing, public accommodations (hotels, restaurants, etc.), insurance, delivery of government benefits such as Social Security and Medicaid, and access to services such as dentistry and nursing home care. Figure 16.1 shows the respective percentages of the types of discrimination. Of all reported incidents of bias, 30 percent of the involved individuals were discriminated against because they were perceived to have been HIV-infected or because they cared for an HIV-infected person. Several examples of cases were cited, and included a Conneticut family being denied housing because an adopted son had AIDS, an Illinois man who was fired from his job after his employer learned that someone the employee knew was HIV-positive, and a Californian who was refused service after he told his dentist that his brother had recently died of AIDS.

According to the ACLU the inconsistencies and gaps in antidiscrimination laws further contribute to the problem. State and local laws vary widely in the United States, and the two federal statutes that prohibit discrimination against disabled people are limited in their coverage. For example, in the same town, a schoolteacher who has AIDS could not be fired because public schools are covered by federal law. However, his mother, who works in a bank, could lose her job, if she is perceived, incorrectly or not, as being HIV-infected. The ACLU report indicated that a company employee with AIDS may be protected from being fired, but a customer with AIDS could be refused service.

From this ACLU report it appears that the discrimination which has been directed against persons ill with AIDS or infected with HIV has been extended to others, despite the fact that numerous studies have shown that HIV cannot be acquired through casual contact.

place a constraint on sexual practices and procreation. It is quite apparent that in the United States and elsewhere, AIDS poses the most profound issues of constitutional law and public health since the Supreme Court approved compulsory immunization against infectious diseases in 1905. Of particular concern and controversy are issues such as testing for antibodies to HIV, confidentiality of test results as well as HIV infection or AIDS, access to housing, schools, and insurance, and the question of isolation and quarantine.

THE BASIS FOR HIV TESTING

Any proposal to test groups of people ought to be examined by asking at least two major questions. The first is, Why test? Before testing a single person or large numbers of people, the purpose of the test and what will be done differently on the basis of the results need to be considered carefully. The second question is, How good is the proposed test? Answering this question involves learning about the test's performance, which includes factors such as

FIGURE 16.1

The types and respective percentages of AIDS-related discrimination as reported by the ACLU.

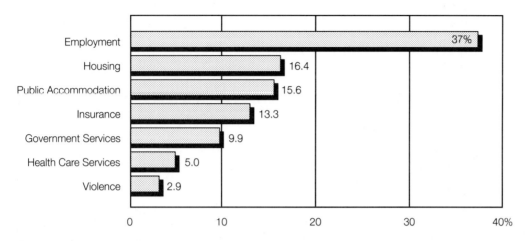

its specificity, its cost, and the ease with which it can be interpreted.

With respect to the first question, several purposes of HIV testing can be suggested. First, donated blood, tissue, organs, and semen can be tested, and infectious material discarded, thereby preventing transmission of the disease agent. This purpose is sound and has been achieved. The screening of blood for antibodies to HIV, combined with self-disqualification by potential donors having a high risk for possible infection, has almost eliminated the transmission of HIV through blood transfusions and the injection of blood products.

Second, the early detection of asymptomatic HIV infection provides an important health benefit to those who are unaware of their infection. Such individuals frequently are not fully educated about the signs and symptoms of the disease, or deny the possibility of contracting HIV-related disease and fail to seek medical attention promptly when symptoms of HIV illness appear. Many persons who may be infected with HIV do not fully recognize that HIV infection is a treatable condition. This is an important point for asymptomatic infected persons to know since early treatment with Zidovudine (AZT) has been shown to delay the progression of HIV infection and to decrease the severity of opportunistic infections. Moreover, starting early treatment specific to opportunistic infections can further benefit

and improve the quality of life of HIV-infected persons. HIV testing can clearly provide the basis for decisions for starting early treatment.

Third, once and/or if HIV antibodies are detected, infected persons can prevent new infections by discontinuing high-risk behaviors that spread the virus. The hope and belief that knowing one's antibody status will encourage behavior change have inspired many policy recommendations for widespread, voluntary testing and associated counseling.

Finally, test results can indicate the prevalence and incidence of infection. Such estimates and projections are important elements in the planning of prevention efforts and health care.

SHOULD THERE BE MANDATORY TESTING?

Some form of mandatory testing for HIV antibodies, like that announced for the U.S. armed forces, may be considered for broader populations. The legality of such a measure is questionable and would depend on medical facts. For example, compulsory testing has long been established for syphilis. Issuing a marriage license only after a blood test for syphilis has been considered to be a reasonable means of limiting the risk of infection to spouses or offspring, although no information is available as to the current contribution of such tests to the control of the STD.

TRAVEL RESTRICTIONS AND AIDS

Travel restrictions to control the spread of infectious diseases have been considered impractical, ineffective, and discriminatory. Furthermore, they have been discouraged and opposed by international organizations. For example, the World Health Organization has urged its member states ". . . to protect human rights and dignity of HIV-infected people and people with AIDS, and of members of population groups, and to avoid discrimination action against and stigmatization of them in provision of services, employment and travel. . . ."

Since it is quite apparent that HIV does not respect national borders or geographic boundaries and that travel has contributed to its initial spread, many countries have imposed or are in the process of developing travel restrictions as a response to the spread of HIV. While in most countries people are free to travel within their own countries and internationally, or do so with minimal restrictions, over fifty countries have now restricted the entry of travellers who are HIV-infected or who have AIDS, for prolonged stays and sometimes for brief visits, including travel to scientific and other types of conferences.*

Among HIV-infected travellers, the most frequently excluded are those applying to immigrate to a country or to reside permanently in it, followed by those planning an extended stay, such as students and migrant laborers. Least frequently excluded are travellers with HIV infection or AIDS, such as tourists, who will not reside in the country. In many countries, existing immigration or public health laws provide a basis for excluding HIV-infected travellers, but in certain countries HIV infection or AIDS have been specified as a criterion for exclusion. Specific grounds used for the exclusion of HIV-infected travellers include: 1) the presence of HIV antibodies; 2) clinical disease (the signs and symptoms of AIDS; 3) possession of the antiviral drug AZT during border searches; and 4) the prevalence of HIV infection in the travellers' country of origin, or in a group or population to which the traveller belongs or is associated.

It is interesting to note that while certain countries are restricting HIV-infected travellers, very few require returning nationals to undergo HIV antibody testing, and none appear to prohibit their own nationals from travelling to areas where HIV is prevalent. However, some countries, such as Australia and Japan, have reacted to this issue in a limited manner by distributing educational information to all their nationals travelling to other countries.

While people infected with HIV remain persistently infectious, they are not at risk for transmitting HIV to others except by practicing high-risk activities such as sexual intercourse and intravenous drug use with uninfected persons. Consequently, travel itself does not create a risk of HIV infection for travellers or for travel industry personnel.

Travel is considered to be the world's largest industry. Moreover, tourism is a major source of revenue for several developing countries. To what extent HIV-related travel restrictions will limit tourism and the investment which follows it, is unknown. In addition, serious harm to national economics, and to cultural and educational exchanges may result. The described restrictions may briefly retard HIV transmission. However, they may also be extremely costly and counterproductive to the control of the infection. A more effective approach to control the worldwide spread of HIV can be found in the suggestion made by an expert committee of the World Health Assembly in 1949: ". . . Each country should develop its internal resistance to disease, rather than rely on measures taken at its frontier. . . ."

*In 1991, the Eighth International AIDS conference scheduled for Boston, Massachusetts in 1992 was canceled as a protest to current U.S. immigration policy. This policy prohibits entry of HIV-positive persons as well as denying them permanent resident status.

An acceptable program of mandatory testing for HIV infection is somewhat more difficult to devise, largely because the usefulness of the test results for purposes other than protecting the blood supply is unknown, and the risk of unreasonable invasions of individual rights is great. Although the HIV tests are good, they should be used only when there are sound, well-defined reasons for doing so, and a reasonable prospect that testing will do more good than harm.

HIV testing should be voluntary and anonymous. Moreover, it should not be used to screen prospective employees, insurance applicants, marriage license applicants, or students. In the event testing is done, every effort should be made to maintain the confidentiality of the results. Revealing the identity of persons tested could result in serious consequences such as fewer people undergoing testing, denying individuals early diagnosis and treatment, and creating a larger group of persons at risk for infection.

In September of 1991, the Centers for Disease Control proposed that all patients entering hospitals be encouraged to undergo testing for HIV infection. This proposal to expand HIV testing represents the first effort to screen hospital patients not necessarily considered to be at risk for HIV infection. Moreover, this policy would be voluntary and not mandatory.

THE ISSUE OF CONFIDENTIALITY

Whether HIV testing is mandatory or voluntary, confidentiality is vital. In the U.S., several states have introduced specific legislation on this subject, and have established principles designed to protect confidentiality and to prevent discrimination against persons who are HIV positive or who have AIDS or AIDS-related complex. In addition, once the responsibility for treating a person with HIV infection or AIDS is accepted by a physician or a hospital it is generally agreed that all facts concerning diagnosis and treatment are confidential. There are, however, some exceptions. For example, all states require that specified "listed" or "notifiable" diseases be reported to public health departments. Since AIDS is considered as a uniformly "notifiable" disease it falls into this situation. A few states expressly require the

reporting of positive HIV-antibody tests. Still others require the reporting of any case, condition, or carrier state relating to notifiable diseases, including AIDS. Currently such reporting does not require the naming of infected persons. However, if the process should change and require the listing of infected parties by name, it is quite possible that such individuals may not seek medical attention because of the fear of disclosure, or fear that physicians may refuse to provide treatment.

Another example of a situation in which some disclosure is proper involves the growing recognition that the physician-patient relation creates a legal obligation on the physician toward an identifiable third party who may be endangered by the patient. In California, for example, "[it] shall be the duty of the physician in attendance on a case considered to be infectious or communicable disease, to give detailed instructions to members of the household in regard to precautionary measures to be taken for preventing the spread of the disease" (California Administrative Code, Title 17, Section 2514). Under such direction the disclosure of a person's illness in tracing the sexual partners of syphilis and gonorrhea cases would be permissible. In cases of AIDS, disclosures of a similar type to spouses or lovers, would not be unlawful on the part of physicians or public health officials. The disclosure of only necessary information is based on a reasonable perception of danger.

A LOOK AT NONDISCRIMINATION LAWS

Because the rights to confidentiality of persons who have been exposed to or who are actually HIV-infected are so compromised in law that their status may become known, they have to invoke related *rights to nondiscrimination* as disabled or handicapped persons. Here are some examples of how rights of nondiscrimination can be applied.

Health Care. Rights to nondiscrimination in health care are particularly important if hospitals and health care facilities test patients for HIV antibodies, and health professionals deny services to seropositive persons. Attending physicians, hospitals, and health facilities in general have duties and responsibilities not to abandon their existing patients; however, when admission to a hospital or health facility is denied and health professionals refuse to provide treatment, nondiscrimination rights become central to the affected person's welfare.

Employment. Keeping a job or being hired may depend on rights of nondiscrimination. If AIDS, or AIDS-related complex, or seropositivity does not interfere with job performance or place other employees or the employer's customers at risk, discrimination on grounds of the condition of health is not justified. Moreover, the fears of other employees working closely with an infected person, that cause a disruption in the workplace also are not sufficient to justify the infected person's dismissal. However, there may be times when courts are sympathetic to an employer's extraordinary hardship because of customer or even co-worker complaints, and rule that an infected employee's condition constitutes "just cause" for dismissal of that employee.

Housing. Infected persons may have to consider their legal rights in order to keep or obtain housing. Public housing is frequently subject to antidiscrimination laws which may also apply to private housing. Their application beyond racial, sexual, and marital status considerations is questionable unless the laws specifically and clearly prohibit handicap or disability discrimination.

Tenants who are HIV-infected or who practice high-risk behaviors actually have no better rights than other tenants to lease renewals, or against eviction for violation of applicable clauses in tenancy agreements. Clauses in tenancy agreements on eviction for misconduct may be used, for example, against criminal drug abusers.

Consumer protection laws may also work to the disadvantage of persons with HIV infection or AIDS. The sale of properties such as homes or apartments formerly occupied by such persons was historically governed by the well-known principle "let the buyer beware." However, some states have developed legislation that requires disclosure to prospective buyers of invisibly unsafe conditions in property and of all related facts that may reduce the property's value. While an HIV-infected occupant as such leaves no risk in a home or similar accommodation that jeopardizes its safety, knowledge of the occupancy by such a person may lower the resale value of the property.

Education. HIV-infected school-aged children and their parents who invoke rights on nondiscrimination under compulsory school attendance laws may be blocked through arguments using public health laws on contagious and infectious diseases. Even though compulsory school attendance laws seem in principle to confer rights of access to public education on all children, picketing and boycotts of schools by uninfected parents and children have been used in attempts to exclude HIV-infected children. Currently, children's rights of school attendance, in the absence of an imminent danger of spreading disease, are based on laws prohibiting discrimination on grounds of handicap and establishing that having HIV antibodies is such a handicap.

Insurance. The ability to obtain insurance protection has been a source of bitter controversy. On the one hand, applicants with HIV antibodies have complained of discrimination when denied insurance coverage, and on the other hand, private insurance companies have complained of exploitation and abuse by persons with AIDS. As discussed earlier in this chapter, health insurance is particularly costly to provide to the population of persons infected with HIV or with AIDS. This is not only because of the high cost of treatment, but also because sufferers tend to be young and have thus not paid premiums long enough to permit insurance companies to accumulate funds with which to cover their expenses. Life insurance is similarly costly, and companies cite cases of persons with full-blown AIDS taking out large policies at high premiums for the short time before they die, at which time their beneficiaries, who may have contributed to payments of premiums, recover high sums from the policies of the insured. The problems of some insurance companies are made worse by their common practice of offering insurance to groups and not requiring individual health examination.

TESTING — HOW ONE INSURER HANDLES THE ISSUE

The livelihood of the insurance industry is dependent on insuring people against the cost of illness, disability, and premature death. The nation's health and life insurers are enormously concerned about the spread of HIV and AIDS and the associated economic costs.

People purchase insurance to provide financial protection for themselves, their families, or others against an event they cannot accurately foresee. Therefore, to price insurance fairly and equitably, insurance companies need to know more about the applicant than just the present state of that person's health. This is an integral part of the insurance business and has been a routine operating philosophy for more than a hundred years.

Comparing the impact on mortality of HIV as against other illnesses illustrates why HIV infection is a significant insurance risk factor. People who have experienced a heart attack present a mortality rate five times higher than the standard rate; diabetes, four times higher; and smokers, twice the standard rate. HIV-infected persons experience a mortality rate twenty-six times higher than standard.

The insurance industry seeks to treat HIV infection and AIDS with the same underwriting principles applied to other insurance risks, and feels strongly that insurers must be allowed to ask applicants questions about AIDS and that they must be allowed to test for HIV infection, just as they test for and inquire about other medical conditions that affect mortality such as heart disease, diabetes, and cancer.

Here is how one company, Metropolitan Life Insurance Company, deals with the problem of HIV testing. This company requires the HIV antibody test when an applicant seeks a substantial amount of coverage and when the applicant has symptoms possibly suggestive of AIDS. No testing is performed without the applicant's consent. If the person declines the test, the application is marked "no action" and filed. An application turned down because of the presence of HIV antibodies is sent to the company's medical director. The information about the applicant is distributed strictly on a need-to-know basis.

To determine if applicants want to know about their positive HIV test, they are first informed that there was a significant blood test result. Then, if they return a signed authorization, the company offers to send the information to them or to their doctors.

How should insurers handle applications from individuals who may be HIV-infected or have AIDS? Some insurers are redesigning their insurance plans to include features such as longer probation periods, limits on benefits that involve many conditions in addition to AIDS, and strict enforcement of clauses that limit coverage for preexisting conditions.

The rights of HIV-infected persons to obtain insurance depend significantly on government regulation of the insurance industry. While such regulation may not permit AIDS-related discrimination such as exclusion from coverage, the use of prohibitive premiums, or the questioning of applicants about their health status, it may permit limits on coverage when health information is not given or applicants do not agree to testing. Conditions may also be established for testing, such as in cases where it is medically indicated and not simply based on lifestyle.

Related Areas of Concern. A large number of additional situations and activities exist that may be subject to laws governing discrimination against persons with HIV infection or AIDS. For example, embalmers, funeral homes, and cemeteries may be reluctant to manage the corpses of persons with AIDS, and thereby may violate the rights of the families of such persons to the proper and prompt disposal of the remains of relatives.

THE LAW AND THE RESPONSIBILITIES OF INFECTED PERSONS

Can an HIV-infected person be charged with murder? Surprisingly, HIV-infected persons are bound by criminal laws that govern offenses ranging from the most monstrous classical crimes to relatively minor modern violations. Some states, such as Florida and Idaho, have introduced a new crime of willfully or knowingly exposing another to HIV. Most other states rely on existing offenses of (attempted) homicide, and assault with a deadly weapon. The latter type of offense was used successfully when an infected prisoner in a Minnesota institution bit two prison guards.

Those individuals who know of their infection but still have sexual relations without taking appropriate preventive measures such as using condoms, and infected drug users who share contaminated needles or syringes may be charged with attempted murder or assault with the intent to kill. If the intent to kill cannot be shown in such cases, the charge generally will be dismissed or at least reduced. Manslaughter, or the unplanned killing of a human being, may be charged against those proved to have caused death when they knew or should have known of their liability to transmit an infectious agent. Risking the transmission of HIV may lead infected persons to also be charged with related offenses. These include prostitution-based crimes, drug offenses, and situations where the law penalizes infected persons' failures to report, to seek testing or treatment, or to remain celibate.

CIVIL LAW—A MEANS TO GET SOME COMPENSATION

Noncriminal or civil law seeks to prevent harmful actions, not by imposing punishment, but by such means as ordering wrongdoers to pay compensation for the injuries they have caused. *Tort law* is frequently used to serve this purpose. Tort law is the private law solution available to the injured person to recover monetary compensation from the person or entity who caused the injury. While most countries have some type of private law system, torts are a uniquely American institution.

An individual seeking compensation is legally required to show that infection was caused by violating the duty or responsibility of the person being sued to inform or otherwise protect sexual partners. Such was the basis of a lawsuit filed by Mark Christian against the estate of the late actor Rock Hudson. The complaint was based in part on the supposed failure of Hudson and others, such as his physicians, to inform Christian that Hudson had AIDS. The lawsuit also claimed that Hudson violated a basic duty or responsibility, associated with their love relationship, to inform Christian about his infection, had exposed him to the risk of contracting AIDS, and that further sexual contact had increased the risk of infection. Aside from the legal aspects of such cases, it is quite clear that HIV carriers have certain moral obligations which include informing their sexual partners sufficiently so that they in turn can take measures to prevent the spread of the infection to others.

Even when causation can be shown, a legal defense exists that implies that the injured party voluntarily accepted the risk of infection. This defense strategy is based on the legal principle that requires persons voluntarily participating in sexual activities and placing themselves at risk for infection to use some form of protection. Many claims for injuries resulting from sexually transmitted diseases have failed on the grounds of this assumption of risk. Some courts make compromised decisions by recognizing a claim for the spread of infection, but reducing the amount of the compensation by finding that the injured person also contributed to the injury.

The legal aspects of sexually transmitted diseases are confusing and difficult to determine or to predict, in part because they affect people on all sides of the syndromes, and because laws are still being made.

INFORMED CONSENT

An individual's right to know if a health care provider has an infectious disease has become another major issue with respect to HIV infection. Since the possibility exists that an HIV-positive surgeon, dentist, or other professional who performs procedures involving blood could under certain conditions expose patients to infection, questions concerning ethical, moral, and legal responsibilities have been raised. The major questions being asked include: should patients be informed of a physician's or dentist's HIV status? Should an HIV-positive health care professional treat patients? Opinions concerning these issues are divided.

PRESSING ISSUES WITH FAR-REACHING IMPLICATIONS

HIV infections and AIDS raise fundamental, very difficult questions concerning the relationship between scientific research and society at large, the responsibilities of physicians to their patients, and the basic rights of both infected and uninfected individuals. The emergence of AIDS has exposed many deficiencies throughout social, legal, and health care systems. Both the tragedy and the ultimate hope of the AIDS crisis is that it will force citizens, patients, health care providers, scientists, clergy, journalists, and politicians to squarely face many pressing issues with far-reaching implications, not just for AIDS, but for other areas of health and disease as well.

TO INFORM OR NOT TO INFORM? THAT IS THE QUESTION

In March 1991 the federal government and the American Academy of Orthopaedic Surgeons began the nation's first large-scale voluntary testing program to determine the percentage of surgeons who are infected with HIV. The testing will be used both for research to help determine the incidence of AIDS in one (high-risk) medical specialty, and as a service to individuals to let those who are infected know of their condition.

The study is the latest development in the highly heated debate over the risks that HIV-infected physicians and other health care personnel pose to their patients, and the related issue of the rights of physicians, particularly surgeons, to require their patients to be tested for the virus. Many physicians, especially those who work in inner-city hospitals or treat emergency accident victims, are concerned about the risk of contracting HIV from their patients.

Most medical groups oppose mandatory testing of physicians for HIV infection. But medical and dental experts disagree about whether doctors who know that they are infected have an obligation to either notify their patients, or to stop performing surgery or other invasive procedures. The concern is that infected surgeons who cut themselves during an operation might bleed into their patients, thereby transmitting the virus.

The Centers for Disease Control (CDC), responding to a Florida case in which a dentist with AIDS apparently infected at least five of his patients, is in the process of formulating national guidelines for HIV-infected health care workers, particularly those who perform invasive or surgical procedures. With the publication of this report, the American Medical and Dental Associations issued recommendations urging physicians and dentists to volunteer to be tested if at risk of HIV infection; and if infected, not to use invasive procedures, to inform their patients of their status, and to proceed only with informed consent. In addition, physicians who are HIV-positive and who must restrict their normal professional activities should have a right to continue their careers in a capacity that poses no identifiable risk to their patients.

The risk of HIV transmission to a patient during a surgical or dental procedure is believed to be small. Precise figures, however, are not available.

The CDC recently estimated that from 1981 to 1990, between 13 and 128 Americans had been infected by either their dentists or surgeons who had been infected by their patients.

Currently, a surgeon is not required to respond to inquiries by patients regarding his or her HIV status unless invasive procedures are to be performed. However, it is generally believed by the health care community that, within the confines of the law, orthopedic surgeons should have access to the HIV status of their patients.

CHAPTER 17

PROSPECTS AND OBSTACLES TO STD PREVENTION AND EDUCATION

We must target preventive programs to those in our society whose behavior exposes them to an increased risk of infection.

—100th Shattuck Lecture
May, 1989

As the news of the California earthquake of 17 October 1989 broke, and as the horrible predictions of lives likely lost on the Nimitz Freeway in Oakland were presented by the news media, hope that anyone who happened to be driving on the lower deck of that highway structure would survive began to fade. Miraculously, four days later, rescue workers found and brought out a single individual who just happened to be wearing his seatbelt when his car was trapped in the falling highway structure. Many of the other drivers and passengers of automobiles also trapped under this freeway who had been rescued in the first few hours following the earthquake were reported to have been saved by their seatbelts which prevented them from being thrown through auto windshields upon impact.

This tragic event, captured repeatedly over a several-day period by both national and international news services, dramatized and made real what most people know—wearing a safety belt greatly reduces the risk of injury or death in an auto accident. It underscored the substantial differences in relative risk of those who do and those who do not practice such simple preventive behaviors on a daily basis.

Quite obviously, individuals have become increasingly aware of preventive behaviors that apply to a number of different situations, and aware that how they live their lives can significantly affect their well-being. The frequency (and often inconsistency) of media-generated and distributed reports of threats to health from various behavioral risk factors and diseases such as those associated with HIV

SEXUAL BEHAVIOR OF COLLEGE WOMEN IN 1975, 1986, AND 1989

The sexual practices in college women before and after the start of the current epidemics of *Chlamydia*, genital herpes, and HIV infections were surveyed in 1975, 1986, and 1989, and reported in 1990 in *The New England Journal of Medicine*. The study was conducted at a large private university in the northeast and was designed to relate sexual practices to the prevalence of selected STDs. The same anonymous questionnaire, which was used for all participants, contained questions dealing with personal sexual development, sexual experiences, and any gynecologic symptoms. The survey involved a total of 779 women (486 in 1975, 161 in 1986, and 132 in 1989). There were no significant differences in age, age at the time menstruation started, or reasons for visiting a gynecologist. The percentage of women in the study group who were sexually experienced were the same in all the three years surveyed. The percentage ranged from 87 to 88.

The survey revealed a number of interesting finds. For example, the methods of birth control used by the participants showed a definite decrease in the use of oral contraceptives. In addition, no significant differences were found among the respective groups as to the number of sex partners or the frequency of oral or anal intercourse. One might have expected that in the years since the first survey (1975), concern about STDs would have resulted in substantial changes in sexual behavior that would have been reflected in the number of lifetime or recent sexual partners. Moreover, it appears that public health education campaigns over a fourteen year period have not had a substantial influence on the habits and behavior of the participants.

The survey did show an increase in the use of condoms as a response to the new and serious STD epidemics. The usage of condoms, however, did not reach 50 percent.

and other STDs have increased the public's concern for better understanding of personal health risks and ways with which to cope with them.

Unfortunately, there is growing evidence that education information and prevention programs aimed at stopping the spread of HIV and various other STDs are not effectively influencing the behavior of certain individuals at highest risk. These specifically include many women, ethnic minorities, teenagers, and drug users who continue to engage in drug use and unprotected sex and are being infected at rising rates. Reasons for the failure of some of these programs include:

- not involving those directly affected in the development of programs;
- not giving sufficient thought to the social and cultural backgrounds of the communities concerned;
- not dealing with or talking about sexual behavior in sufficient and/or explicit detail in order to avoid misconceptions.

Society's wishful thinking that it is enough to tell people how a disease is spread without providing accessible tools with which to avoid it is a major obstacle to STD prevention. This is evidenced by certain public policies that restrict access to addiction treatment programs, or prevent condom or bleach distribution, thus leaving many drug users with information about the risk of HIV infection, but without realistic and immediate ways of avoiding it.

TARGET AUDIENCES FOR EDUCATION AND PREVENTION PROGRAMS

To be effective, STD education must lead to reductions in behaviors that eliminate or substantially reduce the risk of transmission of HIV and other STD agents. Communicating accurate information to everyone at risk of infection is clearly an essential part of any education campaign. However, by itself it is inadequate (fig. 17.1). The affected individual must also have the motivation and the means to effect the desired behavioral changes associated with drug abuse and/or high-risk sexual practices. Maintaining such changes also requires a social environment that reinforces and supports the new pattern of behavior. This type of situation has already occurred among mainstream gay and bisexual men living in large U.S. coastal cities with respect to reductions of high-risk sexual practices. Indications of such changes include sharp decreases in rectal and oral gonorrhea cases, and a substantial increase in the use of condoms. Unfortunately, as mentioned earlier, less risk reduction has been seen in other individuals whose sexual practices may place them at risk for HIV infection and other STDs. Such persons are found among a number of audiences that have been targeted for educational programs. These include:

- all adolescents and young adults;
- infected individuals and their sexual partners;
- individuals living in areas with a high prevalence of STDs;
- individuals practicing high-risk behaviors such as:
- intravenous drug users;

FIGURE 17.1

An example of a comic book approach. In this comic book factual information is presented through the story of a businessman's sexual adventures. (Courtesy of World Health Organization)

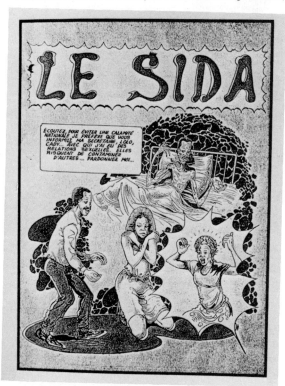

- gay men;
- bisexual men;
- individuals with multiple sexual partners;
- male and female prostitutes; and
- sexual partners of individuals practicing high-risk behavior (fig. 17.2).

Prevention messages and information may also fail to reach some people engaging in high-risk behavior because they do not identify themselves with

FIGURE 17.2

Here is a rather subtle poster that graphically transforms a heart into a skull to stress the point that HIV may be transmitted through sexual relations with people you love. (Courtesy of World Health Organization)

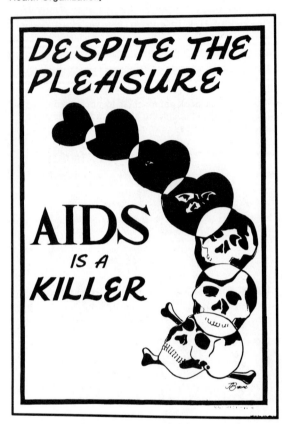

DESPITE THE PLEASURE

AIDS IS A KILLER

the social profile of a given audience. For example, HIV infection or AIDS prevention messages developed for gay men may be ignored by men or women who occasionally participate in homosexual acts, but identify themselves as being heterosexual. Situations of this kind have and continue to pose unique educational challenges. How can the unique educational needs of different population segments with respect to HIV infection and STDs be met?

A LOOK AT SOME OF THE OBSTACLES AND ISSUES

While the environment for the development and establishment of educational programs and strategies for the prevention and control of STDs is much more favorable today than in previous years, there still are obstacles. Examples of such obstacles and related issues will now be explored.

TEACHING SAFER SEX

Information and education programs emphasize avoiding or changing specific risk-related activities. However, many health professionals, teachers, and AIDS service groups experience a fair amount of frustration because of the prejudice and prudery in their respective audiences and other groups. Quite often, to get the message across effectively, the use of sexually explicit, easily understood language specifically tailored to various audiences is needed. For example, teaching about condoms or types of sexual practices that do not result in body fluid exchange is difficult, if not impossible, without mentioning terms such as penis, vagina, rectum, or the intention of having sexual intercourse. The use of appropriate street language rather than, or with, medical terms can be effective for two reasons. First, educated and uneducated people all understand street terms. Second, many people in the target audiences mentioned earlier are more likely to accept and even adopt advice that appears to originate in their own cultural community than that coming from governmental or health authorities. Street language serves this purpose.

The use of drawings and pictures that show safer sex in an erotic light has aroused the most intense controversy. Legislators, various public officials, and others have expressed shock at the language and illustrations used in some educational materials. Based on exposures to a wealth of highly erotic images of unsafe sex in movies, books, discussions with friends, and personal sexual history, a number of people believe that safer sex is unfulfilling, boring, and undersatisfying. Exposures to such unsafe sex situations can undermine the attempts of individuals who are trying to change their sexual behavior. Sex is not primarily a rational activity. Sexual activity may be spontaneous and unplanned and take place when judgment is clouded by alcohol and/or drugs. Thus, while factual information may impart knowledge about what is safe, it does not necessarily change attitudes about what is satisfying and erotic. According to various studies, explicit materials can show some people how to adopt safer sexual practices through a process of adjustment rather than a lifetime of self-sacrifice. The dramatic changes in sexual behavior within the gay community provide support for such findings and argue the point that explicit, culturally tailored materials can benefit public health.

THE QUESTION OF CULTURAL SENSITIVITY

Too often in the past, health education programs for the public have been developed and promoted without giving sufficient thought to their relevance to the social and cultural backgrounds of the communities involved. Fortunately, this situation is changing, especially in the areas of AIDS and STD education (fig. 17.3). Because about 42 percent of reported cases of AIDS have occurred among nonwhites in the United States, racial and ethnic minority groups are becoming increasingly involved in the development of culturally sensitive AIDS education programs and materials for their communities. Such programs and materials go beyond simply presenting the facts of transmission, and address sociocultural and subcultural attitudes and beliefs. Quite clearly, initiating behavior changes and encouraging the motivation to maintain such changes, especially with respect to safer sex practices, do not take place overnight.

MASS MEDIA AND AIDS COVERAGE

The news media serves as the main sources of new information for the public, and thus are considered to be extremely important to the first steps in bringing about changes in behavior: **exposure** and **awareness.** A historical analysis of the media coverage given to AIDS shows that, contrary to what might be expected, the rapid spread of the disease and its high mortality rate did not at first lead to extensive media exposure. In the early years of the pandemic (1981–1982), minimal media attention focused on the disease. After 1983, coverage increased periodically in bursts. Not until 1985, when the movie star Rock Hudson died of AIDS, did media interest increase significantly. Up to this time U.S.

FIGURE 17.3

An example of an informative brochure prepared specifically for targeted audiences. (Courtesy of Gay Men's Health Crisis)

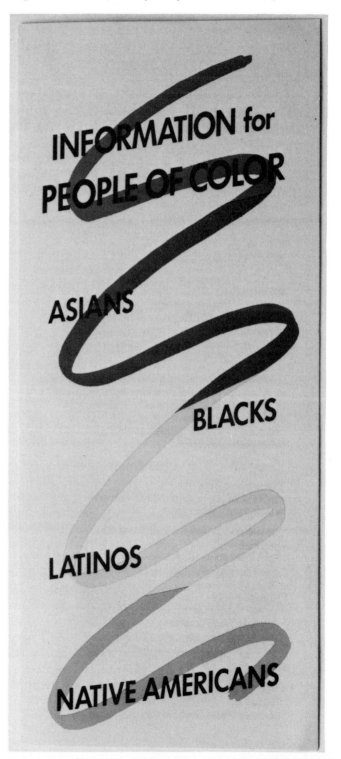

policymakers and the public could have concluded that AIDS was not very important and certainly not a national issue.

Interestingly, the early coverage of AIDS was not comparable to the media treatment given to other epidemic-like health problems such as Legionnaires' disease and Lyme disease. One explanation for the differences in coverage could be a bias on the part of the press in dealing with what was *then* considered a gay plague. Quite often, the most influential factor affecting the press's perception of the news value of a disease or health problem is the number of individuals at risk or the mortality rate. Once it became obvious that HIV infection and AIDS were not limited to any one segment of the population, media coverage exploded onto the television networks and the front pages of newspapers around the country.

Unfortunately, the news media face several barriers to effective reporting. Some of these are externally imposed, while others are self-imposed. For example, the sexual nature of HIV transmission has posed an editorial dilemma for the press. Early coverage of AIDS included only vague terms and phrases such as "exchange of body fluids," "personal contact," and "sexual intimacy." Editors asked themselves, "Would our subscribers like to read about this topic at the breakfast table?" It was only after the deaths of Rock Hudson and other newsworthy persons, and the subsequent increase in coverage and awareness of the disease, that the media began making use of the kind of sexually explicit information that all segments of the population needed to know to avoid spreading HIV infection. Even the well-known newspaper columnist Ann Landers referred directly to "the receiving partner in anal sex." A "Dear Abby" column contained the following information in response to the question: "How is AIDS transmitted? The most important route is by anal sex, oral sex, and 'old-fashioned' sexual intercourse with a person who has been infected by the AIDS virus."

The mass media, especially television, have always been seductive tools for various groups to quickly and inexpensively spread important information to millions of people. AIDS information campaigns have been no exception to this type of approach. In such campaigns public service announcements are distributed to television and radio networks for airing. Unfortunately, television public service announcements have some serious limitations. Because air time is donated rather than purchased, such educational messages are aired at times when few members of a targeted audience are watching. Moreover, public service announcements must be very short, and have to compete with slickly produced commercial advertisements, both for air time and audience attention.

The limitations of public service announcements are increased when the subject is AIDS. For example, local television stations are uneasy about television spots that use explicit terms or mention condoms.

Although it may have taken several years, the general public's awareness of HIV infection and AIDS has been increased significantly by media coverage. Unfortunately, barriers still exist. Thus measures are needed not only to assure continued AIDS coverage, but that coverage is both accurate and complete. Periodic, in-depth updates and reviews of not only AIDS, but of other STDs would be of instrumental value in stimulating conversations between family members and among friends. Such measures will help the public to make wiser personal choices about health risks, and may lead to changes in attitudes, intentions, and ultimately, behavior.

MISSED MESSAGES WITHIN ETHNIC COMMUNITIES

Educational programs and mass media campaigns in the form of public service announcements for television and radio networks have been targeted in inner-city populations toward intravenous drug users and their sexual partners, many of whom are heterosexual, bisexual and/or come from racial and ethnic minority groups. While such approaches have increased the knowledge and awareness about HIV infection and AIDS (figure 17.4), the results of educational programs and media campaigns to bring about long-lasting changes in high-risk behaviors have been rather disappointing. The limited success of such campaigns have in part been associated with

AIDS IN MOVIES AND TV

The trade publication *Daily Variety* regularly runs several obituaries listing AIDS as the cause of death, thus emphasizing how hard this disease has hit the show business community. Despite this dramatic impact, few movie studios have released a movie about AIDS, or for that matter even given approval for an AIDS-related project. This lack of movement is in sharp contrast to the efforts of the television industry, which has been much quicker to respond to dealing with the topic. Television has plunged in where feature filmmakers have feared to tread. Almost every sitcom and soap opera has had a character stricken with AIDS. The subject has even taken its place alongside abortion, child abuse, and wife battering as material for a "movie of the week."

Why is there such a difference between the two media industries? Hollywood has seldom taken the lead in social issues, according to several observers of the industry, because of the amount of money needed for such undertakings. With low operating budgets and even lower box office expectations in connection with investment returns, AIDS films are not only difficult to make but to sell as well. There are certain topics people would watch on TV but would not be willing to go and pay $7.00 or more for. According to Sid Ganis, president of the motion picture group of Paramount Pictures, in defense of the industry, ". . . We're not consciously sweeping it [AIDS] under the rug. But it ain't easy. We're a business and need to have our own assurances that any film we invest in will make a profit. It becomes a business decision wrapped in emotion . . . ."[a] Tragic movies do not do well at the box office. A TV movie costs about $2.5 million, while a feature film for theatres costs at least $15 million to produce and release. Thus, the gamble for television is much less.

The various political aspects of AIDS also have placed a role in the coverage given to the disease. While TV can develop controversial topics relatively quickly and market them effectively as well, the movie industry cannot. Moreover, according to some observers, the movie industry is handicapped by its perceptions of AIDS and homosexuality and audience sensitivities.

Even though TV has a good track record it still has some distance to go. Many but not all of its AIDS projects have focused on children and women as victims of the disease. In the gay-themed AIDS presentations, the TV networks still dilute reality, rather than confront the homosexual element head on. Nevertheless, on balance television has made significant inroads into educating Middle America in a way that movies as yet have not.

[a]Source: E. Dutka, "Fear of AIDS Movies," *Los Angeles Times/Calendar*, 13 May 1990, p. 8

a lack of knowledge and understanding on the part of the target audience.

Experience from public health campaigns suggests that the more precisely a target group is identified, the more effective educational messages are likely to be. Precise group identification makes it easier to deliver a message that tells people exactly what they need to know in their language, through sources they trust and respect. This type of approach requires learning as much as possible about the group in question. Audience makeup, level of education, life-style, attitudes, and behaviors are all important characteristics. Consider the challenges posed by the following particular audiences.

| FOCUS ON STDs |

BEING ABLE TO READ — UNDERSTANDING AIDS

The major aim of AIDS education is to change high-risk sexual and drug abuse behaviors. To achieve their aim, various educational approaches have been used, including the mailing of an informational pamphlet, "Understanding AIDS" (fig. 17.5), to every household in the United States. Since the effectiveness of such educational approaches depends on the literacy of consumers, this 1988 informational pamphlet was studied for its readability by C. Ledbetter and D. Johnson in 1990.

The text of "Understanding AIDS" was divided into sixteen sections according to the specific topic presented in each section. Then the text of each section was analyzed using established formulas appropriate for reading materials from fourth grade to adult reading levels. The analyses of the individual sections concentrated on word and sentence factors such as sentence length, total number of words, total number of sentences, total number of polysyllabic terms, and words with three or more syllables. Table 17.1 summarizes the readability of the pamphlet's sections, expressed in terms of a specific grade level.

While the readability of "Understanding AIDS" ranged from grade levels 6.21 to 9.31, the overall readability was found to be at grade level 7.68. This means that the reader would need at least a seventh grade reading ability to fully understand the general material presented in the pamphlet. Is this good or bad? Well, several studies through the years indicate that at least 20 percent of the people in the United States are functionally unable to read materials written at fourth or fifth grade levels. The problem is compounded by the additional finding that about 50 percent of persons under medical care in health care facilities have difficulty in reading or are unable to read instructional materials written at a fifth grade level.

FIGURE 17.4

Another approach used to emphasize the ways in which HIV can and cannot be spread. These flyers highlight individual pieces of information on the transmission of AIDS taken from a larger, more detailed publication. (Courtesy of World Health Organization)

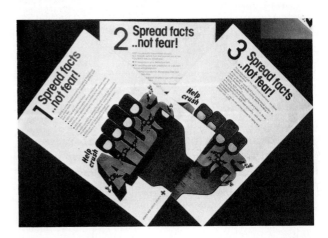

TABLE 17.1   SECTIONS OF THE "UNDERSTANDING AIDS"
PAMPHLET ARRANGED ACCORDING TO RESPECTIVE
READING LEVELS

SECTION TITLE	READING LEVEL
What About Dating?	6.2
The Difference between Giving and Receiving Blood	6.3
AIDS and Babies	6.9
What AIDS Means to You	7.1
Helping a Person with AIDS	7.4
Should You Get an AIDS Test?	7.5
You Won't Get AIDS from Insects, or a Kiss	7.6
What Behavior Puts You at Risk	7.7
A Message from the Surgeon General	8.0
What is All the Talk About Condoms?	8.4
What Does Someone with AIDS Look Like?	8.5
Talking with Kids About AIDS	8.5
The Problem of Drugs and AIDS	8.9
How Do You Get AIDS?	9.6

Issues and Strategies for STD Education among Hispanics. A number of myths concerning HIV infection and AIDS are commonly believed by the Hispanic population in the United States. Among these are the beliefs that AIDS affects only gay, white men and that the disease is transmitted through casual contact. Efforts to correct such misconceptions and to establish effective AIDS prevention programs have met with limited success (fig. 17.6) largely because of certain, widely-held attitudes and values by members of the Hispanic community. Examples of views which may prevent consideration,

let alone accepting the information in AIDS prevention messages, include:

- an unwillingness to discuss human sexuality in the context of the Hispanic family;
- an unwillingness to discuss homosexuality or bisexuality;
- a lack of acceptance of the existence of the gay life-style;
- a refusal to consider that homosexuality may exist among Hispanics;
- an absence of support and training among Hispanic women for negotiating sexual activity with partners; and

FIGURE 17.5

The AIDS brochure sent to every household in 1988 by U.S. Department of Health and Human Services.

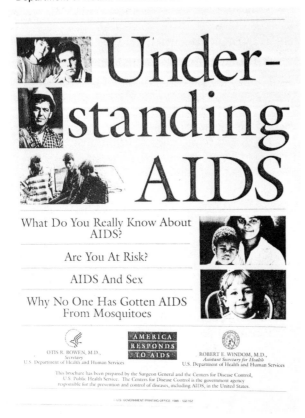

FIGURE 17.6

Dispelling long-held views is difficult. Posters such as the one shown say "You Can't Get AIDS This Way" in Spanish. The poster features photos of everyday activities that many people mistakenly believe transmit AIDS. It also tells that handshaking, dishes, toilets, and doorknobs cannot transmit HIV infection.

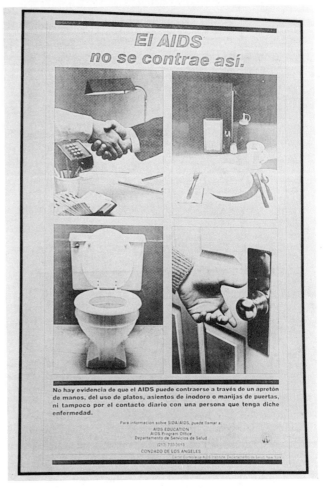

- an unwillingness to discuss drug use, or to admit that a family member may have a drug or alcohol problem.

Since the U.S. Hispanic population is extremely diverse, the development of educational and prevention programs requires an understanding of various characteristics of this population, as well as its socioeconomic and cultural differences. Among the factors to consider in the planning of a preventive education program are national origins, geographic locations, income levels, levels of education, and language. A few examples of selected situations will show how such factors can make the difference between success and failure.

Different regions of the United States have Hispanic populations with different needs. For example, an AIDS brochure developed for the Spanish-speaking population in the New York City area reflects the Spanish vocabulary and language familiar to Puerto Ricans. However, the same brochure might not be appropriate for San Francisco, where many Hispanics from Mexico or Central and South America live. Experience has clearly shown that these cultures have words, experiences, and expressions that are distinctly different.

The educational level of a population also strongly influences the selection of the type of communication medium that should be used for educational and

FIGURE 17.7

In an effort to bring the facts about AIDS to every household, the Centers for Disease Control pamphlet on AIDS was published in both English and Spanish. (Courtesy of U.S. Public Health Service)

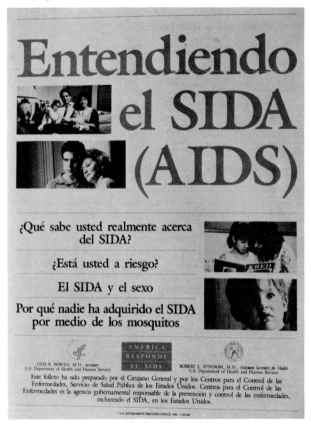

preventive programs. For example, it is far more effective to use television and radio, rather than newspaper ads and articles, to reach Hispanics. Although the print media appeals to some Hispanics, television and radio reach the larger numbers of teenagers, young adults, and older individuals.

Other considerations that are important to the development of effective educational materials include the use of culturally relevant language and symbols (fig. 17.7), as well as the presentation of information at a reading level appropriate to the target audience.

Producing Effective AIDS Educational Materials for Black Communities. In the United States, Black

identity includes African-Americans, early or recent immigrants from Caribbean nations who speak native languages, as well as the languages of their former colonizers—English, French, Spanish, and Dutch—and recent immigrants from African nations who are also greatly separated by language, geography, and national experience. Despite the false perception held by some members of Black communities that AIDS is a "gay, white disease," national statistics demonstrate that the incidence of AIDS and HIV-related diseases continue to increase within the Black population. Although Blacks represent about 12 percent of the American population, approximately 25 percent of the persons diagnosed as having AIDS have been Black. Furthermore, STD rates in general have been and continue to be disproportionately higher in Black teenagers.

Slowing the spread of HIV infection and other STDs within Black communities is critical. In order to do so, effective education and preventive programs and messages are needed. Many of the specific factors described earlier as being relevant to the development of educational and related materials for Hispanic communities also are applicable to Black communities. In addition, such efforts need to particularly take into account such factors as cultural sensitivity and the differences in the language used by Blacks to describe sexual behaviors and methods of drug abuse. Cultural sensitivity here refers to recognition of the dynamics of race and racism, of self-respect and shame, and of failure and faith. Studies have shown that capitalizing the word Black, or choosing figures that are current "core" images of the Black target audience for brochures, billboards, etc., are more effective in getting positive responses.

Blacks at all levels of their respective communities know and use the words everyone else uses. However, some Black people, as well as certain individuals of other ethnic groups who need to be informed and made aware of HIV infection and other STDs do not understand scientific terms such as semen or rectal secretions. The same problem occurs when someone describes the cleaning of "drug paraphernalia" instead of "cooker" and "works." One way out of this type of dilemma is to combine the popular with the scientific version as in, "The virus that causes AIDS can be found in semen ('cum') and in infected blood left in IV drug equipment ('works')." This approach, in a sense, translates different languages used to describe the same things. When education is targeted to a well-defined audience the content of the message can be tailored accordingly.

Adolescents and the "It Can't Happen to Me" Attitude. As the range of STDs has expanded from bacterial diseases such as syphilis and gonorrhea to viral diseases such as genital herpes, genital warts, and HIV infection, the assurance of prompt cures has vanished. While concern about safer sex is growing and some segments of the population are adopting personal protection strategies to reduce their risk of acquiring an STD, this has not been the case for adolescents.

Adolescents are considerably more at risk for several STDs, including HIV infection, than current statistics indicate. For example, although teenagers are informed about AIDS, they frequently have an "It can't happen to me" attitude. They overwhelmingly reject the idea of sexual abstinence and are skeptical about single sexual partners. Many have mixed feelings about condom use. A recent San Francisco study exploring adolescent attitudes and behaviors concerning condom use showed that even though the participants understood that condoms prevented STDs, they did not intend either to use or to increase their use of the protective devices. Similar findings have been reported from other cities.

When adjusted for sexual activity rates, teenagers have the highest reported rates of STDs of any age group. Approximately one in seven teenagers has an STD. This finding reflects the kind of behavior that increases the risk of HIV infection.

Clearly, adolescents present several challenges, in part because they are often sexually active while developing their sense of sexuality and sexual identity. At the same time, they have little sense of their own mortality. Heightened sexual activity, drug experimentation, and the emergence of crack cocaine also have increased the risk of acquiring an STD in adolescents. Associated with the increased use of crack is a growing trend of teenagers exchanging sexual favors for drugs or money to buy drugs. Such adolescents, sometimes called "strawberries," are commonly in or near crackhouses, where they receive a small amount of money for each, often unprotected, sexual encounter. The high incidence of STDs among adolescents underscores the need for concern and effective intervention.

In view of current trends, it is no small wonder that the STD-related knowledge and behaviors among high school students have become a major cause for concern throughout the United States. This is evidenced by the significant increase in the number of surveys being conducted by state, territorial, and local departments of health. The findings of several surveys show that sex education programs have increased the knowledge and decreased the misconceptions of teenagers about sexuality. However, changes in sexual behavior were not evident. Other studies have shown that isolated instructional units on AIDS or STDs, or classes that only emphasize the hazards of STDs and sexual behavior, have little effect on teenage audiences. Programs that help teenagers develop decision-making and refusal skills (to be able to say "no" when appropriate) have been effective. Some of the approaches and techniques used came from established, successful drug abuse and smoking prevention programs.

Effective STD prevention must address a complex group of adolescent risk-taking behaviors and must, in fact, deal with risk-taking as a normal and essential feature of adolescent development. Moreover, the special needs of adolescent sub-populations must be addressed in prevention program planning. Such sub-populations include, gay, lesbian, and bisexual adolescents, abused, exploited, and discarded adolescents, ethnic minorities, emotionally handicapped adolescents, and homeless adolescents. STD prevention programs cannot be narrowly defined, and include strategies to deal with both individual knowledge, attitudes, and behavior, as well as environmental influences such as drug availability and use, community values relating to teen sexuality, and the portrayal of drug abuse and sexual behavior in the mass media. Since such programs cannot exist in a vacuum, effective prevention of STDs among adolescents will require a coordinated community-wide strategy involving all segments of society associated with youth.

Reducing HIV Transmission among and through IV Drug Users. In the United States at least 1.4 million persons inject drugs for other than medical purposes. In this population, the use of contaminated equipment for drug injection serves as a most efficient way to spread HIV to other intravenous drug users (IVDUs), to the sexual partners of IVDUs, and to their unborn children. The results of various approaches currently available to reduce the spread of HIV have had varying degrees of success. Such approaches include community outreach programs designed, first to discourage drug injection and to encourage undergoing treatment and second, to teach those who continue to abuse drugs how to change their injection practices to reduce their risk of acquiring or spreading HIV infection.

Efforts to encourage IVDUs to modify their injection practices usually are met with strong opposition, since the sharing of needles, syringes, and other paraphernalia ("works") is a routine and valued activity in the IVDU culture. The sharing of such drug paraphernalia serves legal, economic, and social functions. Since the possession of drug paraphernalia is legally prohibited in most states, most IVDUs do not carry needles and syringes, in order to avoid the possibility of arrest. Being arrested would result in confinement without drugs and thus withdrawal. Since many IVDUs are poor and cannot afford to buy injection equipment, they rent or borrow what they need in shooting galleries or drug dealers' houses. Such rented needles and syringes are used repeatedly and are discarded only when needles become plugged or too dull to make them usable. Socially, sharing drug paraphernalia among "running partners" can represent a cooperative effort necessary to obtain drugs, and serves to bind users into a temporary but compelling personal relationship. Therefore, efforts to reduce the sharing of needles and syringes usually are strongly opposed by partners, who feel that their closest relations are being attacked.

Various preventive programs and/or campaigns have a number of goals. The most desirable of such goals is to convince individuals to stop abusing drugs and to enter a treatment program. Short of achieving this goal, efforts are directed at changing the behavior that leads to HIV transmission among IVDUs,

and HIV transmission from IVDUs to their sexual partners and offspring. This involves instruction in risk reduction behaviors, counseling on the issues surrounding HIV testing, and possibly the avoidance of pregnancy by women who are or who may become HIV infected.

There is no question that behaviors related to avoiding HIV infection are very difficult for IVDUs to adopt. Their addiction requires that most of their time, energy, and attention be devoted to obtaining and abusing drugs in sufficient quantities to avoid the pain of withdrawal. Thus, drawing attention to the danger of acquiring HIV infection through the use of contaminated drug paraphernalia may have limited effect. If an IVDU begins to experience withdrawal symptoms, for example, he or she is compelled, physically and mentally, to inject a drug as quickly as possible. Under these conditions, IVDUs will typically use any syringe that is available.

Other goals of preventive programs have been to convince IVDUs to use sterile needles and syringes, to use alternate nonintravenous routes to take drugs, and to clean needles and syringes with a bleach solution before injecting drugs. In a wide-scale San Francisco outreach program a comic book type of superhero known as "Bleachman" was used as the center of a campaign to encourage the use of bleach to clean drug paraphernalia and to prevent the spread of HIV (fig. 17.8). Television public service announcements, T-shirts, displays on buses, and posters of various types were used to get the message to IVDUs. The campaign worked fairly well.

Campaigns targeted to IVDUs are incomplete if they cover only the ways necessary to prevent HIV transmission during drug abuse. Though IVDUs now are reporting that they clean their drug paraphernalia much more frequently, few say that they are using safer sex practices with their sexual partners. Thus, many HIV-infected drug abusers who have eliminated the risks associated with drug abuse may nonetheless be spreading HIV by other means.

THE INFLUENCE OF FUNDING ON AIDS AND STD EDUCATION

Despite statements by health agency officials that education is critical to any AIDS prevention strategy, both state and federal funding for information and

SEX, LIES, AND HIV INFECTION

One of the important goals of STD educational and/or counseling programs is to reduce the risk of HIV transmission among sexually active teenagers and young adults. Individuals are advised to select potential sex partners on the basis of a lower risk for HIV infection. One approach to achieving this relationship involves, in part, asking about a partner's risk history. Unfortunately, this type of questioning may not take into account the possibility that individuals may lie about their risk history.

S. D. Cochran and V. M. Mays conducted a study involving a sample of 18-to-25-year-old southern California college students. Their study, summarized in the 15 March 1990 issue of *The New England Journal of Medicine*, casts a dark shadow on the honesty of individuals being questioned about their risk history. A total of 422 young, sexually active adults, anonymously completed an 18–page questionnaire designed to evaluate sexual behavior, HIV-related risk reduction, and personal experiences involving some form of lying when dating. The group was composed of 196 men and 226 women. Table 17.2 lists the types of the questions asked related to having told a lie to have sex, and having been lied to by a date. The responses of the participants also are indicated.

TABLE 17.2 DISHONESTY IN DATING AMONG THE SEXUALLY ACTIVE

	PERCENT	
	MEN	WOMEN
Lied in order to have sex		
1. Told a lie to have sex	34	10
2. Sexually involved with more than one person	32	23
Lied to by a date		
1. Has been lied to for purposes of sex	47	60
2. Partner lied about control of ejaculation or likelihood of pregnancy	34	46

This study produced some interesting and troublesome findings. For example, a significant number of sexually experienced men and women indicated having told a lie to have sex. Moreover, men reported lying more frequently than women, and women indicated they had been lied to more often by a date.

Another aspect of the study involved getting the responses of the group to various fictional situations in which honesty would threaten either the chance to have sex or the stability of an active sexual relationship. Table 17.3 lists the types of questions asked and the responses received.

TABLE 17.3 WILLINGNESS OF DATE TO LIE

	PERCENT	
	MEN	WOMEN
1. Would lie about having had a negative HIV antibody test	20	4
2. Would lie about control of ejaculation	29	—
3. Would lie about possibility of pregnancy	—	2
4. Would lower the number of previous sexual partners	47	42
5. Would tell of other sexual partner(s) to new partner:		
a. never	22	10
b. when safe to do so	34	28
c. only if asked	31	23
d. yes	13	29
6. Would tell of a one-time affair:		
a. never	43	34
b. when safe to do so	21	20
c. only if asked	14	11
d. yes	22	35

In this part of the study, both men and women frequently indicated that they would actively or even passively deceive a date to obtain sex. Again, men were found to be more likely to lie than women.

Even though the possibility exists that the participants were not fully forthright in responding to the questions asked, the implications of the study are quite clear and support the view that safer sex practices are *always* the way to go.

FIGURE 17.8

Bleachman, a superhero character used in a wide-scale
San Francisco outreach campaign to encourage intravenous drug
users to always clean their needles with bleach before injecting
drugs. (Courtesy of GMHC)

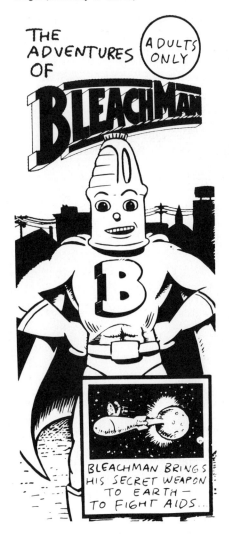
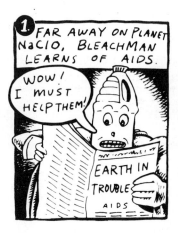
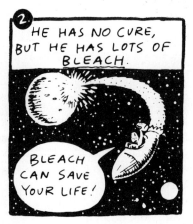
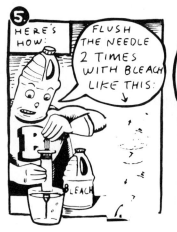
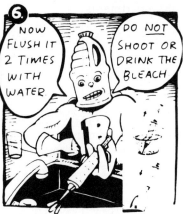

educational programs has been slow and rather limited. Such responses frequently have been influenced by fears of appearing to condone homosexuality and drug use. In addition, in recent administrations a fear also existed that conservative political supporters would be offended by discussions or presentations of sexual and drug abuse practices in educational materials. This type of thinking significantly contributed to the *one-year delay* in mailing a Centers for Disease Control pamphlet on AIDS to every household in the United States (fig. 17.6), and a *two-and-one-half year delay* in the distribution of a National Institute on Alcohol and Drug Abuse pamphlet for sexual partners of intravenous drug users about their high risk for HIV infection. Because of such problems, community-based groups have had to assume a major portion of the responsibility for AIDS education. To date, most educational materials and programs about AIDS have been developed by community-based, often gay-related organizations in association with state and local health departments.

Debates about federally supported approaches to AIDS prevention have been and continue to be issues for governmental agencies and leaders. The development and finalization of most education strategies to prevent AIDS occurs within political and social environments that influence their form, content, and ultimate effectiveness. Moreover, the demand for the distribution of information leads almost inevitably to the setting and possibly to the eventual enforcement of standards. This, in turn, leads to a continuing debate as to what information should be presented to whom, by whom, and how, and what standards should be used in deciding the appropriateness of the information for each target audience. The seriousness of this type of situation can be illustrated by legislation passed in 1987 by the U.S. Senate and House of Representatives that prohibited federal funding for educational materials that "promote or encourage homosexual activities." Funded educational activities and materials were mandated to emphasize "abstinence from sexual activity outside of a sexually monogamous marriage." Even though the final form of the legislation was changed so as not to be interpreted as forbidding descriptions of methods to reduce the risk of HIV transmission, by 1988 certain states had limited their educational efforts that would have benefited gay men. The impact of the 1987 bill was lessened significantly by a later congressional amendment in 1988 that removed any restrictions on the ability of an education program to provide accurate information on reducing the risk of HIV infection.

Whether or not HIV research, prevention, and control efforts will become more effective will depend not only on increased funding, but the efficient use of such funds. This will require the periodic review and honest evaluations of all programs and agencies receiving AIDS funding. Such activities also clearly need to involve target audience representatives.

IT IS WHAT YOU DO AND HOW YOU DO IT

It has taken some time for public health authorities, governmental representatives, AIDS organizations, and especially the news media to realize that it is what you do and how you do it, and not who you are that are central to the prevention of HIV infection and other STDs. Recognizing these facts of life reinforces the finding that STDs do not originate in persons with personal or group characteristics such as sexual orientation, race, ethnicity, or national origin, but rather specific actions that increase the possibility of exposure to STD agents.

CHAPTER | 18 | CONTINUING CHALLENGES OF STDs

> As recently as a decade ago it was widely believed that infectious disease was no longer much of a threat in the developed world.
>
> —*R. C. Gallo and L. Montagnier, 1989*

Epidemics have attracted attention, provoked alarm and sometimes panic throughout recorded history, and doubtlessly will continue to do so in the future. Such epidemics basically result from the creation or the increase of effective opportunities for the transmission of a disease agent to susceptible hosts. It is also possible for an epidemic to develop from the introduction of a disease agent which is new to a population of susceptible hosts, and for which ways for further spread exist. Certainly these situations can be applied to the events associated with the AIDS pandemic (table 18.1) as well as the relative increases in the number of STDs such as genital warts, genital herpes, and the wide variety of chlamydial infections.

While AIDS and HIV infections are receiving a substantial amount of attention on a worldwide basis (fig. 18.1), such attention may pose a serious problem to the control of other sexually transmitted diseases. Public concern and interest need to be increased and directed to the seriousness and dangers associated with all STDs (fig. 18.2).

One central, recurrent, and familiar theme in society is the tendency of both politicians and the public to support public health efforts in response to perceived crises, and to lose interest when such crises either have passed or appear to have passed. This type of complacency is not unusual, especially in the case of STDs.

Unfortunately, many of the STDs are on the increase. The main reasons for the high incidence of such diseases are behavioral and involve the behaviors as well as the attitudes of: 1) individuals who contract and transmit STDs; 2) health care personnel who treat and manage

TABLE 18.1	CDC PROJECTED NUMBERS OF AIDS CASES, AIDS-RELATED DEATHS AND LIVING PERSONS WITH AIDS[a]

	AIDS CASES		
Year	New Cases	Living	Deaths
1989	44,000–50,000	92,000–98,000	31,000–34,000
1990	52,000–57,000	101,000–122,000	37,000–42,000
1991	56,000–71,000	127,000–153,000	43,000–52,000
1992	58,000–85,000	139,000–188,000	49,000–64,000
1993	61,000–98,000	151,000–228,000	53,000–76,000
Through 1993[b]	390,000–480,000		285,000–340,000

[a]These projections are adjusted for unreported AIDS cases by adding 18 percent to the projections from reported cases. The numbers are rounded to the nearest 1,000.
[b]The numbers here are rounded to the nearest 5,000.

FIGURE 18.1

What the future holds as far as AIDS is concerned. According to the results of a survey conducted by the World Health Organization and the Global Programme on AIDS (GPA) predict about nine times more adult AIDS cases for the 1990s than occurred in the 1980s.

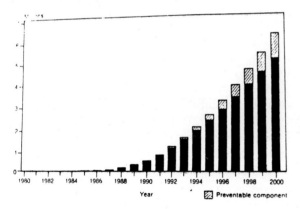

these diseases; and 3) national, state, and community leaders who provide the technical guidance and appropriate the financial support required for the success of prevention and control programs. If STDs are to be brought under control, a number of issues and concerns must be squarely faced, and effective strategies developed and launched to deal with them.

FIGURE 18.2

The rogues' gallery of STD agents. These microscopic forms of life continue to take their toll. (a) Syphilis (From E. E. Quist, L. A. Repesh, R. Zelezniker, and T. J. Fitzgerald, *British Journal of Venereal Disease* (1983) 59:11–20); (b) *Chlamydia;* (c) Papilloma viruses; (d) Hepatitis viruses; and (e) HIV.

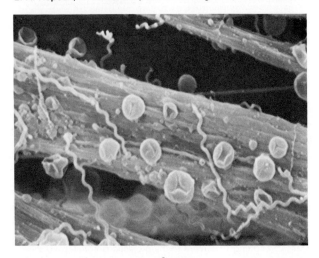

a

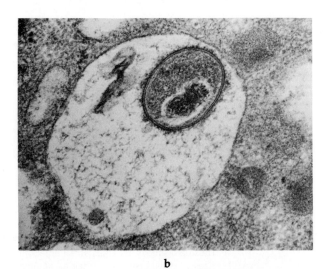

b

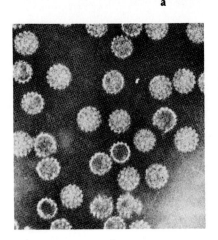

c

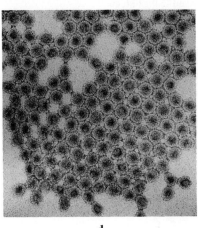

d

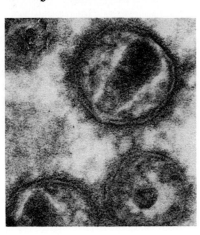

e

Table 18.2	Examples of Cost-Accounting Information Needed to Provide Effective Treatment for STDs

Comparisons of costs of treating STDs at various stages

Cost-effectiveness of current, effective treatments

Comparisons of the costs and benefits of current methods for organizing, delivering, and managing associated health care services in health care facilities and other settings

Comparisons of costs involved with current testing methods

Determination of costs associated with an expanded use of testing methods

Costs involved with providing additional education and training for individuals preparing to become health care professionals

Costs associated with additional training for established health care professionals

ECONOMICS OF PREVENTION AND CONTROL

Awareness of the economic importance of STDs and their complications has increased considerably during the last ten years or so. Of particular concern are the unfavorable outcomes of pregnancy for mother and newborn, neonatal infections, infertility, and genital cancers, in particular of the cervix. While the full economic impact of STDs is not known, no doubt as time passes the picture will become clearer. However, future realistic budget planning for treatment is a pressing matter. It will require the gathering of reliable and accurate information related to the total costs of health, social, and support services for STD infected persons. Table 18.2 lists examples of the types of cost-accounting information that is necessary if approaches to the prevention and control of STDs are to be achieved.

Estimates of the number of persons with HIV infections and other STDs are important, not only to determine future health care needs, but to assess the effectiveness of current prevention and control efforts. It is quite obvious that the financial burden of STDs, especially HIV-related infections, will continue to grow, thus requiring prevention efforts and increased medical and social services.

CHANGING BEHAVIOR?

There are several factors related to human behavior that are important to understanding the reasons for the present STD problem and the difficulty in developing methods of control. The lower age at which an increasingly large segment of the population has sexual intercourse, the increasing number of marriages that break up, increasing sexual freedom and activity of the female (a pattern that was formerly considered predominantly male), are all factors related to an increased risk of acquiring and/or spreading STDs.

A major portion of the population is starting sexual activity before marriage, and there is a significant time lapse between the onset of intercourse and the first use of safer sex practices. This is especially true for preadolescents and adolescents. Many such individuals engage in drug abuse and sexual behavior that place them at risk for various STDs, especially HIV infection. Although adolescents account for only 1 percent of all reported AIDS cases, the number of such cases are doubling annually. Moreover, 20 percent of all AIDS cases have occurred among 20-to-29-year-olds, many of whom presumably became infected during their teenage years.

AIDS AMONG OLDER ADULTS

Who has heard of acquired immune deficiency syndrome occurring in people over fifty? True, Rock Hudson was over fifty, but his youthful image prevented the public from identifying him as a representative of a public health problem in this age group. According to the Centers for Disease Control, 10 percent of all the AIDS cases reported in the United States in 1989 were in people age fifty and over, and 2.9 percent occurred in people over sixty-five. Several hundred more cases of AIDS occurred in the over fifty group in 1989 than in 1988.

There appears to be no end to the articles about AIDS in pregnancy and in the pediatric population. Such coverage is enough to make most people think that these segments of the population are the ones most affected by HIV infection and AIDS.

WHO GETS AIDS AFTER FIFTY?

Only by reading between the lines does the discovery come to light that AIDS is a public health problem in people over fifty. In 1989 six to seven times more cases of AIDS occurred in this age group than in children under five. Statistics from the Centers for Disease Control for transmission categories in AIDS patients over fifty in the United States up to August 1988, shows some interesting differences between this group and the AIDS population in the United States as a whole. Although the percentage of homosexual/bisexual males is almost exactly the same (62 percent over fifty, 63 percent of all ages), the percentage of heterosexual intravenous drug abusers is much less (8 percent over fifty, 19 percent all ages), as is the percentage of homosexual intravenous drug abusers (2 percent over fifty, 7 percent all ages), which reflects the fact that intravenous drug abuse is primarily a disorder of young people. The other major difference is that transfusion-associated AIDS is much more common in this group (16 percent over fifty, 3 percent for all ages), who, as a whole, are much more likely to have received a blood transfusion. These differences are still more obvious in AIDS patients over sixty-five. Only 26 percent of this group have contracted the disease by homosexual transmission, 2 percent are heterosexual intravenous drug abusers, 1 percent are homosexual drug abusers, while transfusion accounts for 55 percent of all AIDS cases.

Certainly, once people have been infected with HIV by any route, they can spread the disease to others by sexual transmission. But do older people have sex often enough to transmit the virus efficiently? According to various studies, older heterosexuals (the overwhelming majority of those who received transfusions) average two to four sexual contacts per month, which may be sufficient for transmission, given the fact that some persons become infected with HIV after a single exposure.

Other factors may increase susceptibility to HIV infection among older persons. These include decreased immune system response with age, and thinning of the vaginal wall in postmenopausal women due to hormonal changes, causing vaginal surface tears during intercourse. Other STDs may also serve as cofactors of HIV transmission in older individuals. Most older homosexuals continue to be sexually active, although their frequency of contacts may decrease with age. AIDS is also being increasingly recognized as the true cause of many diseases of the elderly that were once ascribed to "senility," such as deaths from pneumonia, tuberculosis, as well as dementia and presumed Alzheimer's disease.

It is becoming increasingly obvious that AIDS, like other STDs in persons over fifty, is not at all uncommon, despite the fact that little is written on the subject.

STDs and Victims of Rape

The risk of acquiring an STD as a result of rape is not known, in part because it is difficult to determine whether infections were present before the assault or contracted during it. In a recent study, 204 girls and women were first examined within 72 hours of the rape and again at least one week later. Forty-three percent, or 88 of the study group, were found to have at least one STD. Among the 53 percent, or 109 individuals, who returned for at least one follow-up visit (excluding those who were found to be infected at the first examination, or who were treated as a preventative measure), new infections were found in 37 percent. The accompanying table compares the STD picture in the two groups.

TABLE 18.3 A Comparison of STDs Present in Rape Victims

STD	Percentage of Infected Persons within 72 Hours of Rape	Percentage of Infected Persons Found to Have New Infection after 72 Hours of Rape
Bacterial vaginosis	34	19
Chlamydial infection	10	2
CMV	8	0
Genital herpes	2	0
Gonorrhea	6	4
HIV-positive[a]	1	0
Syphilis[a]	1	0
Trichomonas infection	15	12

[a]Follow-up blood tests were performed in only 26 percent of the individuals examined.

No new cases of CMV, genital herpes, syphilis, or HIV infections were found. The figures for syphilis and HIV, however, are not complete since only 24 of the 109 persons were tested for these STDs.

Even though most of the STDs were present in the victims of rape at the time of the first examination, the results of the study clearly indicate that rape victims have a lower, but substantial additional risk of acquiring an STD from such assaults.

Programs for the prevention of high-risk sexual behaviors, STDs, and drug abuse must clearly deal with adolescents in a variety of settings, including schools, churches, and community organizations. As with other social skills, those skills needed to cope with high-risk sexual experiences must be taught before risky sexual experiences are adopted as normal and routine. This is especially important for women. Current STD prevention programs take into account the fact that the female at risk of acquiring an STD has only one method of protection over which she has some control other than to say "no," and that is self-care. There is clearly a need for women to take an increasingly independent role in maintaining their health and well-being, and using the methods by which they can prevent acquiring an STD.

For the foreseeable future, the major strides in preventing STDs will depend on educational programs emphasizing the widespread use of interventions designed for those who are entering their sexually formative years.

DEALING WITH EMOTIONS MORE EFFECTIVELY

Fear, confusion, and blaming someone or some group when an epidemic strikes is not new, but we need to be able to deal with those emotions more effectively. It was those same fears that branded the newest United States immigrants of 1916 (Italians) as the villains responsible for the poliomyelitis epidemic of that year, and kept children from beaches and the movies during the entire era of polio epidemics in the 1940s and 1950s. Today, such fears keep children from attending classes with HIV-infected classmates, and even caused someone to burn the home of three HIV-infected hemophiliac children in Florida in 1989.

How can the public's perceptions of AIDS be influenced so that there is more compassion towards and less fear of people with HIV infection or AIDS? First and foremost, this will require a strong and lasting commitment by all segments of influence in

society to changing attitudes. As long as some political and religious leaders and health care providers show hostility or indifference towards people with HIV infections or AIDS, there will be enormous difficulties in changing the public's perceptions. This includes those who are preparing to become health care professionals. Little else may do as much good as having religious leaders ask their parishioners to show compassion for persons with AIDS. Likewise, scientists who work in the field of AIDS research, and public health practitioners must become more aware of AIDS-related discrimination and to work against it. The battle involves not only a deadly virus, but also an epidemic of stigmatization. Finally, the mass media must join in this battle by presenting persons with AIDS to the public in a more favorable light. To date, probably most of the public do not know someone with HIV infection or AIDS. Through the mass media, the public may become acquainted with such persons and come to realize that they are not so different from themselves. It is to be hoped that the more familiar the public becomes with persons who have AIDS, the less hostility and fear will be directed towards people with the disease.

STRATEGIES AND CHALLENGES FOR BATTLING STDS

Strategic planning is a process which seeks to set priorities, identify weaknesses, and build on the strengths of existing efforts. Over the next five years, the attention given to HIV infection and AIDS will dominate the STD horizon. However, the interest in and the resources committed to preventing AIDS will also provide unique opportunities to make further inroads to controlling the other STDs (table 18.4).

Factors which influence STD control are complex since they involve interactions of 1) the health care system, 2) governmental agencies, 3) the public's interest in STDs, and 4) resources available for prevention and control programs. Furthermore, strategic planning for such control requires making

TABLE 18.4 | MAJOR RECOMMENDATIONS OF THE NATIONAL COMMISSION ON AIDS

1. Provide "disaster relief" money for cities and states hardest hit by the AIDS epidemic.
2. Provide federal housing assistance to deal with the many problems posed by HIV infection and AIDS.
3. Pass laws forbidding discrimination against HIV-infected persons.
4. Remove federal restrictions that interfere with the effective use of funds for AIDS prevention and education.

FOCUS ON STDs

FREE NEEDLES — POINTS TO CONSIDER

The expanded range of STDs and the responsibilities for providing care has been a two-edged sword. On the one hand, it has stretched limited resources directed to prevent and to control STDs quite thin; on the other hand, it has increased the acceptance of constructive new approaches to reducing STD transmission among high-risk groups. One example of a rather new but controversial approach is the legal availability of free, sterile hypodermic needles and syringes.

As commonly happens with a good catch-phrase, the mention of *free needles* arouses emotions and distorts the discussion. Free needles has been the subject of much public discussion in New York, New Jersey, and California, though none of these states has adopted, or adopted and implemented, any program to provide sterile drug injection equipment to IV drug abusers. Concern about HIV infection among IV drug abusers has also led to increasing the legal availability of sterile injection equipment in France and Sweden, and to the removal of any legalities restricting the availability of sterile needles in Switzerland. Needle exchanges also have been established in the United Kingdom.

Increasing the legal availability of needles has received support among public health officials. However, it has generally been opposed by law enforcement agencies, who predict that the practice of distributing free needles would not be effective because IV drug abusers would not change their behavior, or that it would be too effective and increase the number of IV drug abusers by removing the threat of HIV infection and AIDS.

The actual effects of increasing the legal availability of sterile needles and syringes are unknown. Moreover, considering the controversial nature of the approach, its effectiveness will always be difficult to evaluate.

TABLE 18.5 | ELEVEN STRATEGIES TO STD REDUCTION

1. Design and establish a comprehensive national STD prevention and control program, linked with a global network.

2. Institute mandatory health care employee STD education programs.

3. Monitor and evaluate, on an ongoing basis, the effectiveness of universal precautions in preventing infection. Make immediate changes when appropriate.

4. Link all voluntary STD testing (especially for HIV antibodies) with appropriate counseling.

5. Establish the basis with which to start STD education in elementary schools (both public and private) by the year 1995.

6. Design and initiate special education and service delivery programs to reduce the risk of STDs among, and provide appropriate treatment to, adolescent drug abusers (especially the homeless), runaway, and detained adolescents who exhibit symptoms, and those whose life-styles place them at risk of becoming infected.

7. Develop and enforce laboratory licensing laws to ensure the accuracy of all STD testing results, especially in the case of HIV infection.

8. Establish a functional public health emergency system to get around the bureaucratic obstacles so that public health officials can respond quickly to national medical epidemics.

9. Provide more state and federal funds to pay for STD patients' health care needs.

10. Appropriate state and federal funds to cover the medical expenses of uninsured STD infected persons.

11. Develop and institute a system by which all bona fide agencies involved with STD prevention can be linked in order to prevent duplication of effort and to promote cooperation and coordination.

assumptions about the future and estimating the public health importance and economic consequences of STDs.

STDs will be a continuing public health challenge and problem of immense magnitude throughout the world. The greatest challenge facing all prevention and control programs is to reduce, to the maximum extent possible, the transmission of STD agents. In the absence of effective vaccines for the majority of STDs, national programs will not be able to prevent the millions of STD cases that will occur worldwide over the next decade. During the 1990s the incidence of this group of diseases in any specific segment of the population or country will be a measure of both the commitment and the effectiveness of prevention programs. Table 18.5 lists examples of strategies that will truly evaluate the commitment and effectiveness of efforts to reduce and possibly eliminate certain STDs.

IS THERE A FINAL WORD ON STDs?

The world moves on, and as it moves it becomes less simple. At one time it was appropriate to speak of "venereal diseases," or VD, but some individuals felt that the term "venereal" was misleading since it seemed to exclude marital sexual relations. Thus, the term "sexually transmitted diseases," or STDs, was coined. Not only has the terminology changed in recent years, but so too has the membership of this group of diseases. No longer does it include only syphilis, gonorrhea, and chancroid. The list of disease agents continues to grow. It seems likely that Pandora's box, mentioned in chapter 1, may spring further surprises, and the next decade, indeed the next century, is likely to be no less alarming and challenging than the last in terms of sexually transmitted diseases.

GLOSSARY

A number of important and widely used terms and concepts associated with sexually transmitted diseases (STDs) are included in this glossary. Other terms defined in the text are indicated by page number in the index. Phonetic pronunciations of selected terms also are provided here.

abscess (AB-sess): A localized collection of pus.

acid-fast staining technique: One type of staining procedure used in the identification of microorganisms, such as members of the genus *Mycobacterium.*

active immunity: The state of resistance following exposure to an antigenic stimulus; this form of immunity may be naturally or artificially acquired.

acute (a-KŪT): The term used to indicate the rapid appearance of the signs and symptoms of an illness or disease.

acyclovir (a-SĪ-klō-vir): A drug used in the treatment of herpes simplex virus infections.

aerosol: A fine suspension of particles or liquid droplets sprayed into the air.

AIDS (acquired immune deficiency syndrome): A viral infection caused by the human immunodeficiency virus (HIV), and resulting in a lowering of the host's immune responses. Victims of the condition are more susceptible to opportunistic infections than individuals with normally functioning immune systems.

AIDS-related complex (ARC): A disease state caused by HIV infection. The disease has been defined as exhibiting two clinical conditions and two laboratory abnormalities typical of AIDS.

amphotericin B (am'-fō-TER-i-sin): An antifungal drug used to treat systemic fungal disease.

anamnestic (an-am-NES-tik) *response:* The sudden secondary rise in immunoglobulin (antibody) concentration produced by a second exposure to an immunogen (antigen) some time after the initial exposure.

anemia (ah-NĒ-me-ah): A deficiency of red blood cells, hemoglobin, or both.

anergy (AN-er-jē): An inability to respond to specific antigens; found in immunosuppressed conditions such as AIDS: appears as a lack of response to skin testing substances (antigens).

anoscope (A-nō-skōp): An instrument used to examine the anus and lower rectum.

antibiotics: Chemicals either produced by microorganisms or commercially formed that kill/or inhibit the growth of bacteria, fungi, and certain protozoa; none are currently effective against viruses.

antibody (immunoglobulin): A highly specific protein molecule produced by plasma cells in the immune system; antibodies function in humoral immunity.

antigen: Any substance which when presented to the immune system, stimulates the production of antibodies (immunoglobulins).

asymptomatic: Without symptoms.

attenuated (ah-TEN'-ū-ā-ted): Weakened.

AZT Azidothymidine (a'-zī-dō-THĪ-mi-dēn): Trade name Retrovir. A drug used in the treatment of persons with HIV infection and AIDS. It reduces symptoms of the disease and prolongs the life of the infected.

bacillus (ba-SIL-us): A rod-shaped bacterial cell.

bacteria (bak-TĒ-rē-a): Single-celled microscopic forms of life found in a variety of environments including soil, water, in and on the bodies of animals and plants; several cause a number of diseases.

B cell: A type of lymphocyte (white blood cell) that circulates through the body and is able to detect the presence of foreign agents. Once exposed to an antigen of the agent, these cells develop into plasma cells to produce antibodies (immunoglobulins).

benign (bē-NĪN): Harmless.

bisexual: Refers to an individual having a sexual attraction to persons of either sex.

bubo (BOO-bo): A swollen lymph node.

cancer (KAN'-ser): A broad group of disease states in which harmful or life-threatening growth (tumors) generally develop.

candidiasis (kan-di-DĪ-a-sis): Infection of the skin or mucous membrane with any species of the yeast *Candida.*

capsid (CAP-sid): A shell-like structure, composed of protein subunits, that encloses the nucleic acid of individual virus particles.

capsomere (CAP-soh-mer): Specific protein molecules that represent the building block of a viral capsid.

carrier: An individual harboring a disease agent without showing any obvious symptoms of an associated disease.

cell-mediated immunity: The reaction to antigenic material by specific defensive cells, rather than immunoglobulins.

CD4 protein: A specific protein found on the surfaces of T4 or T helper cells, some macrophages and other body cells; this protein serves as the receptor for human immunodeficiency viruses.

Centers for Disease Control: A branch of the United States Public Health Service responsible for the collection and distribution of epidemiological information and involved with the identification of the causes of major public health problems.

cervicitis (ser-vi-SĪ-tis): Inflammation of the cervix.

cervix: The opening to the uterus, which extends into the upper portion of the vagina.

chancre (SHANG-ker): A circular, purplish sore with a raised edge.

chemotherapy: The treatment of disease by the use of chemicals that inhibit or kill the causative agents, but ideally will not injure the cells or tissues of the host.

chronic: Long-lasting.

chronic disease: A disease that develops slowly. The condition tends to last a long time and requires a long convalescence period.

clinical disease: A disease in which symptoms are obvious.

CNS (Central Nervous System): The CNS is made up of the brain and spinal cord. HIV has been found in the fluid surrounding the CNS and is believed to affect the nerves. Once in the CNS, the virus can cause a variety of symptoms including loss of motor control, headaches, dementia, and vision, hearing, and speech impairment. (Note: Not all viruses are able to pass out of the blood and into the CNS. HIV is attracted to nerves and can move into the CNS.)

coccus (KOK-us): Spherical form of bacterial cell.

colposcope (KOL-pō-skōp): An instrument used for the examination of the vagina and the cervix.

communicable disease: A communicable disease that is transmissable among individuals (hosts).

condom: A barrier device made of a thin latex sheath or animal gut tissue that fits tightly over the penis and prevents the release of semen during sexual activities.

contagious disease: A communicable disease whose causative agent passes easily among hosts.

dementia (dē-MEN-shē-a): Loss of mental function due to damaged brain cells.

deoxyribonucleic acid (DNA): A large biological molecule that contains genetic information coded in specific sequences of chemical subunits.

diarrhea: Excessive loss of fluid from the gastrointestinal tract.

disease: Any change from the general condition of good health.

disseminated: Spreading to neighboring or distant areas.

DNA probe: A highly specific genetic engineering tool consisting of nucleic acid sequences that will match and combine with genetic sequences of material extracted from or left in place in cancer cells, specific microorganisms, or cells from individuals with specific genetic defects.

dose (infectious): The number of pathogenic agents that must be taken into the body in order to establish a disease state.

dormant: Inactive.

douche (doosh): A stream of hot or cold water, medicated or nonmedicated, directed against a body part.

dyspareunia (dis-pa-RŪ-nē-a): The development of pain during sexual intercourse.

dysuria (dis-Ū-rē-a): Painful or difficult urination.

edema (eh-DĒ-ma): An abnormal accumulation of fluids in tissues which causes swelling.

ELISA Test: A laboratory test used to indicate the presence of antibodies to HIV. (Various ELISA tests are used to detect other infections as well.) The HIV ELISA test does not detect the disease AIDS, but only indicates if viral infection has occurred. The test also is used to screen blood and blood supplies, and is utilized in certain research projects.

encephalitis (en-sef′-a-LĪ-tis): An inflammation of the brain.

endemic: Present more or less continuously in a community.

endogenous (en-DOJ-ē-nus): Formed from within a cell.

endotoxin: A form of poison associated with certain bacteria.

envelope: An outer covering of some virus particles.

enzyme: A protein that speeds up or slows down chemical reactions; it causes changes in other substances without undergoing any changes itself.

enzyme-linked immunosorbent assay (ELISA): A laboratory test used to detect the presence of antibodies to infectious disease agents; the test is used to detect HIV infection and to screen blood and blood products.

epidemic: An outbreak of a disease that appears rapidly and attacks a large number of persons in a community at about the same time.

epidemiology (eh-pē-dē-mē-OL-ō-jē): A scientific area of study dealing with when and where diseases occur and how they are spread.

etiology (ē-tē-OL-ō-jē): Cause of a disease.

exogenous (eks-OJ-e-nus): Originating outside of an organ or part.

exotoxin (eks′-ō-TOKS-in): A poison produced by a disease agent and excreted into its surrounding environment.

exudate (EKS-ū-date): Material containing pus that has escaped from blood vessels usually as a result of inflammation.

fetus (FĒ-tus): The later stages of a developing individual within the uterus; usually from the third month of pregnancy to birth.

fomite (FŌ-mi-tē): An inanimate or nonliving object that can spread disease agents.

gene: A segment of a DNA molecule containing specific genetically inherited information for the production of proteins.

gene amplification: A process that causes a gene to be replicated (repeated) several times.

genitalia (jen-i-TĀL-ē-a): Refers to the reproductive organs.

genome (JĒ-nome): The entire set of genetic information of an organism.

glans penis: The enlarged end of the penis.

Gram stain: Specific staining procedure that separates bacteria into the two groups, Gram positive and Gram negative, and is based on the results of color reactions.

granulocyte: A general group of white blood cells containing different types of cytoplasmic granules (e.g., basophil, eosinophil, neutrophil).

gumma (GOO-ma): A tumorlike fleshy mass of tissue (granuloma) found in the late stages of syphilis.

HBsAg: The surface coat, or envelope, of hepatitis B virus.

H chain (heavy chain): One pair of identical proteinlike (polypeptide) chains that form an immunoglobulin molecule.

helper T cells (HT): One type of lymphocyte known for several activities including helping in immunoglobulin production, and the activation of other cells associated with cell-mediated immunity; also known as T_4 cell.

hemorrhage: The escape of blood from blood vessels.

hepatitis: An inflammation of the liver.

high-risk behavior: As it pertains to HIV and AIDS the term is used to describe certain activities that increase the risk of transmitting or acquiring HIV. These include anal and vaginal intercourse without a condom, semen or urine in the mouth, manual-anal penetration, sharing intravenous needles, intimate blood contact, and sharing of sex toys contaminated by body fluids. Such behaviors often are referred to as "unsafe" activities.

HIV: A acronym for the virus that causes AIDS. HIV stands for human immunodeficiency virus. Previously used names include HTLV-III (human T-cell Lymphotropic Virus, Type Three), LAV (lymphadenopathy associated virus), and ARV (AIDS-related retro virus).

host: A form of life infected or attacked by a disease agent.

humoral immunity: One of two types of immune responses; regulated or controlled by immunoglobulins.

IgA: The major immunoglobulin class found in various body secretions.

IgD: A class of immunoglobulin found on B cell surfaces; its function is to assist in antigen recognition.

IgE: The main class of immunoglobulin associated with allergies.

IgG: The major protective immunoglobulin; it is the smallest of the five known Ig classes.

IgM: The first immunoglobulin formed in response to antigen exposure; it is the largest of the known immunoglobulin classes.

immune system: A complex of several specific cell types, including T lymphocytes, B lymphocytes, and macrophages, in the lymph nodes and in blood, that protects against infections, cancers, and other diseases.

immunity: Resistance.

immunization (im-ū-ni-ZA-shun): The process that produces resistance or immunity.

immunocompromized: Refers to the condition in which the parts of the immune system do not function normally.

immunogen (i-MŪ-nō-jen): Any substance that provokes immunoglobulin (antibody) production.

immunosuppression (im'-ū-nō-sū-PRES-shun): Inhibition of the body's immune response to foreign cells and related materials.

incidence: The frequency of occurrence of a disorder or a disease over a period of time and in relation to a segment of the population involved.

incubation (in'-kū-BA-shun) *period:* The time period between exposure to a disease agent and the appearance of the first symptoms.

infection (in-FEK-shun): The condition in which the body or a part of it is attacked by a disease agent.

infectious disease: Any condition caused by the growth and subsequent destruction of body parts by a pathogen or its products.

infertility: Inability to produce offspring.

infestation: The attachment to or invasion of the skin by a parasite.

inflammation: Tissue reaction to injury; a defense mechanism of the body.

interleukins (in-ter-LOO-kins): Small, immunologically nonspecific substances that act on leukocytes; they transmit information related to growth and differentiation among leukocytes.

intravenous (in-tra-VE-nus): Refers to injecting directly into a vein.

in vitro (Latin: *in glass*): Pertains to experiments done outside of the natural environment of living cells or organisms.

in vivo (Latin: *in life*): Pertains to experiments done in living cells or organisms.

invasiveness: The ability of a disease agent to penetrate host tissues and to cause damage.

jaundice (JAWN-dis): Yellowing of body tissues.

Kaposi's sarcoma (KAP-o-shes, sar-KO-ma) (KS): A rare form of cancer. It is recognized by raised, non-tender, purplish skin rash with lesions on any part of the body, notably the upper body and the arms and legs.

killer cells: A form of white blood cell that attacks and destroys cells considered to be foreign by the immune system.

Koch's postulates: A definite sequence of experimental steps that shows the causal relationship between a specific organism and a specific disease.

labia (LA-be-a): Folds of skin lying on either side of the vaginal opening; the female reproductive system has both the *labia majora* and the *labia minora*.

latent (LA-tent): Hidden or not active.

lesion: Refers to a visible wound, sore, rash, or other sign of disease.

leukocyte (LOO-ko-sit): White blood cell.

lithotomy (lith-OT-o-me): In this text, term refers to a specific position used in the physical examination of a female patient.

lymphocyte (LIM-fo-sit): An agranulocytic white blood cell.

lymphokines (LIMF-fo-kins): Soluble products of lymphocytes that are responsible for the multiple effects of a cellular immune reaction.

lymphoma (LIMF-fo-ma): Cancer of lymphoid tissue.

macrophage (MAK-ro-faj): A phagocytic mononuclear cell that originates from bone marrow monocytes and serves various roles in cellular immunity.

macule (MAK-yuhl): A red spot on the skin.

major histocompatibility complex (MHC): A number of genes located close to one another that determine histocompatibility tissue antigens of members of a species; MHC codes for the majority of cell-surface antigens that guide antigen recognition and cell interactions, especially by T cells.

malaise (ma-LAZ): A feeling of general discomfort.

malignant (ma-LIG-nant): Cancerous.

medium: Liquid or solid nutrient preparation used for the cultivation of microorganisms.

memory cells: Cells derived from B and T lymphocytes that react rapidly to second and later exosures to antigens.

meningitis (men-in-JI-tis): An inflammation of the coverings (meninges) of the brain and spinal cord.

menstruation (men-stroo-A-shun): The periodic discharge of blood from the uterus; occurs at more or less regular intervals during the reproductive period of women.

microbiota: The populations of microorganisms normally found in various areas of the body.

mold: A form of fungus consisting of microscopic cells that form visible cottony growths.

molecule: A combination of atoms forming a specific chemical.

mons pubis: The anatomical fleshy projection in the pubic area of a female.

morbidity rate: The number of cases of a disease per 1,000 of the population within a given time period.

mortality rate: The percentage of individuals dying from a specific disease.

mutation: A sudden change in the genetic code of an organism, resulting in a hereditable (permanent) property differing from the parent cell.

neonate (NĒ-ō-nāt): A newborn up to six weeks of age.

neoplasm (NĒ-ō-plazm): A new and abnormal tissue formation.

NK cells (natural killer cells): Cytotoxic cells belonging to the T cell subpopulation, responsible for cellular injury and destruction.

nucleocapsid: The capsid and the enclosed nucleic acid core of a virus particle.

opportunist: A form of life that causes infection only under especially favorable conditions (e.g., when host defense mechanisms are not fully functioning).

pandemic: Affecting the majority of the population of a large region, or concurrent epidemics in many different parts of the world.

papule (PAP-ūl): A small, firm, generally round, elevated skin lesion.

parasite: An organism that lives within or upon another form of life.

passive immunization: The transfer of antibodies from an immunized donor to a nonimmune recipient.

Pap smear: A stained preparation of material collected from the cervix and vagina.

pathogenic: Capable of producing disease.

pathogenicity: The ability of an organism to produce disease.

pelvic inflammatory disease (PID): Inflammation of the female pelvic organs, especially the ovaries, fallopian tubes, and uterus.

person with AIDS (PWA): Preferred designation for an individual with the signs and symptoms of AIDS.

placenta: The internal organ that develops in the uterus with pregnancy and through which the fetus absorbs oxygen and nutrients, and excretes wastes.

plasma: The liquid portion of blood.

plasma cells: Fully differentiated antibody-forming cells that are derived from B lymphocytes.

prepuce (PRE-pus): The foreskin or fold of skin over the glans penis in the male.

prevalence (PREV-a-lens): The number of cases of a disorder or disease occurring in a specific population at a specific time.

prion (PRE-ahn): An infectious disease agent that is neither virus nor viroid, and consists only of protein.

proctitis (prok'-TĪ-tis): Inflammation of the rectum and anus.

prodromal (prō-DRŌ-mal): Pertains to the initial stage of a disease.

prognosis (prog-NŌ-sis): Prediction as to the course, end of a disease, and the chance for a recovery.

pustule: A small elevated skin lesion containing pus.

pyogenic (pī-oh-GEN-ik): Pus-producing.

reverse transcriptase: An enzyme involved in the formation of DNA complementary to an RNA pattern or template.

salpingitis (sal-pin-JĪ-tis): Inflammation of the uterine (fallopian) tube.

sarcoma (sar-CŌ-mah): A solid tumor developing from connective tissue, bone, muscle, and fat.

scrotum (SKRŌ-tum): A fleshy pouch or sac located outside of the body that contains the male sex organs, the testes.

semen: The secretion of the male reproductive organs, which is ejaculated from the penis during an orgasm; contains sperm cells, products of accessory glands, and some white blood cells.

seroconversion: The process by which a person who has been infected with HIV converts to testing positive for HIV antibodies.

sexual reproduction: The formation of an organism from the union of two different sex cells (gametes).

sexually transmitted diseases (STDs): Any disease spread through sexual activities.

sign: An obvious feature of a disease or disorder.

slim disease: A disease characterized by general body weakness, severe weight loss, long-lasting diarrhea, and a persistent cough.

spirillum: A twisted- or curved-shaped bacterial cell.

spirochete (spi-rō-KĒT): A curved bacterial cell resembling a compressed corkscrew.

sputum (SPŪ-tum): The thick mucous secreted by irritated tissues in the lower respiratory tract and expelled.

sterile: Unable to produce young.

submicroscopic: Beyond the range of a regular microscope; electron microscopes are needed for viewing submicroscopic materials.

suppressor T cells: A subset of T lymphocytes that suppress antibody synthesis by B cells or inhibit other cellular activities such as those of T helper cells.

symptom: Refers to any change in a body part or activity that can be observed or felt by the person.

syndrome: Specific signs and symptoms that occur together and characterize a specific disease.

systemic: Pertaining to or affecting the body as a whole.

T cell (T lymphocyte): A thymus-derived cell that participates in a variety of cell-mediated (controlled) immune reactions; four subsets of T cells are known.

thymus: The central lymphoid organ, which is present in the thorax and controls the development of T lymphocytes.

toxin: A poisonous substance.

toxoid: A converted toxin; the resulting preparation is nontoxic, but still is capable of provoking immunoglobulin production.

transcriptase: An enzyme that catalyzes the flow of genetic information from DNA to RNA.

transcription: The formation of a complementary copy of a DNA or RNA template pattern strand.

ulcer: An irregularly shaped sore or area of tissue destruction.

urethra (ū-RĒ-thra): A canal or tube used to eliminate urine.

urethritis (ū-rē-THRĪ-tis): Inflammation of the urethra.

uterine tube: One of two small tubes attached to either side of the uterus and leading from the area of the ovary.

uterus (U-ter-us): The pear-shaped hollow organ with muscular walls of a female that can contain a developing human.

vaginitis (vaj-in-Ī-tis): Inflammation of the vagina.

venereal (vē-NĒ-rē-al) *disease:* A disease, such as gonorrhea or syphilis, which is spread by sexual contact and involves parts of the genitourinary system.

viroid: Small fragments of nucleic acids capable of causing disease.

virulence (VIR-ū-lens): The capacity to produce disease; it is a function of microbial invasiveness and toxicity and is measured with reference to a particular host.

virus: Submicroscopic, noncellular disease agents generally consisting of one type of nucleic acid and surrounded by some form of protein covering.

Western blot test: A blood test used to detect antibodies to HIV. Compared to the ELISA test, the Western blot is more accurate, more detailed, and more expensive. It is used to confirm the results of the ELISA test. The test may occasionally be negative even though a person is infected with HIV, particularly in the first few months, but when it is positive it is very accurate—the person is almost surely infected with HIV.

yeast: A type of fungus that is single-celled.

Index

A

Abnormal growth, 11
Abnormal masses, 228
Abscess formation, 91
Accessory sex glands, 44
Acid-fast stain, 196
ACLU. *See* American Civil
  Liberties Union (ACLU)
Acquired forms of immunity,
  summary of, 254
Acquired immune deficiency
  syndrome (AIDS), 11, 17,
  20, 23, 26, 27, 28, 37
  ADC. *See* AIDS dementia
    complex (ADC)
  and AIDS-related infections,
    187, 199, 209
  ARC. *See* AIDS-related
    complex (ARC)
  ARD. *See* AIDS-related
    dementia (ARD)
  and cats, cattle, horses,
    monkeys, and sheep, 204,
    205
  and causative agents, 57
  consequences of, 59–61
  and *Cryptococcus*, 186
  and fashion industry, 266
  and HIV spectrum, 163, 199
  and immunodeficiency
    diseases, 178
  and incubation period, 228
  introduced, 1, 2, 3
  and Kaposi's sarcoma. *See*
    Kaposi's sarcoma (KS)
  in movies and television,
    301
  and newer STD, 58
  and Norwegian scabies, 156,
    158–61
  occupations and exposure,
    267–73

and opportunistic infection
  and immunocompromised
  host, 180, 182–83
  pediatric AIDS (PAIDS). *See*
    Pediatric AIDS (PAIDS)
  preventing spread of, 247–49
  and reading, 302–3
  vaccines for, 250–62
  women with, 230
Acquired immunity, 251–53
Acquired immunodeficiency
  diseases, 178–79
Active immunity, 173, 251–52,
  253
Acute disease, 14
Acyclovir, 65, 129, 192
ADC. *See* AIDS dementia
  complex (ADC)
Adjuvant, 259
Adolescents, 306
Adrenal glands, 126
Adult T cell leukemia/
  lymphoma (ATLL), 203
African sleeping sickness, 17,
  19
Agar, 15
Agranulocytes, 168
AIDS. *See* Acquired immune
  deficiency syndrome
  (AIDS)
AIDS dementia complex
  (ADC), 57, 224
AIDS-related complex (ARC),
  37, 57, 224, 226, 227, 229,
  240, 245
AIDS-related dementia (ARD),
  224, 226, 237–38
Albumins, 167
Allergies, 176
Alpha interferon, 243
Amantadine, 65
Amebiasis, 57
Amebic dysentery, 17, 58, 198

American Association of
  Physicians for Human
  Rights, 247
American Civil Liberties
  Union (ACLU), 286
Amphotericin, 185
Anamnestic response, 173, 177
Anemia, 167
Anne Klein, 266
Anogenital, 135, 139
Anorectal areas, 59
Anoscope, 52
Anoscopic examination, 52
Antibodies, 167, 175–76
Antibody molecule, 176
Antigen attachment, 175
Antigens, 166, 185, 217, 251
Anti-idiotype vaccines, 260
Antiretroviral therapy, 218
Antitoxins, 254
Antiviral drugs, 65
Apollo, 78
ARC. *See* AIDS-related
  complex (ARC)
ARD. *See* AIDS-related
  dementia (ARD)
Areola, 46, 47
"Aristotle Contemplating the
  Bust of Homer," 79
Art, and syphilis, 79–80
Artificially acquired active
  immunity, 253
Artificially acquired passive
  immunity, 253
Aspergillosis, 187
Aspergillus, 187
Asymptomatic, 72, 190
Asymptomatic condition, 6
Asymptomatic genital disease,
  89
Athlete's foot, 17, 19
ATLL. *See* Adult T cell
  leukemia/lymphoma
  (ATLL)

Attachment, 214
Audiences, for education and prevention, 297–98
Awareness, 299
Azidothymidine (AZT), 65, 204, 234, 238, 241, 244, 245, 287
AZT. *See* Azidothymidine (AZT)

B

Bacillus, 15
Bacteria, 12, 14, 15–17, 57, 69, 183
Bacterial infections, 194–98
Bacterial pathogens, 205
Bacterial vaginosis (BV), 69, 71
 cause and transmission of, 113
 diagnosis of, 114
 and genital warts, 138
 signs and symptoms of, 113–14
 treatment and prevention of, 114–15
Balanitis, 57, 58, 149
Bank of America, 265
Bartholinitis, 91
Bartholin's glands, 45, 49
Basophils, 168, 170
Bassereau, P., 107
Bateman, 141
B cells, 173, 174
Beethoven, Ludwig van, 77
Behavior, changing, 315–18. *See also* Sexual behavior
Benign, 10
Benign tertiary syphilis, 83
Benign tumors, 135
Beta interferon, 243
Betaseron, 243
Bimanual examination, 51
Binding sites, 175
Biological transmission, 33, 34
Biological vector, 33
BIT. *See* Burrow ink tests (BIT)
BIV. *See* Bovine immunodeficiency virus (BIV)

Black communities, 305–6
Black Death, 21, 22, 24
Bleachman, 310
Blindness, 120
Blister, 47
Blood, 167–70, 171
 components of, 167–68
 and leukocytes and body defenses, 168–70
 and lymphatic system, 170–71
 overview, 167–70, 171
 and blood tests, 62, 64
 and blood vessels, 167
B lymphocytes, 170, 173, 174, 184
Body, of uterus, 45
Body defenses, and leukocytes, 168–70
Body lice, 158–61
Bovine immunodeficiency virus (BIV), 204
Breasts, 46, 47, 54–55
Buboes, 102
Bubonic plague, 21
Budding process, 217
Bulbourethral glands, 44
Burnet, Macfarlane, 166
Burrow ink tests (BIT), 158
BV. *See* Bacterial vaginosis (BV)

C

Calvin Klein, 266
Calymmatobacterium granulomatis, 110
Cancer, 5, 10
 cervical, 10, 138
 and herpes, 133
 and HIV, 228
Candida albicans, 149, 150, 151, 153, 182
Candida infections, 185–87
Candidate vaccines, 255, 258–60
Candidiasis, 148, 234, 235
Capone, Al, 77
Capsid, 17, 20

Carcinomas, 228
Cardiovascular syphilis, 83
Carriers, 32, 208
Cats, and AIDS, 204, 205
Cattle, and AIDS, 204
Cautery, 140
CDC. *See* Centers for Disease Control (CDC)
CD4 markers, 175
Ceftriaxone, 92
Cellini, Benvenuto, 77
Cell-mediated immunity (CMI), 173, 177–78
Centers for Disease Control (CDC), 30, 225, 228, 229–30, 239, 311, 316
Centers for Disease Control Classification System, 229–30
Central nervous system (CNS), and HIV, 239
CERVEX-BRUSH, 32
Cervical cancer, 10, 138
Cervicitis, 57, 99
Cervix, 45
Cesarean section, 122
Chagas, C., 188
Chain of events, for infectious diseases, 36
Chancre, 6, 7, 80
Chancroid, 28, 57, 61, 94, 107–10
Charles VII of France, 77
Chicago Health Department of Health, 28
Chicken pox, 13, 20, 192
Chlamydia, 58, 138, 178, 296
 basic features, 95–96
 life cycle, 95
 unsuspected infection, 97–100
Chlamydial cervicitis, 99
Chlamydial infections, 94–116
Chlamydia trachomatis, 94, 96–100, 101
 diagnosis, 100
 epidemiology of, 96–97
 and LGV, 101, 102, 106

prevention and management, 100
signs and symptoms of, 97
transmission of, 96
treatment, 100
who should be tested for, 101
Cholera, 21
Christian, Mark, 292
Chronic disease, 14
CID. *See* Cytomegalic inclusion disease (CID)
Cilia, 45
Circumcision, 44
Cirrhosis, 145
Civil law, 292–93
Clap, 87
Classification system. *See* Centers for Disease Control Classification System
Clinical history, 47
Clinical signs, of HIV, 239–40
Clitoris, 45, 46
CMI. *See* Cell-mediated immunity (CMI)
CMV. *See* Cytomegalovirus (CMV)
CNS. *See* Central nervous system (CNS)
Cocaine, 93
Coccidioides immitis, 187
Coccidioidomycosis, 187
Coccus, 15
Cochran, S. D., 308
Cofactors, 59, 60
Coinfections, 195
Coitus, 37
Cold sores, 119, 120
Colonies, 15
Colostrum, 253
Colposcope, 50, 138
Common sense, 275–76
Communicable diseases, 12
Communion cup, 274
Communities, ethnic, 300–307, 310
  Black, 305–6
  Hispanic, 303–5
Complement, 172
Compromised host, defined, 184–85
Computed tomography, 190

Condom, 61, 64–66, 67, 68, 211
Condylomas, 135
Condylomata acuminata, 57, 135–41
Condylomata lata, 83
Confidentiality, 289
Congenital defects, 10
Congenital diseases, 8, 9–10
Congenital syphilis, 84–85
Conjunctivitis, 86, 97
Consent, informed, 293
Consequences, of STD, 59–61
Contact, direct and indirect, 33
Contact transmission, 33
Contagious, and noncontagious, 12
Contagious diseases, general approaches to control of, 35–36
Control
  of chancroid, 109
  of contagious diseases, 35–36
  economics of, 315
  of genital warts, 141
  of LGV, 106
  of scabies, 158
  of TSS, 116
  of tuberculosis, 197
Convalescence phase, 13
Convalescent carrier, 32
Costs, 280–83
Counseling, and genital herpes, 129–30
Cowper's glands, 44
Cowpox, 252
Crab lice, 158–61
Crabs, 158–61
Crack cocaine, 93
Crusted scabies, 157
Cryosurgery, 140
Cryptococcosis, 185, 186
Cryptococcus neoformans, 182, 185
Cryptosporidiosis, 188, 190–92
Cryptosporidium, 182, 191
Cultural sensitivity, 299
Culture, 53
Cultures, 15
Culturing, 15
Cycloserine, 198

Cytomegalic inclusion disease (CID), 133
Cytomegalovirus (CMV), 57, 118, 130–33, 183, 185

D

Daily Variety, 301
Dane particle, 144
d'Aragona, Maria, 59, 60
Dating, and honesty, 308–9
ddA, 243
ddC, 243
Defense mechanisms, host, 184
de Gama, Vasco, 77
Degenerative diseases, 8, 10
de Lairesse, Gerard, 79, 80
de Maupassant, Guy, 77
Deoxyribonucleic acid (DNA), 17, 119, 136, 141, 143–44, 200, 214–17, 220, 229, 259–60
Destructive techniques, 140
DGI. *See* Disseminated gonococcal infection (DGI)
Diagnosis
  of bacterial vaginosis (BV), 114
  of candida infections, 187
  of chancroid, 109
  of *Chlamydia trachomatis*, 100
  of CMV, 132
  of *Cryptococcosis*, 185
  of cryptosporidiosis, 192
  differential, 52
  of genital candidiasis, 151–52
  of genital herpes, 127–28
  of genital warts, 138
  of gonorrhea, 92
  of granuloma inguinale, 112–13
  of HBV, 146
  of herpes simplex virus, 121
  of HIV, 239
  of isosporiasis, 192
  of Kaposi's sarcoma, 233
  of LGV, 106
  of molluscum contagiosum, 143

of *Mycobacterium avium-intracellulare* infections, 197–98
of Norwegian scabies, 160
of pneumocystis pneumonia, 189
of scabies, 158
of STD, 62–63
of syphilis, 85
of toxoplasmosis, 190
of trichomoniasis, 154
of TSS, 116
of tuberculosis, 196
Diathermy, 140
Dideoxyadenosine, 243
Dideoxycytidine, 65, 243
Differential diagnosis, 52
Digestive system disorders, 10
Dilation and curettage, 69
Diphtheria, 29
Direct contact, 33
Discrimination, and human rights, 284–92
Diseases, 6
  acute and chronic, 14
  and causative agents, 57–58
  communicable and noncommunicable, 12
  congenital. *See* Congenital diseases
  contagious and noncontagious, 12
  defined, 6
  degenerative. *See* Degenerative diseases
  endemic, epidemic, pandemic, and sporadic patterns, 26–30
  general approaches to control of, 35–36
  and helminths (worms), 18–20
  hereditary. *See* Hereditary diseases
  immunological diseases. *See* Immunological diseases
  infectious. *See* Infectious diseases
  metabolic diseases. *See* Metabolic diseases
  microbial world of, 14–18

neoplastic. *See* Neoplastic diseases
patterns of occurrence, 26–30
PID. *See* Pelvic inflammatory disease (PID)
signs, symptoms, and syndromes, 6–8
spread of, 21–36
transmission mechanisms, 32–35
tropical. *See* Tropical diseases
types of, 8–14
VD. *See* Venereal disease (VD)
Dishonesty, and dating, 308–9
Disseminated gonococcal infection (DGI), 89, 91
DNA. *See* Deoxyribonucleic acid (DNA)
Donovanosis, 110, 111, 112
"Don't Give A Dose," 94
Dose, 32, 94
Douche, 48
Down's syndrome, 9
Drugs
  antiviral, 65
  and HIV, 241, 243, 244
  See also Intravenous drug user (IVDU) *and* Investigational new drug (IND)
Ducrey, A., 107
Durer, Albrecht, 77
Dysentery, 17, 58, 198

E

EB. *See* Elementary body (EB)
Economics
  and ethical and political issues, 279–94
  of prevention and control, 315
Ectoparasites, 58, 148, 154–61
Ectopic pregnancy, 91
Education
  and nondiscrimination, 290
  and prevention, 295–311
  programs, 265–67

Egg, 42
Egg cell, 45
Ehrlich, Paul, 63
EIA. *See* Enzyme immunoassay (EIA)
Ejaculation, 42
Ejaculatory ducts, 44
Elementary body (EB), 95
Elements, formed, 167
Elephantiasis, 106
ELISA. *See* Enzyme-linked immunosorbent assay (ELISA)
Embryonic defects, 10
Embryonic period, 9
Emotions, dealing with, 318
Employee education programs, 265–67
Employment, and nondiscrimination, 290
Encephalitis, 190
Endemic, disease pattern, 27–30
Endocrine disorders, 10
End stage renal disease (ESRD), 236–37
Entry, portals of, 32
Enzyme immunoassay (EIA), 218
Enzyme-linked immunosorbent assay (ELISA), 219, 220, 228, 239
Enzymes, 10
Eosinophils, 168, 170
Epidemics, 21, 22, 24, 25
  disease pattern, 27–30
  silent, 1
Epidemiological eyeglass model, of infectious disease, 30
Epidemiology, 25, 26
  of chancroid, 107
  of *Chlamydia trachomatis*, 96–97
  of CMV, 131–32
  of genital candidiasis, 149
  of genital herpes, 122–23
  of genital warts, 136
  of gonorrhea, 88–89
  of granuloma inguinale, 110
  of HBV, 144–45

of HIV, 219–24
of LGV, 101
of Norwegian scabies, 158
of syphilis, 78–79
Epididymis, 44
Epididymitis, 57
Epithelial tissue cells, 228
Epstein-Barr virus, 57, 118, 131, 183
Equine infectious anemia virus, 204
Erythrocytes, 167, 170
ESRD. *See* End stage renal disease (ESRD)
Ethambutol, 196, 198
Ethical, economic, and political issues, 279–94
Ethnic communities, 300–307, 310
Etiology, 6
Examination
  anoscopic, 52
  bimanual, 51
  female physical, 48–52
  male physical, 48, 51–52
  rectal, 51–52
  of reproductive system, 41–55
  and self-examination. *See* Self-examination
  for STD, 46–51
Exit, portals of, 32
Exposure, 299
External genitalia, 42, 43, 45–46, 48–51
Extrapulmonary, 194
Eyeglass model, of infectious disease, 30
Eyes, 92, 132

F

Farr, William, 5
Fashion industry, and AIDS, 266
FDA. *See* Federal Drug Administration (FDA)
Fear, 263
Feces, 33, 34
Federal Drug Administration (FDA), 241

Feline immunodeficiency virus (FIV), 204, 205
Fellatio, 58, 91
Female nonspecific genital infections, 69–71
Female physical examination, 48–52
Female reproductive system, 44–47
  breasts (mammary glands), 46, 47
  external genitalia, 45–46
  organs of, 44–45
Females
  sexual behavior of, 296
  with AIDS, 230
Female self-examination, 54–55
Ferner, J., 41
Fertilization, 9, 42
Fetal period, 9
Fever, 172
Fever blisters, 119, 120
Fibrinogen, 167
Fingers, 33, 34
FIV. *See* Feline immunodeficiency virus (FIV)
Five Fs, 33, 34
Flea, 22, 24
Flies, 33, 34
Flucytosine, 185
Fomites, 33, 34
Food, 33, 34
Foreign factors, 167
Foreskin, 44, 53
Formed elements, 167
Foscarnet, 243
Fracastorius, Girolamo, 78
Frederick the Great, 77
Free needles, 319
Friel, Patrick, 199
Funding, 307–11
Fungi, 12, 14, 17, 18, 57, 182, 185

G

Galen, 87
Gallo, R. C., 312
Gametes, 42

Gamma globulin, 167
Ganciclovir, 132
Ganis, Sid, 301
Garden of Eden, 5
Gardnerella vaginalis, 69, 113–15, 138, 152
Gastrointestinal infections, 198
Gauguin, Paul, 77
Gc. *See* Gonorrhea (Gc)
Genetic disorder, 9
Genital candidiasis, 149–53
Genital chlamydial infections, 94–116
Genital herpes, 10, 57, 121–30
Genitalia, 42, 43, 45–46, 48–51
Genital infections, nonspecific. *See* Nonspecific genital infections
Genital sores, causes of, 210
Genital thrush, 150
Genital ulcers, 61
Genital warts, 57, 58, 134, 135–41
Genital yeast infection candidiasis, 151
Genitourinary system, 31
Genitourinary tract, 47
Genome, of HIV, 212, 213
German measles, 10
Giardiasis, 57, 198
Glands, accessory sex, 44
Glans, 53
Glans penis, 44
Global Programme on AIDS of the World Health Organization, 220
Globulins, 167, 254
Glossary, 321–27
Golden Age, 5, 21
Gonococcal pelvic inflammatory disease, 89
Gonococcus, 86, 88, 92
Gonorrhea (Gc), 1, 57, 58, 86–93
  background of, 87–88
  cause and transmission of, 86–87
  diagnosis of, 92
  epidemiology of, 88–89

highs and lows of, 93
incubation period of, 90
prevention of, 93
signs and symptoms of,
89–92
and syphilis, 75–93
treatment of, 92–93
Gonorrhea, oral gonorrhea, 91
Gottlieb, M. J., 225
Gram stain, 92
Granulocytes, 167
Granuloma inguinale, 56, 57,
110–13
Great pox, 23, 211
Groin, 47
Groove sign, 102, 103
Growing, of bacteria, 15
Growth, abnormal, 11
Gumma, 83
Gynecologic history, 47

H

Haemophilus ducreyi, 107, 108
Hairy leukoplakia, 194, 234,
236
HBcAg, 144, 146
HBeAg, 144
HBsAg, 144, 146
HBV. *See* Hepatitis B virus
(HBV) infections
Head lice, 158–61
Health, public. *See* Public
health
Health care, and
nondiscrimination, 289–90
Health care workers, 267–71
Healthy carrier, 32
Heart, 167
Heart attack, 10
Heat, 11
Heine, Heinrich, 77
Helminths. *See* Worms
Hemoglobin, 167
Hemophilia, 205
Henry III of France, 77
Heparin, 169
Hepatitis, 57
Hepatitis B immune globulin,
146

Hepatitis B virus (HBV)
infections, 58, 134, 143–46,
147
Herbert, A. P., 180
Hereditary diseases, 8, 9–10
Herpes, 48, 57, 133, 293. *See
also* Genital herpes
Herpes febralis, 119
Herpes labialis, 117
Herpes progenitalis, 57
Herpes simplex virus (HSV),
58, 119–21, 183
Herpes viruses, 117–33
and cancer connection, 133
introduction, 117–18
Herpes zoster, 192–93
Hispanic communities, 303–5
Histamine, 169
Histoplasma capsulatum, 187
Histoplasmosis, 187
History. *See* Clinical history
and Gynecologic history
HIV. *See* Human
immunodeficiency virus
(HIV)
HIVAN. *See* HIV-associated
nephropathy (HIVAN)
HIV-associated nephropathy
(HIVAN), 236–37
Holy Communion, and
infection, 274
Home care providers, 273
Home hygienic practices,
275–76
Hominis, 154
Honesty, and dating, 308–9
Hood, 54
Horizontal transmission,
34–35
Hormonal disorders, 10
Hormones, 10
Horses, and AIDS, 204
Host, 20. *See also*
Immunocompromised host
Host defense mechanisms, 184
Host-microorganism
relationships, 20
House of Representatives. *See*
United States House of
Representatives

Housing, and
nondiscrimination, 290
HPV. *See* Papilloma viruses
(HPV)
HSV. *See* Herpes simplex
virus (HSV)
HTLV-III, 200
Hudson, Rock, 292, 316
Human immunodeficiency
virus (HIV), 1, 17, 24, 27,
28, 31, 32, 37, 163–276
and antiviral drugs, 65
and associated conditions,
228
and cancers, 228
classification system for
related illness, 228–30
clinical signs of, 239–40
and CNS, 239
consequences of, 59–61
detection of, 217–18
diagnosis of, 239
drugs and, 241, 243, 244
epidemiology of, 219–24
genome of, 212, 213
historical aspects and
geographic distribution of,
203–6, 212–13
and HIV-1, 203–12
and HIV-2, 212–13
incubation period, 228
and kidney disease, 236–37
life cycle of, 214–17
in movies and television,
301
occupations and exposure,
267–73
and opportunistic infection
and immunocompromised
host, 180
and oral involvement,
234–36
preventing spread of, 247–49
and psychological impact,
237–39
and reading, 302–3
and related infections,
199–224
replication cycle of, 216
risk factors (cofactors), 60

scope of infection, 227–28
spectrum of, 163, 225–49
tests for, 218–19
transmission of, 206–11, 213
treatment of, 240–44
and tropical diseases, 195
vaccines for, 250–62
virus structure and
organization of, 212
and the workplace, 263–76
Human papilloma virus
(HPV). *See* Papilloma virus
(HPV)
Human retroviruses. *See*
Retroviruses
Human rights, 284–92
Human T cell lymphotropic
virus, 200
Humoral immunity, 173–77
Hunter, John, 88
Hutchinson's teeth, 84
Hybrid, 216
Hygienic practices, 275–76

I

IB. *See* Initial body (IB)
Idiotype, 260
IgA, 176
IgD, 176
IgE, 176
IgG, 176
IgM, 176
Immune globulins, 254
Immune responses, 11
Immune system, 166–79
  and blood and its functions,
    167–70, 171
  and humoral immunity,
    173–77
  and immune responses, 171
  and immunodeficiency
    diseases, 178–79
  and lymphatic system,
    170–71
  and nonspecific immunity,
    171–72
  and specific immunity,
    172–73
Immunity, 28, 166
  acquired, 251–53

active and passive, 173,
  251–53
cell-mediated (CMI). *See*
  Cell-mediated immunity
  (CMI)
humoral. *See* Humoral
  immunity
nonspecific. *See* Nonspecific
  immunity
specific. *See* Specific
  immunity
summary of acquired forms
  of, 254
Immunization, 35–36, 251, 253
Immunocompromised host,
  132, 156
  defined, 184–85
  and opportunistic infection,
    180–98
Immunodeficiencies, primary
  and secondary, 11
Immunodeficiency diseases,
  178–79
Immunoglobulin molecule,
  176
Immunoglobulins, 53, 62, 167
Immunoglobulin vaccines,
  260
Immunological diseases, 8,
  10–11
Immunology, 35
Immunomodulators, 241
Inactivated vaccines, 255
Incidence, 26
Inclusion body, 130
Incubation period, 13, 228
Incubatory carrier, 32
IND. *See* Investigational new
  drug (IND)
Index sex partner, 61
Indirect contact, 33
Infections, 6, 48
  chlamydial. *See* Chlamydial
    infections
  and coinfections, 195
  and communion cup, 274
  HBV. *See* Hepatitis B virus
    (HBV) infections
  nonspecific genital. *See*
    Nonspecific genital
    infections

opportunistic. *See*
  Opportunistic infection
and reinfection, 63
reservoirs of, 31–32
unsuspected, 97–100
vaginal, 69
Infectious diseases, 11–14
  causes, detection, and
    control of, 1–36
  chain of events for, 36
  concept of, 14
  course of, 13–14
  epidemiological eyeglass
    model of, 30
  general approaches to
    control of, 35–36
  introduction to, 5–20
  microbial world of, 14–18
  reservoirs of infection, 31–32
  sources, 31
  spreading factors, 31–35
  STD. *See* Sexually
    transmitted disease (STD)
  success factors of, 14
Infectious dose, 32
Infective balanitis, 57
Infestation, 154
Inflammation, 10–11, 172. *See
  also* Pelvic inflammatory
  disease (PID)
Influenza virus, 7, 23, 28
Informed consent, 293
Informing, 294
Initial body (IB), 95
Inoculation, 251
In One Day, 75
Insurance, 282, 290–91
Interferon, 65, 140, 172, 243
Intergrase, 217
Intermittent carrier, 32
Interstitial cells, 43
Intravenous drug user
  (IVDU), 265, 282, 307, 310
Invasive phase, 13
Invasive techniques, 140
Investigational new drug
  (IND), 244
Iodoxuridine, 65
Isolation, 35
  of bacteria, 15
  of persons with AIDS, 285

Isoniazid, 196
Isospora belli, 182
Isosporiasis, 188, 192
Issues, economic, ethical and political, 279–94
Isthmus, 45
Italian mummy, and syphilis, 59, 60
Itch, 154
Ivan the Terrible, 77
IVDU. *See* Intravenous drug user (IVDU)

J

Jarisch-Herxheimer reaction, 85
Jaundice, 131
Jenner, Edward, 252
Johnson, D., 302

K

Kaposi's sarcoma (KS), 228, 231–34, 235
Karlen, Arno, 148
Kidney disease, and HIV, 236–37
Kidney disorders, 10
Koch, Robert, 14
KS. *See* Kaposi's sarcoma (KS)

L

Labia majora, 45, 46, 54
Labia minora, 45, 46, 54
Laboratory tests, 53
Ladies Home Journal, 38
Laparoscope, 70
Latent syphilis, 83
Late syphilis, 80, 83, 84
LAV. *See* Lymphoadenopathy virus (LAV)
Law, 292–93
Lawrence, D. H., 56
Ledbetter, C., 302
Legislation, 311
Lentivirus, 202, 204
Lesions, 6
Leukemia, 203
Leukocytes, 167

Leukoplakia, 194, 234, 236
Levine, Alexander, 260
Levi Strauss Company, 265
LGV. *See* Lymphogranuloma venereum (LGV)
Liability, and vaccines, 257
Lice, 158–61
Lies, and dating, 308–9
Life cycles
of *Chlamydia*, 95
of HIV, 214–17
Lithotomy position, 49
Live vaccines, 255
Local heat, 11
Lockjaw, 12, 254
Look Back and Laugh, 180
Lymphadenopathy, PGL. *See* Persistent generalized lymphadenopathy (PGL)
Lymphatic system, 170–71
Lymphoadenopathy virus (LAV), 200
Lymphocytes, 11
and body defenses, 168–70
B and T, 170, 173, 174, 184
Lymphogranuloma venereum (LGV), 56, 57, 94, 97, 100–107
Lymphoid malignancy, 203
Lymphokines, 175
Lymphoma, 203, 232
Lymphotropic virus, 200

M

Mcleod, K., 110
Macrophages, 169, 184
Macules, 123
Major lips, 45, 46, 54
Malaria, 17, 21
Male nonspecific genital infections, 71–73
Male physical examination, 48, 51–52
Male reproductive system, 42–44
Male self-examination, 53–54
Male sex cells, 43
Malignancy, 203
Malignant, 10
Malignant syphilis, 79
Mammary glands, 46, 47

Management
of ARD, 238
of *Chlamydia trachomatis*, 100
of herpes simplex virus, 121
Mantoux, 196
Marlowe, Christopher, 77
Marriage, and VD, 42, 64
Masses, abnormal, 228
Mass media, 299–300
Mast cells, 169
Mays, V. M., 308
Measles, 10, 23, 28, 29
Mechanical transmission, 33
Mechanical vector, 33
Mechanisms of disease transmission, 32–35
Media, mass. *See* Mass media
Medium, 15, 16, 53
Megakaryocytes, 168
Memory, 173, 254
Memory cells, 170, 174, 178
Men. *See Male entries*
Meningitis, 185
Menstrual flow, 47
Menstruation, 47
Messenger ribonucleic acid (mRNA), 200
Metabolic diseases, 8, 10
Metronidazole, 114–15
Metropolitan Museum of Art, 79
MHA-TP. *See* Micro-hemagglutination *Treponema pallidum* (MHA-TP) test
Microbial world, introduction to, 14–18
Microbiota, 11, 69
Micro-hemagglutination *Treponema pallidum* (MHA-TP) test, 85
Microorganisms, 14–18, 17
and host-microorganism relationships, 20
and immunity, 253
Mignard, Pierre, 22
Minor lips, 45, 46, 54
Mites, 154
Miticides, 158
Molds, 17, 18
Molluscum contagiosum, 57, 134, 141–43

Robert Lehman Collection, 79
RPR. *See* Rapid plasma reagin (RPR) test
RT. *See* Reverse transcriptase (RT)
Rubber. *See* Condom
Rubella, 10

S

Safer sex, 61, 64, 67, 298–99
Salk vaccine, 254
Salpingitis, 57, 71
Salvarsan, 63
Sarcoma. *See* Kaposi's sarcoma (KS)
Sarcoptes scabies, 154
Scabicides, 158
Scabies, 58, 148, 154–61
Schopenhauer, Arthur, 77
Schumann, Robert, 77
Scrotum, 43, 53, 54
Scybala, 158
Sebaceous glands, 62
Secondary immunodeficiencies, 11
Secondary immunodeficiency diseases, 178–79
Secondary response, 176–77
Secondary syphilis, 80–83
Self-care, 273–75, 276
Self-examination, 41, 53–55
Semen, 42, 44
Seminal vesicles, 43, 44
Seminiferous tubules, 43
Senate. *See* United States Senate
Sensitivity, cultural, 299
Sequelae, 7
Seroconversion, 217
Serological tests, 53, 62
Serum, 167
Sex, lies, and HIV infection, 308–9. *See also* Oral sex *and* Safer sex
Sex cells, 43
Sex glands, accessory, 44
Sex partner, index. *See* Index sex partner
Sexual behavior, 74, 296

Sexually transmitted disease (STD), 1, 37–161
and antiviral drugs, 65
consequences of, 59–61
continuing challenges, 312–20
diagnosis of, 62–63
diseases according to causative agents, 57–58
introduction to, 56–74
newer, 58
and nonspecific genital infections, 66–73
physical examination for, 46–47
and pregnancy, 66
prevention and education, 64, 67, 295–311
and rape victims, 317
strategies for battling, 318–20
symptoms of, 62
treatment of, 63–64
Sexually transmitted ectoparasites, 58, 148, 154–61
Shamrock Safety Blood Collection Set, 272
Shape, of bacteria, 15
Sheep, and AIDS, 204
Shingles, 13, 118, 192–93
Signs
of ARD, 238
of bacterial vaginosis (BV), 113–14
of candida infections, 186
of chancroid, 107–9
of *Chlamydia trachomatis*, 97
of *Cryptococcosis*, 185
of cryptosporidiosis, 191
and disease, 6–8
of genital candidiasis, 149–51
of genital herpes, 123–27
of genital warts, 137–38
of gonorrhea, 89–92
of granuloma inguinale, 110–12
of HBV, 145–46, 147
of herpes simplex virus, 119–21

of HIV, 239–40
of isosporiasis, 192
of LGV, 102–6
of molluscum contagiosum, 141–43
of *Mycobacterium avium-intracellulare* infections, 197
of Norwegian scabies, 158–60
of PAIDS, 246–47
of pneumocystic pneumonia, 188
of scabies, 156–57
of syphilis, 80–84
of toxoplasmosis, 190
of trichomoniasis, 154
of TSS, 116
of tuberculosis, 194–96
Silent epidemic, 1
Silverstein, Shel, 94
Simian immunodeficiency virus (SIV), 204
SIV. *See* Simian immunodeficiency virus (SIV)
Skin burrow, 156
Sleeping sickness, 17, 19
Smallpox, 5, 6, 23
Smith, Sidney, 21
Sneezing, 33
Society's responsibilities, and public health, 277–320
Soft chancre, 107, 108
Sources, 31, 35, 208
Spatula, 50
Specific immunity, 172–73
Specific response, 251
Speculum, 49, 51
Sperm, 42, 43
Spiramycin, 192
Spirillum, 15
Spirochete, 15, 76
Sporadic, disease pattern, 27–30
Spores, 18
Spumivirus, 201–3
Staphylococcus aureus, 115, 116
STD. *See* Sexually transmitted disease (STD)
Stirrups, 49
Strategy, for battling STD, 318–20

of molluscum contagiosum, 141
of Norwegian scabies, 158
of PAIDS, 246
perinatal, 206
of pneumocystic pneumonia, 188
of scabies, 154–56
and syphilis, 76
of toxoplasmosis, 189–90
of trichomoniasis, 154
of TSS, 115–16
Travel restrictions, and AIDS, 288
Treatment
of bacterial vaginosis (BV), 114–15
of candida infections, 187
of chancroid, 109
of *Chlamydia trachomatis*, 100
of CMV, 132–33
of *Cryptococcosis*, 185
of cryptosporidiosis, 192
of genital candidiasis, 152
of genital herpes, 128–29
of genital warts, 138–41
of gonorrhea, 92–93
of granuloma inguinale, 113
of herpes simplex virus, 121
of HIV, 240–44
of isosporiasis, 192
of Kaposi's sarcoma, 233–34
of LGV, 106
of molluscum contagiosum, 143
of *Mycobacterium avium-intracellulare* infections, 197–98
of Norwegian scabies, 161
of pneumocystis pneumonia, 189
of scabies, 158
of STD, 63–64
of syphilis, 85
of toxoplasmosis, 190
of trichomoniasis, 154
of TSS, 116
of tuberculosis, 196
versus prevention, 282–83
Treponemal tests, 85
Treponema pallidum, 31, 76, 78, 80, 83, 84, 85

Trichloroacetic acid, 140
Trichomonas infection, 58, 138, 149, 151, 152–54
Trichomonas vaginalis, 151, 152
Trichomoniasis, 57, 148, 152–54, 155
Trifluridine, 65
Trimethoprim-sulfamethoxazole, 188
Trisodium phosphonoformate, 243
Tropical diseases, and HIV, 195
T suppressor cells, 175, 178
Tubercle bacillus, 194
Tuberculosis (TB), 28, 194–97
Tumors, 10, 11, 228

U

Ulcers, 61, 123
"Understanding AIDS," 302–3, 304
United Nations, 36
United States House of Representatives, 311
United States Senate, 311
Universal Declaration of Human Rights, 285
Universal precautions, 267, 269–71
University of Pisa, 59
Ureaplasma urealyticum, 99
Urethra, and urethral opening, 44, 53, 54
Urethral syndrome, 72
Urethritis, 57, 72–73, 94, 97. *See also* Nongonococcal urethritis (NGU)
Uterine tubes, 44
Uterus, 42, 44, 45

V

Vaccines, 250–62
and AIDS, 256–61
and anti-idiotype vaccines, 260
and candidate vaccines, 255, 258–60
developmental stages, 255–56

and immunoglobulin vaccines, 260
liability for, 257
live versus inactivated, 255
and preparation of representative vaccines, 253–55
and recombinant DNA, 259–60
safety of, 255
and sub-unit vaccines, 259–60
Vagina, 42, 44
Vaginal candidiasis, 149
Vaginal infections, 69
Vaginalis, 151
Vaginal opening, 45
Vaginal speculum, 49, 51
Vaginitis, 57, 69, 70–71, 149, 152
Vaginosis, 57, 69, 71, 113–15. *See also* Bacterial vaginosis (BV)
van Gogh, Vincent, 77
Varicella-zoster virus, 117–18, 183
Variolation, 251
Vas deferens, 44
VD. *See* Venereal disease (VD)
VDRL. *See* Venereal disease research laboratory (VDRL) test
Vector, 33, 34, 35
Venereal disease (VD), 38, 42, 56, 64
Venereal disease research laboratory (VDRL) test, 85
Venereal warts, 135, 137
Venus, 56
Vertical transmission, 34–35
Vesicles, 123
Vestibule, 45
Vidarabadine, 65
Viral RNA, 200
Virazole, 243
Virions, 17, 20
Virulence, 12
Viruses, 12, 13, 14, 17–18, 57, 183
and antiviral drugs, 65
cultivation, 18
herpes. *See* Herpes viruses

herpes simplex. *See* Herpes simplex virus (HSV)

HPV. *See* Papilloma viruses (HPV)

influenza, 7

and retroviruses. *See* Retroviruses

structure and shape, 17, 18

and virus infections, 192–94

Visna virus, 204

Vulva, 45

Vulvitis, 57

Vulvovaginal candidiasis (VVC), 57, 149, 153

Vulvovaginitis, 57, 152

VVC. *See* Vulvovaginal candidiasis (VVC)

W

Warts, 57, 58. *See also* Genital warts *and* Venereal warts

Watkins, James D., 284

WB. *See* Western blot (WB) assay

Wellferon, 243

Western blot (WB) assay, 218, 219, 220

White blood cells, 167

WHO. *See* World Health Organization (WHO)

Whooping cough, 29

Wilde, Oscar, 77

Wolf, Hugo, 77

Women. *See Female entries*

Workplace, and HIV infection, 263–76

World Health Organization (WHO), 36, 37, 161, 163, 219, 225, 226, 230, 278

World War II, 38

Worms, 12, 17, 18–20, 58, 198

Y

Yaws, 77

Yeasts, 17, 18, 148–61

Yellow fever, 21

Yves Saint Laurent, 266

Z

Zidovudine. *See* Azidothymidine (AZT)

Zoster, 118, 192–93

Zygote, 42